Greinix / Knobler
Extracorporeal Photopheresis

Hildegard T. Greinix and Robert Knobler

Extracorporeal Photopheresis

Cellular Photoimmunotherapy

Edited by Hildegard T. Greinix and Robert Knobler

DE GRUYTER

Editors
Univ.-Prof. Dr. Hildegard T. Greinix
Medical University of Vienna
Department of Internal Medicine I
Währinger Gürtel 18-20
1090 Vienna, Austria
e-mail: Hildegard.greinix@meduniwien.ac.at

Univ.-Prof. Dr. Robert Knobler
Medical University of Vienna
Department of Dermatology
Währinger Gürtel 18-20
1090 Vienna, Austria
e-mail: Robert.knobler@meduniwien.ac.at

The book contains 50 figures and 16 tables.

ISBN 978-3-11-027594-0
e-ISBN 978-3-11-027613-8

Library of Congress Cataloging-in-Publication data
A CIP catalog record for this book has been applied for at the Library of Congress.

Bibliographic information published by the Deutsche Nationalbibliothek
The Deutsche Nationalbibliothek lists this publication in the Deutsche Nationalbibliografie; detailed bibliographic data are available in the Internet at http://dnb.d-nb.de.

© 2012 Walter de Gruyter GmbH & Co. KG, Berlin/Boston.
The publisher, together with the authors and editors, has taken great pains to ensure that all information presented in this work (programs, applications, amounts, dosages, etc.) reflects the standard of knowledge at the time of publication. Despite careful manuscript preparation and proof correction, errors can nevertheless occur. Authors, editors and publisher disclaim all responsibility and for any errors or omissions or liability for the results obtained from use of the information, or parts thereof, contained in this work.
The citation of registered names, trade names, trademarks, etc. in this work does not imply, even in the absence of a specific statement, that such names are exempt from laws and regulations protecting trademarks etc. and therefore free for general use.

Typesetting: Medien Profis GmbH, Leipzig
Printing: Hubert & Co. GmbH und Co. KG, Göttingen
Cover image: Steve Gschmeisser/SPL/Getty images
∞ Printed on acid-free paper
Printed in Germany
www.degruyter.com

Preface

Extracorporeal photopheresis (ECP) is a leukapheresis-based therapy incorporating ex vivo mononuclear cell incubation with the photosensitizing agent 8-methoxypsoralen followed by irradiation with ultraviolet-A light. Based on results of a prospective, multicentre, international clinical study in patients with cutaneous T cell lymphoma ECP was approved by the FDA as the first cellular immunotherapy for cancer in 1988. During the following 25 years ECP has been investigated worldwide for prevention and treatment of a variety of T cell-mediated diseases including acute and chronic graft-versus-host disease (GVHD), solid organ and tissue transplantation, systemic sclerosis, systemic lupus erythematodes, rheumatoid arthritis, Crohn's disease and diabetes mellitus. Administering ECP to patients suffering from these diseases revealed promising results initially in retrospective and increasingly in recent years also in prospective single and multicentre clinical trials. Recent preclinical and clinical research provides insight into its mechanisms of action revealing induction of apoptosis of treated mononuclear cells, modulation of cytokine production, effects on antigen presenting cells and T cells and generation of regulatory T cells after ECP therapy. Preclinical hypersensitivity and GVHD models provided important insights on the effects induced by ECP in various diseases and support clinical findings excellently.

ECP has received wide and increasing acceptance from clinical investigators, policy makers and afflicted patients worldwide. Over 750 000 treatments have been performed attesting to its safety and excellent tolerance. Due to the favourable risk-benefit profile of ECP in adults and children and the increasing number of clinical trial results available to the scientific community, many clinical investigators as well as scientific organizations place ECP within the accepted and recommended therapeutic modalities.

New technical developments allow its use in children and substantially shortened treatment times. The excitement generated by this therapeutic modality, a development and expansion from classical PUVA photomedicine, from the outset and shared by prominent and numerous preclinical and clinical researchers worldwide will hopefully enable us to further extend the value of ECP into the future. Additional knowledge gained from further understanding the complexities of its mechanisms of action as well as extension of its clinical use in the coming years should contribute to cement its safe use for the benefit of patients around the world in a multi-disciplinary manner.

We would like to thank all co-authors for their valuable contributions and co-workers from De Gruyters Publishers for their excellent support in writing this book. We apologize to those colleagues whose work could not be cited because of space restrictions.

Vienna, June 2012
Hildegard T. Greinix and Robert Knobler

Content

1	**History of Extracorporeal Photopheresis —— 2**	
1.1	First Clinical Studies Using ECP —— 2	
1.2	ECP for Treatment of CTCL and Other Diseases —— 3	
1.3	Technical Developments in Use of ECP —— 3	
1.4	Current Role of ECP 5	
2	**Technical Aspects —— 8**	
2.1	ECP in Children and Adolescents —— 8	
2.1.1	Introduction —— 8	
2.1.2	ECP Methodology and Instrumentation —— 9	
2.1.3	Summary —— 20	
2.2	ECP in Patients with Bleeding Risks —— 22	
2.2.1	Anticoagulation with Heparin —— 22	
2.2.2	Anticoagulation with Acid Citrate Dextrose —— 24	
2.2.3	Anticoagulation during ECP in Patients with Bleeding Risks —— 25	
2.2.4	Anticoagulation during ECP in Patients with Absolute Contraindications for Heparin Use —— 26	
2.2.5	Vienna Experience on ECP with ACD-A —— 26	
2.2.6	Recommendations and Conclusions —— 28	
2.3	ECP with Central Venous Access —— 30	
2.3.1	Arteriovenous Fistulas (AVFs) or Arteriovenous Grafts (AVGs) —— 30	
2.3.2	Central Venous Catheters (CVCs) —— 31	
2.3.3	Totally Implantable Central Venous Access Systems (Ports) —— 33	
2.3.4	Summary/Conclusions —— 35	
2.4	New Technical Developments —— 38	
2.4.1	Extracorporeal Photopheresis Regulatory Recommendations —— 38	
2.4.2	The Closed System's New Technical Developments —— 39	
2.4.3	Conclusions —— 45	
3	**Mechanisms of Action of ECP —— 48**	
3.1	Preclinical GVHD Model —— 48	
3.1.1	Introduction —— 48	
3.1.2	Results —— 48	
3.1.3	Discussion —— 53	
3.2	Preclinical Hypersensitivity Models —— 59	
3.2.1	Introduction —— 59	
3.2.2	The Experimental Model —— 59	
3.2.3	Characterization of ECP/PUVA-Induced Treg —— 60	
3.2.4	Interleukin-10 is a Crucial Mediator —— 60	
3.2.5	Other Models and Data Indicating a Role of Treg in ECP —— 62

3.2.6	Conclusion —— **62**	
3.3	Mechanism of Action of ECP – Clinical Evidence —— **65**	
3.3.1	Introduction —— **65**	
3.3.2	Cellular Vaccination Hypothesis —— **65**	
3.3.3	Apoptosis of ECP-Treated Lymphocytes —— **66**	
3.3.4	Direct Effect of ECP on Effector Cells —— **67**	
3.3.5	ECP Modulation of Peripheral Blood Monocytes and Dendritic Cells —— **69**	
3.3.6	Distal Effects on Untreated Lymphocytes in GVHD —— **70**	
3.3.7	Emergence of Regulatory T cell Populations during ECP Treatment —— **72**	
3.3.8	Dysregulation of B Cell Homeostasis and Hallmarks of Improvement in ECP Treatment in GVHD —— **73**	
4	**Extracorporeal Photopheresis in Acute Graft-versus-Host Disease —— 84**	
4.1	First-Line Therapy of Acute GVHD —— **84**	
4.1.1	When to Start First-Line Therapy —— **84**	
4.1.2	What First-Line Therapy to Use —— **84**	
4.1.3	Duration of First-Line Therapy and Response —— **85**	
4.1.4	Combination First-Line Therapy —— **85**	
4.2	Predicting GVHD Severity —— **86**	
4.3	Second-line Therapy of Corticosteroid-Refractory Acute GVHD —— **86**	
4.3.1	Defining Steroid-Refractory Acute GVHD —— **86**	
4.3.2	Second-Line Therapy with Immunosuppressive Agents —— **86**	
4.3.3	ECP in Corticosteroid-Refractory Acute GVHD —— **87**	
4.4	Conclusions on the Use of ECP in Acute GVHD —— **93**	
5	**Extracorporeal Photopheresis in Chronic Graft-versus-Host Disease —— 98**	
5.1	Results of ECP in Cutaneous Manifestations of Chronic GVHD —— **98**	
5.1.1	Cutaneous Manifestations of Chronic GVHD —— **98**	
5.1.2	Results of Phase II Studies with Non-ECP Therapies for Cutaneous Chronic GVHD —— **99**	
5.1.3	Results of Phase II Studies with ECP Treatment for Cutaneous Chronic GVHD —— **99**	
5.1.4	Results of Two Phase II Randomized, Single-Blind, Multicenter Studies of ECP for Treatment of Cutaneous Chronic GVHD —— **100**	
5.1.5	Summary —— **104**	
5.2	Results of ECP in Extracutaneous Manifestations of Chronic GVHD —— **107**	
5.2.1	Introduction —— **107**	
5.2.2	Liver and Gastrointestinal (GI) GVHD —— **107**	
5.2.3	Ocular and Oral GVHD —— **111**	

5.2.4	Chronic GVHD of the Lungs —— 114	
5.2.5	Summary —— 116	
5.3	ECP in Chronic GVHD: Steroid-Sparing Effect —— 122	
5.3.1	Introduction —— 122	
5.3.2	Corticosteroids and Other Immunosuppressive Agents in Chronic GVHD —— 122	
5.3.3	Overview of ECP in Chronic GVHD and its Steroid-Sparing Effect —— 124	
5.3.4	Conclusions —— 125	
5.4	Prediction of Response to ECP —— 128	
5.4.1	Identification of Biomarkers in Chronic Graft-versus-Host Disease —— 128	
5.4.2	Biomarkers for Prediction of Response to ECP —— 130	
5.4.3	Conclusions —— 133	
6	**ECP for the Prevention of Graft-versus-Host Disease —— 136**	
6.1	Introduction —— 136	
6.2	Standard GVHD Prevention Strategies —— 136	
6.2.1	Methotrexate —— 136	
6.2.2	Cyclophosphamide —— 137	
6.2.3	Calcineurin Inhibitors —— 137	
6.2.4	Mycophenolate Mofetil —— 138	
6.2.5	Sirolimus —— 138	
6.3	GVHD Prevention with ECP: Potential Mechanism of Action —— 139	
6.3.1	Targeting Dendritic Cells —— 139	
6.3.2	Targeting Regulatory T Cells —— 141	
6.3.3	Targeting Dendritic Cells and Regulatory T Cells —— 143	
6.4	Extracorporeal Photopheresis during HCT Preparative Regimens —— 144	
6.5	ECP for Prevention of Solid Organ Rejection —— 145	
6.6	ECP for GVHD Prevention: Tolerogeneic DC and Treg Induction —— 146	
6.7	Conclusions —— 147	
7	**ECP in Cutaneous T Cell Lymphoma —— 152**	
7.1	ECP for Treatment of CTCL —— 152	
7.1.1	Treatment Schedule —— 154	
7.1.2	Recommendations —— 155	
7.2	Predictors of Response —— 158	
7.3	Adjuvant Therapy —— 158	
7.4	Monitoring during ECP Therapy —— 158	
7.5	Conclusion —— 159	
8	**ECP in Scleroderma and Other Skin Diseases —— 164**	
8.1	Systemic Sclerosis —— 164	
8.1.1	ECP in Systemic Sclerosis —— 164	

8.2	ECP in Localized Scleroderma/Morphea —— **166**
8.3	ECP in Autoimmune Bullous Diseases —— **167**
8.4	Atopic Dermatitis —— **167**

9	**ECP in Crohn's Disease —— 170**
9.1	Results on ECP in Crohn's Disease —— **170**
9.2	Conclusions —— **171**

10	**Extracorporeal Photopheresis after Solid Organ/ Tissue Transplantation —— 174**
10.1	Prevention and Treatment of Solid Organ Transplant Rejection —— **174**
10.1.1	Introduction —— **174**
10.1.2	Immune Mechanisms of Acute and Chronic Allograft Rejection —— **175**
10.1.3	Potential Mechanisms of Action of Photopheresis in the Treatment of Allograft Rejection —— **177**
10.1.4	ECP in Lung Transplantation —— **179**
10.1.5	ECP in Cardiac Transplantation —— **182**
10.1.6	ECP in Renal Transplantation —— **185**
10.2	ECP after Facial Transplantation —— **191**
10.2.1	Introduction —— **191**
10.2.2	Immunosuppression in Organ and Tissue Transplantation —— **191**
10.2.3	Case Description —— **192**
10.2.4	Conclusions —— **194**

11	**ECP in Diabetes Mellitus —— 200**
11.1	Introduction —— **200**
11.2	Prospective, Placebo-Controlled Clinical Study on Use of ECP —— **201**
11.3	Results —— **202**
11.3.1	Discussion of Study Results —— **202**
11.4	Conclusions —— **205**

12	**Side Effects of Extracorporeal Photopheresis —— 208**
12.1	Side Effects Concerning the Apheresis Procedure —— **208**
12.2	Side Effects Concerning 8-Methoxypsoralen —— **209**
12.3	Miscellaneous —— **210**

13	**Summary —— 214**

Authors Index

Section 1
Prof. Robert Knobler
Medical University of Vienna
Department of Dermatology
Währinger Gürtel 18–20
1090 Vienna
Austria
robert.knobler@meduniwien.ac.at

Section 2
Chapter 2.1
Prof. David Jacobsohn and **Dr. Edward Wong**
Children's National Medical Center
Sheikh Zayed Campus for
Advanced Children's Medicine
111 Michigan Avenue, NW
Washington, DC 20010
United States of America
dajacobs@cnmc.org | ewong@cnmc.org

Chapter 2.2
Prof. Nina Worel
Medical University of Vienna
Department of Blood Group Serology and
Transfusion Medicine
Währinger Gürtel 18–20
1090 Vienna
Austria
Nina.worel@meduniwien.ac.at

Chapter 2.3
Dr. Kristina Hölig
University Hospital Carl Gustav Carus Dresden
Department of Transfusion Medicine
Fetscherstrasse 74
01307 Dresden
Germany
kristina.hoelig@uniklinikum-dresden.de

Chapter 2.4
Prof. Alain Bohbot, Vincent Liu, Bruno Lioure, Karin Bilger, Dr. Annegret Laplace and **Dr. Raoul Herbrecht**
Centre Hospitalier Universitaire (CHU) Strasbourg
Hôpital CHRU de Hautepierre
Département d'Hématologie et d'Oncologie
1 Avenue Molière
67098 Strasbourg CEDEX
France
alain.bohbot@chru-strasbourg.fr

Section 3
Chapter 3.1
Prof. James LM Ferrara and **Dr. Erin Gatza**
University Michigan Cancer Center
Bone Marrow Transplant Program
1500 E Med Ctr Dr, CCC 6303
Ann Arbor, MI 48109-0942
United States of America
ferrara@med.umich.edu | egatza@gmail.com

Chapter 3.2
Prof. Thomas Schwarz
Christian-Albrechts-University Kiel
Department of Dermatology and Allergology
Schittenhelmstrasse 7
24105 Kiel
Germany
tschwarz@dermatology.uni-kiel.de

Chapter 3.3
Prof. Peter C. Taylor and **Dr. Rob M. Whittle**
Rotherham District General Hospital
Moorgate Road
Rotherham S60 2UD
United Kingdom
peter.taylor@rothgen.nhs.uk
rob.whittle@rothgen.nhs.uk

Section 4

Prof. Hildegard T. Greinix
Medical University of Vienna
Department of Internal Medicine I
Währinger Gürtel 18–20
1090 Vienna
Austria
hildegard.greinix@meduniwien.ac.at

Prof. Andrea Bacigalupo
Ospedale San Martino
Department of Hematology II
L. go R. Benzi 10
16132 Genova
Italy
andrea.bacigalupo@hsanmartino.it

Section 5

Chapter 5.1

Prof. Mary E.D. Flowers and **Dr. Yoshiro Inamoto**
Fred Hutchinson Cancer Research Center
1100 Fairview Avenue N D5-290
Seattle WA 98109-4433
United States of America
mflowers@fhcrc.org | yinamoto@fhcrc.org

Chapter 5.2

Prof. Madan Jagasia
Vanderbilt University Medical Center
Section of Hematology-SCT
2665 TVC; 1301 22nd Ave S
Nashville TN 37232-5505
United States of America
madan.jagasia@vanderbilt.edu

Dr. Kavita Raj
Kings Health Partners, Guys& St Thomas' and
Kings College Hospital
Department of Hematology
Kings College Hospital
Denmark Hill SE5 9RS
United Kingdom
Kavita.Raj@gstt.nhs.uk

Dr. Emma Das-Gupta
University of Nottingham
Division of Epidemiology and Public Health
Clinical Sciences Building,
Nottingham City Hospital
Hucknall Road
Nottingham, NG5 1PB
United Kingdom
emma.dasgupta@nuh.nhs.uk

Chapter 5.3

Prof. Daniel Couriel and **Kari Zureki, NP**
University Michigan Cancer Center
Bone Marrow Transplant Program
1500 E Med Ctr Dr, CCC 6303
Ann Arbor, MI 48109-0942
United States of America
dcouriel@med.umich.edu

Chapter 5.4

Prof. Hildegard T. Greinix
Medical University of Vienna
Department of Internal Medicine I
Währinger Gürtel 18–20
1090 Vienna
Austria
hildegard.greinix@meduniwien.ac.at

Section 6

Prof. John E. Levine and **Carrie Kitko**
University Michigan Cancer Center
Bone Marrow Transplant Program
1500 E Med Ctr Dr, CCC 6303
Ann Arbor, MI 48109-0942
United States of America
jelevine@umich.edu

Section 7

Dr. Julia Scarisbrick
John Radcliffe Hospital
Headley Way
Headington
Oxford OX3 9DU
United Kingdom
juliascarisbrick@doctors.net.uk

Priv.-Doz. Chalid Assaf
Helios Hospital Krefeld
Department of Dermatology and Venerology
Lutherplatz 40
47805 Krefeld
Germany
chalid.assaf@helios-kliniken.de

Section 8
Dr. Ulrike Just
Medical University of Vienna
Department of Dermatology
Währinger Gürtel 18–20
1090 Vienna
Austria
ulrike.just@meduniwien.ac.at

Section 9
Prof. Walter Reinisch
Medical University of Vienna
Department of Internal Medicine III
Division of Gastroenterology and Hepatology
University Hospital of Internal Medicine
Währinger Gürtel 18–20
1090 Vienna
Austria
walter.reinisch@meduniwien.ac.at

Section 10
Chapter 10.1
Prof. John A. Zic
Vanderbilt University School of Medicine
215 Light Hall
Nashville, TN 37232-0685
United States of America
john.zic@vanderbilt.edu

Chapter 10.2
Prof. Mauricette Michallet
Hopital E. Herriot
BMT Unit Pavillon E
5 Place d'Arsonval
69437 Lyon Cedex 03
France
mauricette.michallet@chu-lyon.fr

Mohamad Sobh
Department of Hematology
Centre Hospitalier Lyon Sud
69495 Pierre Bénite
France

Section 11
Prof. Gösta Berlin
Linköping University
Department of Clinical Immunology and Transfusion
SE-581 85 Linköping
Sweden
gosta.berlin@liu.se

Prof. Johnny Ludvigsson
Linköping University
Division of Pediatrics
Department of Clinical and Experimental Medicine
Faculty of Health Sciences
SE-581 85 Linköping
Sweden
johnny.ludvigsson@liu.se

Section 12
Priv.-Doz. Uwe Hillen
University Hospital of Essen
Department of Dermatology
Hufelandstrasse 55
45147 Essen
Germany
uwe.hillen@uk-essen.de

Section 13
Prof. Hildegard T. Greinix
Medical University of Vienna
Department of Internal Medicine I
Währinger Gürtel 18–20
1090 Vienna
Austria
hildegard.greinix@meduniwien.ac.at

Section 1: History of Extracorporeal Photopheresis

Robert Knobler
1 History of Extracorporeal Photopheresis

The history of extracorporeal photopheresis (ECP) can essentially be traced back to the origins of two well-known treatment modalities in dermatology: the one modality known as "PUVA" (a combination of the photosensitizing drug 8-methoxypsoralen (8-MOP) and the photoactivating agent ultraviolet light type-A [UVA]) and the other "leukapheresis" (removal of nucleated cells from the patients' blood). The origins of basic PUVA therapy can be traced back 2000 years ago to what was then called "heliotherapy". Used for the treatment of a disfiguring pigment disorder called vitiligo this therapy originally consisted of the ingestion of a boiled extract that was derived from a weed named "Ammimajus L", originally identified growing in the Nile Delta Region in Egypt, and subsequent exposure to natural sunlight. This therapeutic approach is considered the origin of what we today call PUVA.

1.1 First Clinical Studies Using ECP

Photochemotherapy over time has been identified to be of significant clinical value in the treatment of psoriasis, vitiligo, cutaneous T cell lymphoma, localized scleroderma, and more than 30 other diseases. The introduction of modern PUVA photochemotherapy that made this a more suitable and reproducible therapeutic modality in the clinical setting came in the early to mid 1970's when the exposure to natural sunlight, after ingestion of the drug, was replaced by the use of sophisticated computerized UVA irradiators. The original UVA radiators were designed to deliver uniform irradiation from specially designed fluorescent tubes and the delivery of energy was designated in joules. Directly related to the initial concept for the development of photopheresis was the important observation by Edelson and co-workers in 1974 [1] that patients with the Sezary syndrome variant of cutaneous T cell lymphoma (CTCL) could be effectively treated by leukapheresis and in 1979 by Gilchrest that PUVA therapy could be used in palliative treatment of cutaneous T cell lymphoma [2]. Based on these observations and the initial intention to deliver "site-directed chemotherapy" so that this therapy would only be active in the cells where the presence of the drug could be activated directly by UVA light Edelson and co-workers took this PUVA therapy one step further and combined it with leukapheresis. Then, in 1982, to their surprise they made a key observation that can be considered the true origin of extracorporeal photopheresis as we understand it today: [3] Two of their first five phase I leukemic CTCL patients went into remission after treatment of less than 5 percent of their estimated total body burden of malignant cells. That meant that 95 percent of the cells that had not been exposed to this treatment were also eliminated, suggesting that this therapy had triggered a very specific and strong immune response against malignant cells.

With the excitement provided by these observations and in order to confirm their observations Edelson and co-workers, then at the Department of Dermatology at Columbia College of physicians and surgeons initiated a prospective international multicentre clinical trial. The results of this trial were subsequently published in 1987 and confirmed their initial observations [4]. In this study twenty-seven of 37 patients with otherwise therapy-refractory cutaneous T cell lymphoma responded to the treatment modality. The group of the 27 responders included 8 of 10 patients with lymph-node involvement, 24 of 29 with exfoliative erythroderma, and 20 of 28 whose disease was resistant to standard chemotherapy. Heald and co-workers subsequently published a study suggesting that ECP may also increase survival of these patients when compared to historical controls [5]. A key observation that since has been confirmed in multiple subsequent trials was the very low side effect profile which is otherwise seen with standard chemotherapy, such as bone marrow suppression, gastrointestinal erosions, and hair loss which did not occur.

1.2 ECP for Treatment of CTCL and Other Diseases

Improvement of the delivery of the drug from oral ingestion to direct addition to the leukapheresis cells has further increased its reproducibility to reach consistently the appropriate serum levels and reduce some of the critical problems associated with oral intake of the drug [6]. In 1988, based on the studies and observations by Edelson and co-workers ECP received expedited approval by the US Food and Drug Administration (FDA) as the first sanctioned cellular immunotherapy for any cancer. It is in this light and its assumed potential to initiate also profound changes in the immune response that ECP in the years that followed and up to the present has found its application far beyond its initial indication. With confirmation of its efficacy and safety in the treatment of CTCL, exploration for ECP's potential additional application and use reached other areas of T cell mediated diseases that include rheumatoid arthritis [7, 8], systemic sclerosis [9], systemic lupus erythematosus [10], pemphigus vulgaris [11] and more recently solid organ graft rejection, especially acute cardiac and lung graft rejection [12, 13] and graft-versus-host disease [14, 15]. The present most widely used and accepted indication for ECP has become both the treatment and possible prevention of acute and chronic graft-versus-host disease after allogeneic bone marrow and blood stem cell transplantation.

1.3 Technical Developments in Use of ECP

After the success with the first experimental instrument which basically consisted of a locally constructed very large radiation chamber and what in those times was a standard "extracorporeal" blood circulating system used in dialysis (Later Therakos

Inc., a Johnson and Johnson subsidiary) the initially "closed" system went through a number of significant technical changes (Figure 1.1) that have made this therapy more reproducible and feasible within the premises of numerous specialties beyond dermatology. Outside of the United States a number of socalled "open" systems have been put into use particularly within the confines of specific centers such as blood banks.

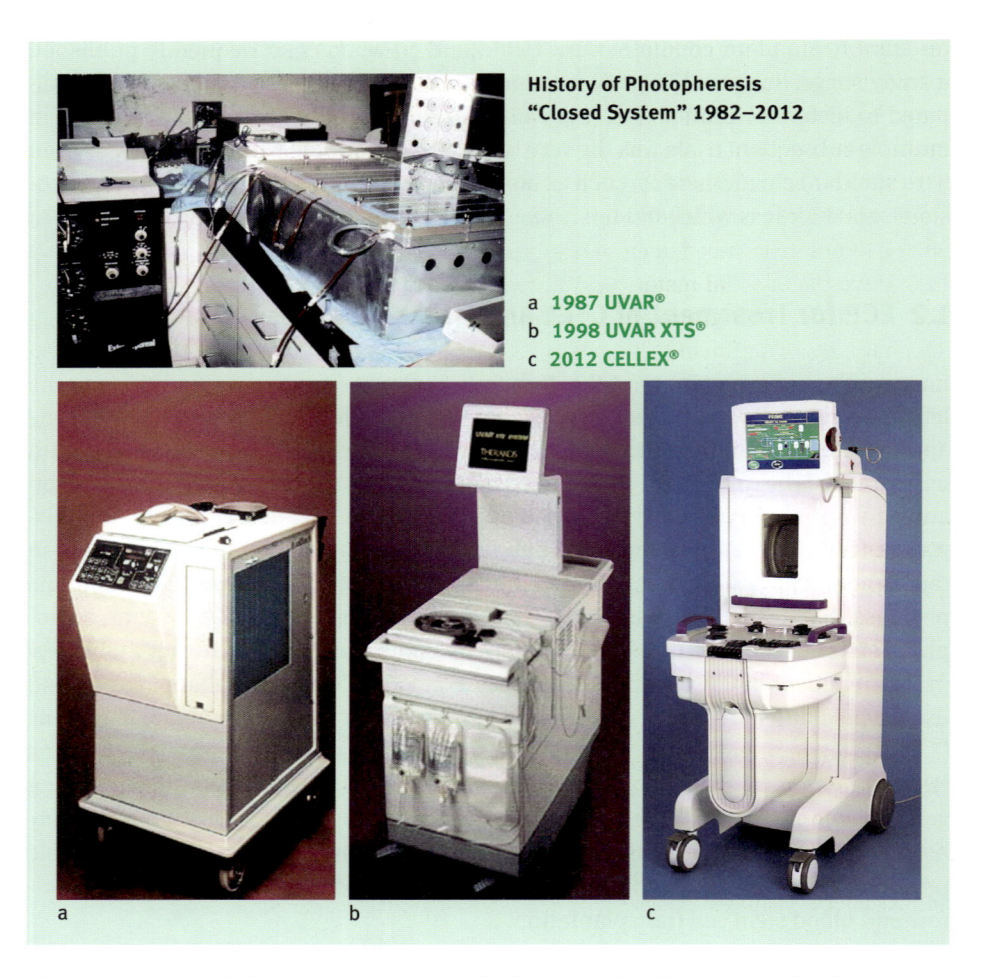

History of Photopheresis
"Closed System" 1982–2012

a 1987 UVAR®
b 1998 UVAR XTS®
c 2012 CELLEX®

Fig. 1.1. 1982: Original Photopheresis Device Combining an Existing "Extracorporeal Unit" and a One of a Kind Produced Irradiation Chamber Used at Columbia University by the Inventor Richard Edelson. The Subsequent "Closed System" Models were Developed by Therakos Inc. and Concentrated on Improving Efficacy of Cell Separation and Handling (UVAR®, UVAR XTS®) and Treatment Time as Well as Accessibility to Low Body Weight Patients (CELLEX®).

1.4 Current Role of ECP

Taking these observations further and based on an increasing pool of knowledge on the possible mechanisms of action Edelson and co-workers [16] proceeded to propose an extended form of ECP defined as "transimmunisation" in which the PUVA-treated cells are incubated over one night before reinfusion into the patient.

Over the past 25 years the use of ECP has received wide and increasing acceptance from investigators, policy makers and afflicted patients both in the USA as well as in Europe and other countries across the world. Over 750,000 treatments have been performed worldwide attesting to its safety within the indications used. Some indications have received sufficient acceptance that recently multiple consensus statements have been published placing the therapy within that widely accepted framework [17–20]. The guidelines of the European Dermatology Forum, summarizing all of the available evidence in dermatological and non-dermatological indications should provide a template for needed evidence-based studies in the coming years.

Since the original historical observations by Edelson and the subsequent observations made by his group and many others enormous strides into understanding the mechanisms of action of ECP have been made and many additional indications have been explored and documented in prospective clinical trials [15, 21–24]. Still, many of the exact mechanisms of action that explain all of its impact into the various indications of ECP remain to be unraveled in the exciting years ahead.

References

[1] Edelson R, Facktor M, Andrews A, Lutzner M, Schein P. Successful management of the Sézary Syndrome – Mobilization and removal of extravascular neoplastic T cells by leukapheresis. N Engl J Med 1974; 291:293–4.

[2] Gilchrest BA. Methoxsalen photochemotherapy for mycosis fungoides. Cancer Treat Rep 1979; 63:663–7.

[3] Edelson R in Extracorporeal Photochemotherapy and transfusion medicine, F Heshmati Editor, Dixit Medical In Haemapheresis, p. 2, 2008.

[4] Edelson R, Berger C, Gasparro F, et al. Treatment of cutaneous T-cell lymphoma by extracorporeal photochemotherapy. N Engl J Med 1987;316:297–303.

[5] Heald P, Rook A, Perez MI, et al. Treatment of erythrodermic cutaneous T-cell lymphoma with extracorporeal photochemotherapy. J Am Acad Dermatol 1993;28:1023–4.

[6] Knobler R, Trautinger F, Graninger W, et al. Parenteral administration of 8-methoxypsoralen in photopheresis. J Am Acad Derm 1993;28:580–4.

[7] Malawista S, Trock D, Edelson R. Treatment of rheumatoid arthritis by extracorporeal photochemotherapy. A pilot study. Arthritis &Rheumatism 1991;34:646–54.

[8] Menkes CJ, Andreu J, Heshmati F, Hilliquin P. Treatment of refractory rheumatoid arthritis by extracorporeal photochemotherapy. Brit J Rheumatol 1992;31:789–90.

[9] Rook AH, Freundich B, Jegasothy BV, et al. Treatment of systemic sclerosis with extracorporeal photochemotherapy. Results of a multicenter trial. Arch Dermatol 1992;128:337–46.

[10] Knobler RM. Extracorporeal photochemotherapy for the treatment of lupus erythematosus: preliminary observations. Springer Semin Immunopathol 1994;16:323–5.

[11] Rook AH, Jegasothy BV, Heald P, et al. Extracorporeal photochemotherapy for drug resistant pemphigus vulgaris. Ann Int Med 1990;112:303–5.
[12] Costanzo M, Nordin MR, Hubbel EA, et al. Photopheresis versus corticosteroids in the therapy of heart transplant rejection. Circulation 1992;86:242–50.
[13] Barr ML, Meiser BM, Eisen HJ, et al. Photopheresis for the prevention of rejecton in cardiac transplantation. N Engl J Med 1998;339:1744–51.
[14] Greinix HT, Volc-Platzer B, Rabitsch W, et al. Successful use of extracorporeal photochemotherapy in the treatment of severe acute and chronic graft-versus-host disease. Blood 1998; 92:3098–3104.
[15] Flowers ME, Apperley JF, van Besien K, et al. A multicenter prospective phase 2 randomized study of extracorporeal photopheresis for treatment of chronic graft-versus-host disease. Blood 2008;112:2667–74.
[16] Berger CL, Hanlon D, Kanada D, Girardi M, Edelson RL. Transimmunization, a novel approach for tumor immunotherapy. Transfus Apher Sci 2002;26:205–16.
[17] Trautinger F, Knobler R, Willemze R, et al. EORTC consensus recommendations for the treatment of mycosis fungoides/Sézary syndrome. Eur J Cancer 2006;42:1014–30.
[18] Scarisbrick JJ, Taylor P, Holtick U, et al. Photopheresis Expert Group.U.K. Consensus statement on the use of extracorporeal photopheresis for treatment of cutaneous T-cell lymphoma and chronic graft-versus-host disease. Br J Dermatol 2008;158:659–78.
[19] Wolff D, Gerbitz A, Ayuk F et al. Consensus conference on clinical practice in chronic graft-versus-host disease (GVHD): First-line and topical treatment of chronic GVHD. Biol Blood Marrow Transplant 2010;16:1611–28.
[20] Wolff D, Schleuning M, von Harsdorf S et al. Consensus conference on clinical practice in chronic GVHD: Second-line treatment of chronic graft-versus-host disease. Biol Blood Marrow Transplant 2011;17:1–17.
[21] Abreu MT, von Tirpitz C, Hardi R, et al. Crohn's Disease Photopheresis Study Group. Extracorporeal photopheresis for the treatment of refractory Crohn's disease: results of an open-label pilot study. Inflamm Bowel Dis 2009;15:829–36.
[22] Bisaccia E, Klainer AS, Gonzalez J, et al. Feasibility of photopheresis to reduce the occurrence of restenosis after percutaneous transluminal coronary angioplasty: A clinical pilot study. Am Heart J 2001;142:461–5.
[23] Ludvigsson J, Samuelson U, Ernerudh J, Johansson C, Stenhammer L, Berlin G. Photopheresis at onset of type 1 diabetes: a randomised, double blind, placebo controlled trial. Arch Dis Childhood 2001;85:149–54.
[24] Reinisch W, Nahavandi H, Santella R, et al. Extracorporeal photochemotherapy in patients with steroid-dependent Crohn's disease: a prospective pilot study. Aliment Pharmacol & Therap 2001;15:1313–22.

Section 2: **Technical Aspects**

2 Technical Aspects

Edward C.C. Wong and David Jacobsohn

2.1 ECP in Children and Adolescents

2.1.1 Introduction

The history of extracorporeal photopheresis (ECP) has been dependent on the development of cell separation devices using discontinuous and continuous methodologies [1]. Extracorporeal photopheresis has been used as adjunctive therapy for acute and chronic graft-versus-host disease (GVHD), cardiac rejection, and other autoimmune cell-mediated diseases in adults and as main therapy for cutaneous T cell lymphoma [2–4]. In contrast, the use of extracorporeal photopheresis in children has been limited because of their unique physiology and small size. However, predominant use of ECP in children has been for acute and chronic GVHD (Table 2.1). With rare exceptions (e.g. type I diabetes) potential indications for children largely follow diseases seen in adults, if occurring also in children. Because of the physiologic challenges in children, the technical use of ECP requires special consideration. This chapter will describe the unique physiologic and technical considerations in performing ECP in children and adolescents.

Disease	Frequency
Cutaneous T cell lymphoma	
– Erythrodermic[a]	Frequent
– Non-erythrodermic	Frequent
Graft-versus-host disease	
– Skin (chronic)[a]	Frequent
– Skin (acute)	Frequent
– Non-skin (acute and chronic)	Limited
Heart transplantation	
– Rejection[a]	Limited
– Prophylaxis	Rare
Lung transplantation	Limited
Liver transplantation	Rare
Kidney transplant rejection	Rare
Scleroderma (progressive systemic sclerosis)	Limited
Crohn's disease	Limited
Nephrogenic systemic fibrosis	Rare

Disease	Frequency
Pemphigus vulgaris	Limited
Rheumatoid arthritis	Rare
Other solid organ transplantation (including face)	Rare
Diabetes mellitus (Type I)	Rare reports (children)

[a]Note: Approved for reimbursement by the US Department of Health and Human Services, Centers for Medicare and Medicaid Services, provided there is refractoriness to standard immunosuppressive therapy. National Coverage Decision Memo 12/9/2006.

Table 2.1. Reported Use of Extracorporeal Photopheresis Based on Pubmed Search (2005–2011).

2.1.2 ECP Methodology and Instrumentation

The technique relies on the initial collection of mononuclear cells (MNCs) using either continuous or discontinuous cell separators, then ex-vivo exposure to a photosensitizing agent (8-methoxypsoralen), followed by photoactivation with UV-A irradiation, and then re-infusion of the photoactivated product. In children, this process can be performed using either separate cell separation and UV-A irradiation devices (e. g. two-step methods) or having both performed within the same instrument (i. e. "one-step" methods). Current techniques are summarized in Table 2.2.

Methodology	Automated	Weight Limit	Cell Separator Extracorporeal Volumes	Cell Separator Technology
One-Step Methods				
CELLEX® (THERAKOS®, Inc)	Yes (Double Needle)	RBC prime needed if >115% ECV	Variable, dependent on Hct, blood volume processed, return bag threshold (lower than UVAR XTS®)	IFC (continuous buffy coat collection with intermittent fluid return) (Latham Bowl)
	Yes (Single Needle)	RBC prime needed if >115% ECV	Variable, dependent on Hct, blood volumes processed (higher than Double Needle method)	CFC (Latham Bowl)
UVAR XTS® (THERAKOS®, Inc)	Yes (Single Needle)	>40 kg (need to satisfy ECV limits)	Variable, dependent on Hct, number of cycles and bowl size (225 or 125 mL)	IFC (Latham Bowl)

Methodology	Automated	Weight Limit	Cell Separator Extracorporeal Volumes	Cell Separator Technology
Two-Step Methods[b]				
COBE Spectra (Terumo BCT) and UV-A irradiator	Yes (only cell separation)	None	282 mL (MNC procedure, Version 4.7) 165 mL (AutoPBSC procedure, Version 6.0)	CFC
Mini-buffy coat and UV-A Irradiator	No	Smaller children	None, but limited to 5–8 mL/kg whole blood draw	Standard manual buffy centrifugation technique
Three-Step Methods[c]				
COBE Spectra (Terumo BCT) & UVAR XTS®	Yes (only cell separation)	None	See above for MNC and AutoPBSC procedure	CFC

ECV, extracorporeal cell volume; IFC, intermittent flow centrifugation; CFC continuous flow centrifugation; MNC, mononuclear cell, Hct, hematocrit.

[a] Data from Table 4-1 Burgstaler EA, Current instrumentation for apheresis. In: McLeod BC, Szczepiorkowski ZM, Weinstein R, Winters JL, eds. Apheresis: principles and practice, 3rd edition. Bethesda, MD: AABB Press, 2010:76; Table 21-1 Kim HC, Therapeutic apheresis in pediatric patients. In: McLeod BC, Szczepiorkowski ZM, Weinstein R, Winters JL, eds. Apheresis: principles and practice, 3rd edition. Bethesda, MD: AABB Press, 2010:446; and COBE Spectra, CELLEX® and UVAR XTS® Operator's manuals [1, 5, 19, 23].

[b] Only cell separation is automated while the UV-A irradiator is operated manually. Other dedicated continuous or intermittent cell separators may also be used such as Amicus (Fenwal, MNC kit), AS104 (Fresenius Kabi) which has extracorporeal volumes of 163 and 175 mL, respectively.

[c] Three-step methods involve standard mononuclear cell collection using dedicated continuous cell separators, followed by red blood cell priming of UVAR XTS® instrument and photoactivation treatment of the 8-methoxypsoralen treated mononuclear cells within the UVAR XTS® instrument after programming the instrument that the last ECP cycle has occurred. Has been in use at several U.S. Centers [8, 9].

Table 2.2. ECP Approaches Currently Used In Children[a].

2.1.2.1 Venous Access

In both adults and children, dedicated continuous cell separators (e. g. COBE Spectra, Terumo BCT) have been used successfully to collect mononuclear cells. Using this technique, mononuclear cells are separated on basis of density via centrifugation and/or elutriation [1]. Once a stable interface is achieved, the mononuclear cells are collected into sterile plastic containers.

Main advantages of using dedicated continuous cell separators include:
1. the familiarity with these instruments in many centers performing therapeutic apheresis,

2. ability to specifically target the number of mononuclear cells desired,
3. lower kit costs, and
4. ability to use this instrument in very small children (< 15 kg).

Main disadvantages include:
1. the need for an additional dedicated UV-A irradiator,
2. increased risk of microbial contamination of the product because of the open system configuration, and
3. potential off-label device use (e. g. no U.S. Food and Drug Administration approved UV-A irradiator), and
4. need for relatively high dual access flow rates.

Since relatively high flow rates are needed for continuous flow cell separators in order to achieve a stable interface for mononuclear cell collection, large, stiff, double lumen, central venous catheters suitable for apheresis or double-lumen Vortex ports (Angiodynamics) may have to be inserted [5]. Alternatively, the use of stiff peripherally placed (located as close as possible to the superior vena cava/right atrium) central catheters (PICCs) for draw, and a single lumen broviac (greater than 6 Fr) [6], (K. Capocelli, University of Denver Children's Hospital, personal communication), or for the smallest children, an epicranial needle for return [7], may be considered. Use of a PICC for draw with a broviac-type line for return may be preferred because it avoids a large indwelling catheter (associated with higher risk of infection and thrombosis), and if a Vortex port is used, the need for analgesia, delay in use (usually a 2–3 week healing period is required) and double needle access [6] (W. Paul, Children's National Medical Center, personal communication). These PICCs need to be 20 gauge or 4 Fr or greater in size and placed as close as possible near the superior vena cava/right atrium junction for adequate flow. In addition, the selection of adequate venous access is critical because of relatively long procedural times which can be 2–3 times longer in children compared to adults who often have adequate venous access. (W. Paul, Children's National Medical Center, personal communication). Although antecubital peripheral access using 18 gauge needles or larger may be attempted, this would only be suitable for non-continuous cell separators, given that a dual-arm technique is unlikely because of the need for adequate antecubital veins in both arms. Furthermore, considering the continuous use of steroids in these patients, repeat venous access (often two consecutive days) could result in increased hematoma formation and skin break down. Thus, venous access in children needs to be customized taking into account the method of cell separation, patient psychological and social needs, and patient's available access.

2.1.2.2 Mononuclear Cell Collection and UVA Irradiation

Once venous access has been achieved, if a two-step method is used, the mononuclear cell collection is typically performed using the standard MNC program (COBE Spectra, Terumo BCT) to collect greater than 1×10^7 lymphocytes/kg or 10 mL/kg body weight collected while performing a leukapheresis at 1 mL/kg/min [6], or by processing 2–3 blood volumes [7, 8]. 8-methoxypsoralen is then added to the mononuclear cells for a final concentration of 200 ng/mL. The treated cells are then transferred to a UV-A permeable bag, irradiated at 2 J/cm² (365 nm) in a UV-A irradiator and then re-infused back into the patient. A variation of this method (often called a "three-step" method) is to place the mononuclear suspension into the UVAR XTS® machine for UV-A irradiation after first priming the bowl with red blood cells (RBCs) before the addition of 8-methoxypsoralen. This is followed by re-infusion into the patient. The two step technique is primarily used in Italy and France [9], while the latter technique has been reported from some U.S. centers [10, 11]. The two-step (or three-step) technique is preferred by some centers because of the theoretical possibility of improved ECP efficacy by the delivery of larger doses of reinfused cells [12, 13]. In addition, because cells can be potentially frozen, thawed and then treated with 8-methoxypsoralen and UV-A irradiation, the use of dedicated continuous cell separators can allow for the freezing of mononuclear cells, similar to the process seen with autologous peripheral blood stem cell collection, potentially adding flexibility to the treatment schedules for patients, decreasing the number of visits for mononuclear cell collection and allowing for potential manipulation or analysis of the product prior to reinfusion [14, 15].

An alternative to two-step or three-step methods includes the use of instruments which have either single needle (discontinuous) or double needle, continuous cell separation coupled to an internal UV-A irradiation device. The advantages of these systems include: 1) decreased risk of microbial contamination due to closed system configuration, 2) integrated mononuclear cell collection and 8-methoxypsoralen/UV-A irradiation processing, and 3) regulatory agency approval of the devices. Disadvantages include: 1) need for a dedicated device (higher initial instrument cost startup), 2) higher kit costs, and 3) potential patient size limitations. Both the CELLEX® and UVAR XTS® (THERAKOS®, Inc) use a microprocessor controlled, modified Latham bowl methodology, which allows for the elutriation of mononuclear cells once the bowl is sufficiently filled with RBCs. The UVAR XTS® instrument is recommended for patients weighing more than 40 kg, while the CELLEX® instrument can be used safely in patients weighing less than 25 kg provided an RBC prime is used.

Because of extracorporeal volume limitations and venous access difficulty and for those patients in whom conventional ECP using cell separation is contraindicated (i.e. critically ill patients), manual buffy coat preparations as a source of mononuclear cells has been proposed. This entails the withdrawal of 5 to 8 mL/kg whole blood, followed by ex-vivo exposure to 8-methoxypsoralen and UV-A irradiation [16]. Although this approach may be useful in smaller children, clinical follow-up has yet to be reported; however, white blood cell (WBC) apoptosis and lymphocyte proliferation inhibition were seen to be similar when compared to standard ECP treated cells [16].

2.1.2.3 Physiologic Considerations

In order to perform ECP safely in children, one has to consider their blood volumes. Table 2.3 shows the change in blood volume (mL/kg) as a function of age [17]. Although the differences do not seem to be very impressive, when kg body weight is considered, the differences in blood volume can be dramatic. For example, a 24-month old girl (with an average blood volume of approximately 80 mL/kg) has a blood volume that can range from 976 to 1168 mL (5th and 95th percentiles respectively, using 12.2 kg and 14.6 kg, representing the 5th and 95th percentile for age), respectively [18]. Extracorporeal volumes of the COBE Spectra cell separator seen in Table 2.2, can be a significantly large percentage of a child's total blood volume. Thus, if there is no immediate fluid return as often seen in discontinuous dedicated cell separators for ECP (e.g. discontinuous/intermittent single needle mode for CELLEX® and single needle mode for UVAR XTS® instruments), pediatric patients can experience repeated cycles of symptomatic and potentially life-threatening hypo- and hypervolemia. Table 2.4 shows the dramatic changes in extracorporeal blood volume during discontinuous cell separation that occur with the UVAR XTS® instrument as function of hematocrit and cycle number [19]. These changes do not include the manual return of residual red cells within the instrument nor the return of psoralen treated, UV-A irradiated, buffy coat cells which can make a significant positive contribution to a child's fluid balance. At our institution, patients weighing 25 to 30 kg and receiving 3 cycles of ECP by UVAR XTS®, typically have positive fluid balances ranging from 500 to 600 mL.

Several studies and reviews have strongly suggested that when there is rapid loss of blood volume or conversely a rapid increase in blood volume (approximately 15% of total blood volume) modifications must be made to the apheresis procedure in order to make the procedure as safe as possible [5, 20–22]. Initial signs and symptoms typically include anxiety, tachycardia, pallor, light-headedness and orthostatic hypotension evolving to more serious signs and symptoms such as shock and loss of consciousness. These considerations become even more important in critically ill patients and therefore, it is preferable to use techniques that allow for continuous cell separation.

Maneuvers to Mitigate Extracorporeal Volume Shifts

For use of dedicated continuous cell separators performing the initial leukapheresis step (two or three step methods), technical alterations to the procedure to improve safety for children include: 1) not performing the initial saline divert or performing divert only when the divert volume is less than 15% of the total blood volume, and 2) avoiding partial or total rinse back if the return volume is greater than 15% of the total blood volume [21]. Taking these considerations into account, treatment of patients as small as 13 kg has been reported [6]. However, theoretically even smaller patients may be treated. For use of dedicated discontinuous ECP machines (i.e. UVAR XTS® or single needle mode CELLEX®), because the starting hematocrit greatly influences the amount of plasma drawn (and therefore the amount of volume removed from the patient before buffy coat collection), transfusion of RBCs or the use of erythropoietin to raise the hematocrit may be desirable in order to avoid the removal of large volumes of plasma and subsequent symptomatic hypovolemia. For the UVAR XTS®, the use of the smaller Latham bowl (125 mL) is recommended in children and performing fewer cycles (typically 3) of buffy coat collection in order to decrease extracorporeal volume shifts; while adults or children greater than 40 kg can typically undergo 6 cycles using the UVAR XTS®. However, it should be noted that the manufacturer cautions against too high a transfusion target (>40% hematocrit) because of the potential difficulty of buffy coat separation at these high hematocrits. Table 2.4 shows extracorporeal volumes (ECVs) seen in patients as a function of hematocrit and cycle number using the UVAR XTS® instrument [19], while Figure 2.1 shows corresponding ECVs using the CELLEX® instrument for processing of 1500 mL of blood volume. Operation of the CELLEX® in double needle mode (continuous separation and fluid return) dramatically decreases the ECV compared to single needle mode (continuous separation and discontinuous return mode) which is dependent on the bag return thresholds. Thus, the CELLEX® is ideally suited for younger children [23]. Furthermore, one disadvantage of the UVAR XTS® instrument is its inability to undergo RBC priming for patients who have unacceptably low hematocrits. Thus, patients have to be transfused prior to ECP treatment if the predicted ECV based on a pre-transfusion hematocrit cannot be tolerated. In contrast, the CELLEX® can undergo RBC priming, obviating the need for pre-treatment RBC transfusion. However, it should be noted that a patient hematocrit >27% is required per manufacturer for CELLEX®. Dedicated continuous cell separators similarly have the ability to undergo RBC priming per manufacturer's recommendations.

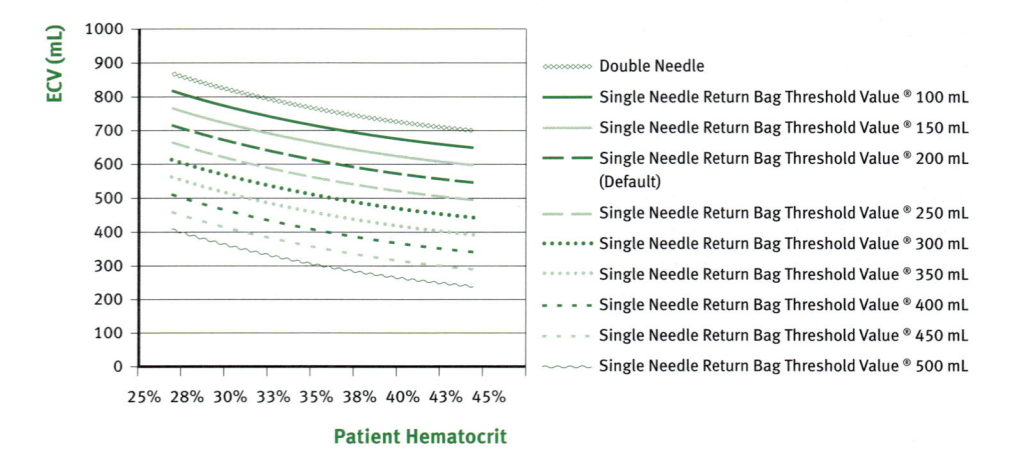

Fig. 2.1. Estimated Extracorporeal Volumes Using CELLEX® (THERAKOS®, Inc.).
ECV is extracorporeal volume. Note: for each additional cycle processed, the patient's extracorporeal volume will increase approximately between 100 and 280 mL.
Section 10-4. THERAKOS® CELLEX® Photopheresis, Operator's Manual. (© THERAKOS®, Inc. 2012).

Compounded on the concern for hypo- or hypervolemia are changes in hematocrit, which may or may not be tolerable particularly in critically ill, small children. This is of particular concern in continuous cell separation devices with relatively large extracorporeal volumes. For example a 25 kg child with a blood volume of 80 mL/kg × 10 kg (2000 mL) who undergoes leukapheresis using a continuous cell separator with an extracorporeal cell volume of 285 mL can reduce his/her hematocrit from 25.0 to 21.9 % during the procedure if no red cell prime is performed. Discontinuous dedicated ECP devices (UVAR XTS®, THERAKOS®, Inc), in addition, are not primed with RBCs or whole blood, so that hemodilution increases with each cycle of buffy coat/mononuclear cell collection because of the additional fluid given to patients as part of the anticoagulation protocol during each cycle. As mentioned above, patients weighing 25 to 30 kg, can easily be hemodiluted given the large positive fluid balances experienced despite manual return of the residual RBCs in the instrument. On average approximately a hematocrit drop of 2–4 % is what we see in patients weighing between 25 and 30 kg using the UVAR XTS® instrument (CNMC experience, data not shown). In addition, this hemodilution can be exacerbated with successive ECP treatments. Kanold et al, 2007 [6] similarly have reported decreases in mean hemoglobin between 12.5 and 16 g/L using continuous cell separators; however, it is unknown if these patients were given rinse back (to return RBCs) at the end of collection.

Schneiderman et al [22] have recently published their technical experience in using fluid boluses to mitigate hypovolemic symptoms in children weighing between 25 and 40 kg and less than 25 kg using the UVAR XTS® instrument. For patients between 25 and 40 kg, they have successfully pioneered the use of fluid boluses to mitigate symptomatic hypovolemia. This is done by giving boluses using the following formula: the difference of 15 % of the total blood volume of the patient and the extracorporeal volume of the circuit (determined by the bowl size and the hematocrit of the patient). For example, if a patient is 30 kg with total blood volume of 2250 mL, has a hematocrit of 28 %, the patient's extracorporeal volume (UVAR XTS®) will be 400 mL. Given that 15 % of 2,250 mL is 338 mL, the amount of saline needed to bolus the patient to avoid potential symptomatic hypovolemia would be 400 mL minus 338 mL or 62 mL. Depending on the patient's symptoms, a repeat bolus may be necessary. For patients less than 25 kg, the authors advocate the use of 5 % albumin instead of normal saline for better oncotic effect. Only three cycles of buffy coat preparation are performed if the maximal ECV exceeds 15 % total body volume (TBV) in the first cycle. The authors report successful use of this protocol in a patient as small as 19 kg.

2.1.2.4 Anticoagulation

Mononuclear cell collection by continuous cell separators is performed using either systemic heparin or regional citrate anticoagulation (Table 2.5). A variety of protocols have been published [5] indicating institutional preferences and patients' considerations. Similarly, patients who undergo ECP using one-step methods have a variety

Patient	Representative Weight (kg)	Blood Volume (mL/kg Body Weight)	Total Blood Volume (mL)
Newborn, 15–30 min. of age	3	76.5	230
Newborn, 24 hours	2.8	83.3	233
Children, 3 months	4	87	438
Children, 6 months	7	86	602
Children, 1 year	10	80	800
Children, 6 years	20	80	1600
Children, 10 years	35	75	2625
Children, 15 years	60	71	4260
Adult men	70	71	4970
Adult women	65	70	4550

[a]Values for mean blood volume (mL/Kg) in children, men and women (Geigy Scientific Tables, 7th Ed; 1971) [17]

Table 2.3. Blood Volumes in Children and Adults as a Function of mL/Kg with Representative Total Blood Volumes[a].

% Hematocrit	Cycle 1	2	3	4	5	6
27	435	376	417	464	511	438
28	423	365	406	453	500	428
29	411	355	395	442	489	418
30	401	345	385	432	479	410
31	391	336	375	422	469	401
32	381	327	366	413	460	393
33	372	305	358	405	451	386
34	364	312	350	397	443	378
35	356	305	342	389	435	372
36	348	298	335	382	427	365
37	341	291	328	375	420	359
38	334	285	321	368	413	353
39	327	279	315	361	407	347
40	321	273	309			
41	315	268	303			
42	309	263	297			
43	304	258	292			

Note: technical difficulties may prevent collecting more than 3 cycles when the patient's hematocrit is greater than 40 %.

[a]modified from Table 10. THERAKOS® UVAR XTS® Photopheresis, Operator's Manual (© THERAKOS®, Inc. 2012).

Table 2.4. Estimated Extracorporeal Volume Changes During UVAR XTS® (THERAKOS®, Inc.) Using 125 Bowl as a Function of Patient Hematocrit and Cycle Number.[a]

of anticoagulation choices. At our institution, using the UVAR XTS® instrument, patients with low risk of bleeding are placed typically on standard heparin anticoagulation (10,000 units of heparin in 500 mL of normal saline) which is infused at a whole blood to anticoagulant ratio of 8:1. In contrast, patients with high risk of bleeding or with gastrointestinal bleeding may be placed on citrate anticoagulation (infused at a whole blood ratio of 12:1) or low dose heparin anticoagulation (5,000 units of heparin in 500 mL of normal saline, infused at a whole blood to anticoagulant ratio of 8:1). Patients with moderate or severe thrombocytopenia should have post-procedure complete blood counts to monitor for potential bleeding and the degree of post-procedure platelet count decrement. Figure 2.2 shows the pre and post-ECP procedure (UVAR XTS®) platelet counts seen in an 11 year old female after matched unrelated hematopoietic stem cell transplantation for sickle cell disease at our institution. Median decrease was 19.4 % with 5th to 95th percentile decrease of 40.8 % and 8.1 %, respectively. Given expected drops in platelet counts post-procedure, some centers may elect to transfuse platelets prior to getting the results. This decrease in platelet count is not limited to dedicated one step ECP devices, but is also seen with two-step methods using dedicated continuous cell separators. Reported decreases have ranged between 0–71 % with higher average decreases significantly different between patients greater than 25 kg (21 %) versus patients less than or equal to 25 kg (14 %) [6].

Citrate toxicity occurs as a result of citrate chelation of divalent cations such as Ca^{2+} which leads to signs and symptoms such as mild perioral and/or peripheral paresthesias, dysgeusia (unusual taste), nausea, hypotension, continuous muscle contractions (initially involuntary carpopedal spasm, then life-threatening laryngospasm), neuromuscular irritability (as evidenced by Chvostek's and/or Trousseau's sign), EKG changes (e. g. prolonged QT interval) and rarely cardiac arrhymias [24]. Furthermore, in the liver citrate is metabolized to bicarbonate resulting in a metabolic alkalosis which, in turn, may also cause hypokalemia. The development of alkalosis might render patients susceptible to symptoms related to hypocalcemia. Thus, in patients with the potential for citrate toxicity, it is advisable to monitor ionized calcium and/or provide a calcium drip, and monitor magnesium and potassium levels. A relatively safe prophylactic protocol established at our institution is the use of 20 mg/mL calcium gluconate drip at 1 mL/kg/hr which can be given through either central or peripheral lines, including the apheresis return line. In critically ill patients, it is advisable to correct hypomagnesemia and hypokalemia when encountered prior to start of the ECP procedure when citrate anticoagulation is used. However, it should be noted that the development of alkalosis and hypokalemia is less pronounced with ECP procedures because of the relatively smaller blood volumes processed compared to mononuclear cell collection procedures for stem cell harvesting where routinely more blood volumes are processed.

One Step Methods (UVAR XTS®, CELLEX®)[a]

Heparin (unfractionated)
Standard Dose
Anticoagulant: 10,000 units heparin/500 mL normal saline
Infusion rate: WB:AC ratio of 8:1 to 10:1

Low Dose
Anticoagulant: 5,000 units heparin/500 mL normal saline
Infusion rate: WB:AC ratio of 8:1 to 10:1

Citrate
Anticoagulant: ACD-A
Infusion rate: WB:AC ratio of 11:1 to 12:1

Two Step Methods (Cell Separation only)

Heparin
Heparin/ACD-A Methods (COBE Spectra, Terumo BCT)

Bolus Heparin (separate)/Continuous ACD-A Method
Anticoagulant: Heparin separately from ACD-A
Bolus 50 units/kg, then after 1 hour 10 units/kg every 30 minutes
Infusion rate (ACD-A only): WB to AC ratio of 20:1 to 30:1 (aPTT monitoring recommended; alternatively activated clotting time of 180 to 220 seconds can be targeted)

Continuous Heparin/ACD-A Method
Anticoagulant: 5,000 units heparin in 500 units of ACD-A
Infusion rate: WB to AC ratio of 30:1 (activated clotting time or aPTT monitoring not required)

Modified Continuous Heparin/ACD-A Method
Anticoagulant: 5,000 units heparin in 500 units of ACD-A
Infusion rate: WB to AC ratio of 30:1 to 50:1 (dependent on blood volumes processed, activated clotting time or aPTT monitoring not required, Spectra Version 4.7)

Citrate (Same as one-step method)

WB is whole blood; AC is anticoagulant
[a]Note: THERAKOS® recommends heparin dose of 150 units/kg to 250 units/kg

Table 2.5. Anticoagulation Approaches for Children Undergoing ECP.

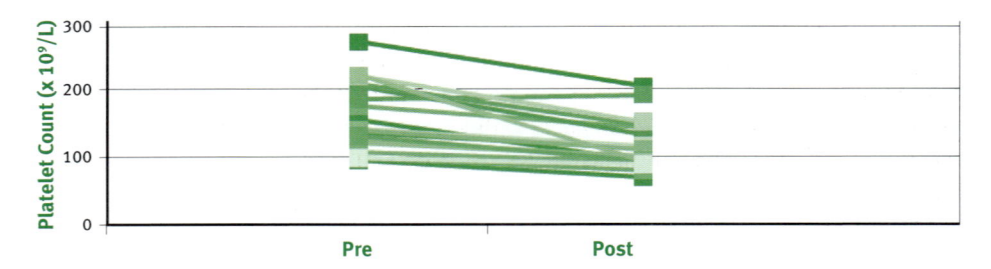

Fig. 2.2. Comparison of Pre- and Post-Procedure Platelet Count (x 10^9/L) Changes (n=18) seen in a Representative Patient Using UVAR XTS® (THERAKOS®, Inc.) over a 5 Month Period.

2.1.2.5 Limitations to the ECP Procedure

Patients first and foremost must be hemodynamically stable and capable of tolerating reinfusion of a photoactivated mononuclear cell preparation as well as potential swings in volume during the procedure. This is of particular concern when using discontinuous ECP techniques. Both the development of allergy to 8-methoxypsoralen and heparin induced thrombocytopenia (rare in immunocompromised children after hematopoietic stem cell transplantation) are an absolute contraindication (the latter of which can be mitigated by the use of regional citrate anticoagulation). In patients with low platelet counts, alterations to anticoagulation can be made to reduce the risk of bleeding as described previously. Patients should furthermore avoid the ingestion of fatty foods 24 hours prior to the start of ECP because of the risk of erroneous early detection of the buffy coat layer due to lipemia which would cause negative fluid shifts. Similar concerns occur when patients have elevations in bilirubin levels and reticulocyte counts or abnormally shaped RBCs, again potentially causing erroneous early detection of the buffy coat layer. These interferences may be less of a problem when performing two-step methods, using dedicated continuous cell separators or use of CELLEX® instrument. Patients with very low WBC counts ($<1\times10^9$/L) may also not benefit due to the low number of cells collected, treated and reinfused. Some centers have limited ECP to patients with WBC count $>1\times10^9$/L and ANC >0.5 to 1.0×10^9/L using either single or two-step methods [7, 25, 26].

2.1.2.6 Scheduling of Procedures

Historically, ECP procedures were originally derived from treatment schedules in patients with cutaneous T cell lymphoma. These treatments involved the ingestion of 8-methoxypsoralen followed by tandem two day mononuclear cell collections and subsequent UV-A irradiation of each day's product, with infusion of the irradiated product back to the patient on the same day of collection. The procedure was also developed to accommodate patients who often traveled long distances for the treatment. Current ECP treatments, however, involve the ex-vivo exposure of 8-methoxypsoralen. Thus, scheduling tandem day treatments is likely more of a historical hold over, than based on scientific evidence of proven efficacy of tandem procedures. Some centers for the convenience of patients, who may have to travel long distances to get to an ECP center, schedule tandem day procedures. However, other studies have reported other ECP treatment schedules such as a MWF schedule [6]. Further immunological monitoring trials are needed to determine the best treatment schedule in these patients. This will likely be based on future careful studies of biological markers and corresponding clinical findings.

2.1.3 Summary

Extracorporeal photopheresis can be safely performed in children provided there is adequate consideration of small total blood volumes, venous access, potential for extracorporeal volume shifts, hemodilution and anticoagulation issues. ECP techniques that utilize continuous cell separation methodologies provide the most hemodynamically safe approaches for mononuclear cell collection and can be utilized in the smallest children. The use of the CELLEX® should mitigate a number of these issues and further improve the safety and tolerability of ECP in children. Further proof of ECP utility in children will require studies of biomarkers that correlate with efficacy.

References

[1] Burgstaler EA. Current instrumentation for apheresis. In: McLeod BC, Szczepiorkowski ZM, Weinstein R, Winters JL, eds. Apheresis: principles and practice, 3rd edition. Bethesda, MD: AABB Press, 2010:71–109.
[2] Ward DM. Extracorporeal photopheresis: how, when, and why. J Clin Apher 2011;26:276–85.
[3] Voss CY, Fry TJ, Coppes MJ, Blajchman MA. Extending the horizon for cell-based immunotherapy by understanding the mechanisms of action of photopheresis. Transfus Med Rev 2010;24: 22–32.
[4] Szodoray P, Papp G, Nakken B, Harangi M, Zeher M. The molecular and clinical rationale of extracorporeal photochemotherapy in autoimmune diseases, malignancies and transplantation. Autoimmun Rev 2010;9:459–64.
[5] Kim HC. Therapeutic apheresis in pediatric patients. In: McLeod BC, Szczepiorkowski ZM, Weinstein R, Winters JL, eds. Apheresis: principles and practice, 3rd edition. Bethesda, MD: AABB Press, 2010:445–64.
[6] Kanold J, Merlin E, Halle P, et al. Photopheresis in pediatric graft-versus-host disease after allogeneic marrow transplantation: clinical practice guidelines based on field experience and review of the literature. Transfusion 2007;47:2276–89.
[7] Salvaneschi L, Perotti C, Zecca M, et al. Extracorporeal photochemotherapy for treatment of acute and chronic GVHD in childhood. Transfusion 2001;41:1299–305.
[8] Berger M, Pessolano R, Albiani R, et al. Extracorporeal photopheresis for steroid resistant graft versus host disease in pediatric patients: a pilot single institution report. J Pediatr Hematol Oncol 2007;29:678–87.
[9] Klassen J. The role of photopheresis in the treatment of graft-versus-host disease. Curr Oncol 2010;17:55–8.
[10] Linenberger M, Murtaugh A, Jarosek B, Guthrie K, Sanders J, Zhu Q. A novel 2-process, 3-step method for extracorporeal photochemotherapy in small body weight children with steroid resistant graft-versus-host disease: processing efficiencies, treated cell doses and clinical experience. J Clin Apher 2005;20:18 (abst 28).
[11] Huang ST, Moon P, Marques MB. Photopheresis in small child using the UVAR XTS® system. Transfusion 2001;41(9S):42S.
[12] Kanold J, Paillard C, Halle P, D'Incan M, Bordigoni P, Deméocq F. Extracorporeal photochemotherapy for graft versus host disease in pediatric patients. Transfus Apher Sci 2003;28:71–80.
[13] Perseghin P, Incontri A. Mononuclear cell collection in patients treated with extracorporeal photochemotherapy by using the off-line method: a comparison between COBE Spectra AutoPbsc version 6.1 and Amicus cell separators. J Clin Apher 2010;25:310–4.

[14] Merlin E, Jacomet F, D'Incan M, et al. Use of cryopreserved autologous cells for extracorporeal photochemotherapy: clinical applications. Transfusion 2011;51:1296–9.
[15] Merlin E, Hannani D, Veyrat-Masson R, et al. Cryopreservation of mononuclear cells before extracorporeal photochemotherapy does not impair their anti-proliferative capabilities. Cytotherapy 2011;13:248–55.
[16] Hackstein H, Misterek J, Nockher A, Reiter A, Bein G, Woessmann W. Mini buffy coat photopheresis for children and critically ill patients with extracorporeal photopheresis contraindications. Transfusion 2009;49:2366–73.
[17] Values for mean blood volume (mL/Kg) in children, men and women. Geigy Scientific Tables, 7th Ed; 1971.
[18] UVAR XTS® Instrument Operator's Manual.
[19] 2000 CDC Growth Charts for the United States: Methods and Development. Department of Health and Human Services, Center for Disease Control and Prevention. National Center for Health Statistics. Vital and Health Statistics Series 11, No. 246, May 2002.
[20] Collins JA. Hemorrhage, shock and burns. In: Petz LD and Swisher SN, editors. New York: Churchill Livingston, Inc., 1981:425–53.
[21] Gorlin JB. Therapeutic plasma exchange and cytapheresis in pediatric patients. Transfus Sci 1999;21:21–39.
[22] Schneiderman J, Jacobsohn DA, Collins J, Thormann K, Kletzel M. The use of fluid boluses to safely perform extracorporeal photopheresis (ECP) in low-weight children: a novel procedure. J Clin Apher 2010;25:63–9.
[23] CELLEX® Instrument Operator's Manual.
[24] Crookston KP, Novak DJ. Physiology of Apheresis. In: McLeod BC, Szczepiorkowski ZM, Weinstein R, Winters JL, eds. Apheresis: principles and practice, 3rd edition. Bethesda, MD: AABB Press, 2010:45–70.
[25] Perotti C, Torretta L, Viarengo G, et al. Feasibility and safety of a new technique of extracorporeal photochemotherapy: experience of 240 procedures. Haematologica 1999;84:237–41.
[26] Messina C, Locatelli F, Lanino E, et al. Extracorporeal photochemotherapy for paediatric patients with graft-versus-host disease after haematopoietic stem cell transplantation. Br J Haematol 2003;122:118–27.

Nina Worel
2.2 ECP in Patients with Bleeding Risks

Extracorporeal photopheresis (ECP) consists of two steps: a leukapheresis procedure collecting approximately 3–5% of circulating mononuclear cells and photoactivation by 8-methoxypsoralen (8-MOP) and ultraviolet A light (UVA, 1–2 J cm^{-2}). The treated cells are then reinfused into the patient. Two concepts of photopheresis do currently exist: a single unit apheresis device (THERAKOS® UVAR XTS® or THERAKOS® CELLEX®; Therakos Inc. USA; Figure 2.3) and an "offline" system requiring three separate processing steps (leukocyte collection, addition of psoralen plus UVA irradiation and reinfusion of treated cells).

To prevent coagulation in the extracorporeal circuit anticoagulants have to be used during therapeutic apheresis and are usually limited to citrate anticoagulants. The advantage of citrate is that any amount returned to the patients will be rapidly metabolized and never leads to any systemic anticoagulation. On the other hand, prevention of clotting is related not only to the anticoagulant itself but also to the flow rate – a slow flow promotes clotting. Therefore, some authors recommend the addition of heparin to citrate for anticoagulation [1].

Special caution using heparin is advisable in patients with low platelet counts, renal and/or hepatic dysfunction as those have a higher risk for bleeding. Moreover, patients with mucous membrane lesions of the intestine can experience severe bleeding under systemic anticoagulation with heparin.

2.2.1 Anticoagulation with Heparin

The current FDA-approved protocol for extracorporeal photopheresis performed with the technology developed by Therakos (Johnson and Johnson, New Jersey, USA) requires the use of heparin during priming and as anticoagulation fluid. To prevent clotting in the extracorporeal circuit approximately 10.000 units of heparin are applied extracorporeally and reinfused into the patient together with plasma, red blood cells and leukocytes. This results in systemic anticoagulation of the patient for a longer time period due to the half-life of heparin.

After intravenous application about 40% of unfractionated heparin is initially eliminated fast resulting in a half-life of 5–15 minutes due to rapid binding to surface receptors on endothelial cells and macrophages. This elimination is followed by a slower, renal clearance leading to a half-life of 60–90 minutes. After saturation of all binding sites the dose-response relationship becomes linear and therapeutic plasma levels can be reached. The main complication of heparin anticoagulation is bleeding: major bleeding is reported to occur in up to 7% of patients and fatal bleeding in up to 3% [2]. Other complications include heparin-induced thrombocytopenia (HIT) in

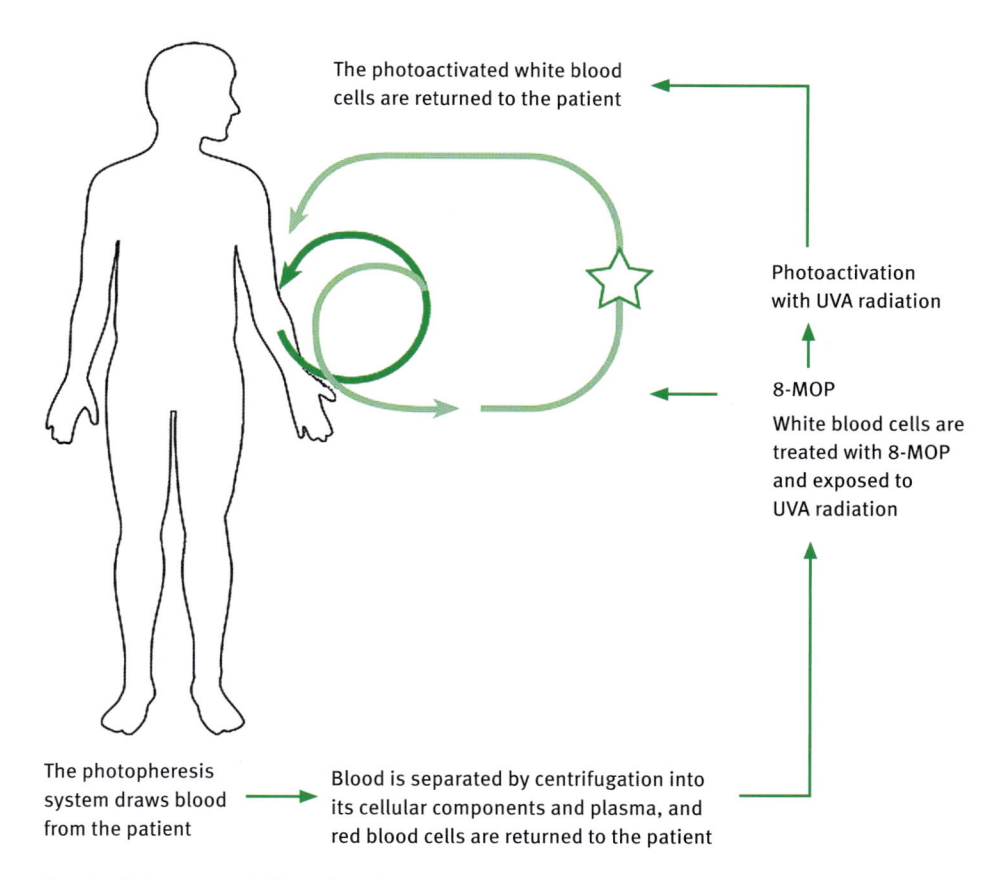

Fig. 2.3. Extracorporeal Photopheresis.
During extracorporeal photopheresis (ECP) whole blood is drawn from the patient and separated into plasma and different cell fractions. Mononuclear cells are collected, incubated with 8-methoxypsoralen (8-MOP), photoactivated with ultraviolet A light (UVA) and reinfused into the patient.

1–5%, which is a life-threatening event caused by antibodies directed to complexes containing heparin and an autologous platelet protein, platelet factor 4 [3].

In a study of Ivancic and colleagues the extent of heparin anticoagulant activity after ECP was determined by monitoring activated partial thromboplastin time (aPTT) and anti-factor Xa [4]. Before treatment, aPTT levels were normal in all patients (mean of 35.76 ± 2.63 sec; normal values 27.0–41.0 sec), but increased significantly to a mean of 135.91 sec (± 35.77) measured 1 hour after end of ECP. APTT levels dropped over time and returned to normal in the majority of patients within 4 hours.

However, patients with relative contraindications to heparin such as low platelet counts, overt or occult bleeding or risk factors for bleeding, severe hypertension and impaired renal function may benefit from an alternative anticoagulation protocol.

Additionally, alternative anticoagulation is needed especially in patients with absolute contraindications to heparin such as heparin-induced thrombocytopenia.

2.2.2 Anticoagulation with Acid Citrate Dextrose

Acid citrate dextrose (ACD-A) is recommended and routinely used in apheresis procedures during cell separation to collect blood components and in therapeutic procedures such as plasma exchange, immunoadsorption and cell depletion [5]. Citrate is naturally present in the blood at low concentrations and is an important substrate in the metabolism of cells. When added to the blood in significantly higher concentrations, citrate combines with ionized calcium (Ca^{2+}) to form a soluble complex, which reduces the concentration of Ca^{2+} in the plasma. The process of coagulation requires Ca^{2+} and is inhibited when enough citrate is present. While citrate also combines with other cations, for example ionized magnesium, binding with ionized calcium is believed to be the most important anticoagulatory effect [6].

The concentration of citrate in the anticoagulated plasma of the extracorporeal circuit of apheresis systems (15 to 20 mmol/L) causes a decrease in Ca^{2+} from about 1.1 mmol/L, the normal concentration in the circulation, to 50 to 100 µmol/L, i.e. a 10- to 20-fold decrease. Because the volume and flow rate through the extracorporeal circuit are small in comparison to the total blood volume and cardiac output of the donor or patient undergoing apheresis, return of this anticoagulated blood containing elevated levels of citrate has little effect on the ionized calcium concentration in the circulation. However, as citrate containing blood is returned to the patient, chelation of cations can continue in the systemic circulation. Consequently, metabolic complications ensue (hypocalcemia, hypomagnesemia, metabolic alkalosis, and other electrolyte derangements) and are accompanied by symptoms which are usually modest. Nevertheless, if citrate is added too rapidly or over a long time period, the ionized calcium in the circulation may drop low enough to cause noticeable sensations or symptoms in the patient [1]. Citrate related complications have been reported to occur in 1.2% of donors during voluntary donations [7], 7.8% of patients undergoing therapeutic plasma exchange procedures [8], and 48% of patients undergoing large volume leukapheresis during peripheral blood progenitor cell collection [9]. Symptoms occur variably when ionized Ca^{2+} levels fall below normal range (<1.1 mmol/L) and can be categorized as mild, moderate, or severe (Figure 2.4).

To prevent discomfort, it is important to control the rate of citrate infusion into the patient and to take into account the duration of the procedure. Before start of therapeutic apheresis, ionized Ca^{2+} levels should be measured. Depending on the kind of procedure (duration, amount of whole blood processed) calcium replacement can be contemplated and administrated orally or intravenously for prophylactic, intermittent, or continuous supplementation [1].

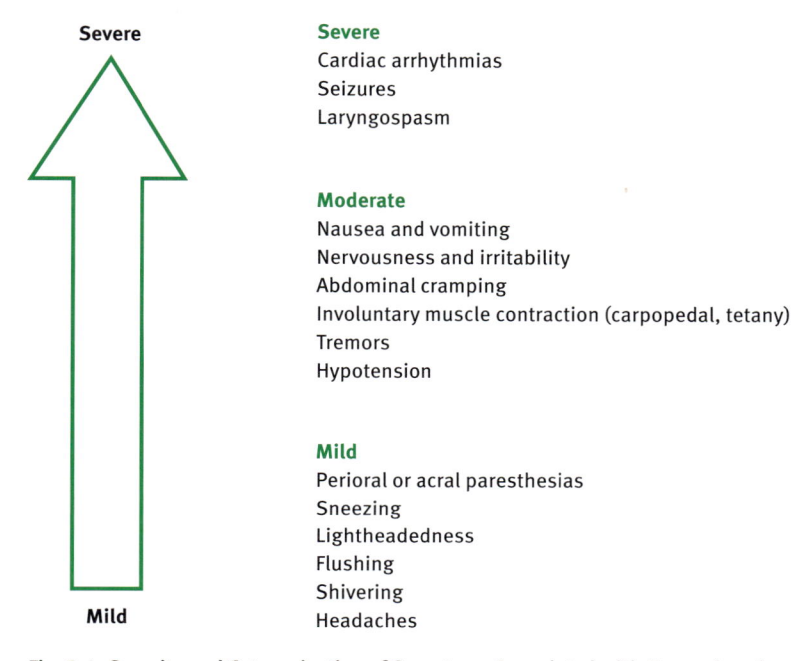

Severe
Cardiac arrhythmias
Seizures
Laryngospasm

Moderate
Nausea and vomiting
Nervousness and irritability
Abdominal cramping
Involuntary muscle contraction (carpopedal, tetany)
Tremors
Hypotension

Mild
Perioral or acral paresthesias
Sneezing
Lightheadedness
Flushing
Shivering
Headaches

Fig. 2.4. Severity and Categorization of Symptoms Associated with Hypocalcemia.

2.2.3 Anticoagulation during ECP in Patients with Bleeding Risks

The fact that increasing numbers of ECP treatments nowadays are performed in patients with acute graft-versus-host disease (GVHD) who have in parts insufficiently regenerated platelet counts and/or patients with severe GVHD of the gastrointestinal tract and/or impaired renal or hepatic function highlights the need for alternate anticoagulation protocols. For these patients, anticoagulation using acid citrate dextrose has been infrequently used in small patient cohorts [10, 11].

Apsner and colleagues compared two anticoagulation protocols in a study on 55 patients with different diagnoses including 21 patients with GVHD [10]. A total of 404 ECP treatments were performed with citrate and 278 ones with heparin anticoagulation, respectively. In both procedures priming of the extracorporeal circuit consisted of saline containing 30.000 IU/L of heparin of which 1.500 IU of heparin were infused. Thereafter, either ACD-A or sodium/heparin (30.000 IU/L) was added at a ratio of 1:10 to whole blood during the apheresis procedure. Calculation of the infused anticoagulant revealed that patients received either an average amount of 12.500 IU of heparin or 1.600 IU of heparin and an average of 288 mL of ACD-A during priming and treatment. Citrate anticoagulation was well tolerated and citrate reactions occurred in 1.7 % (7 of 404) of procedures. Bleeding complications were only documented in the group of patients with heparin anticoagulation (3 of 278 procedures, 1.08 %) but not after citrate use (0 of 404) [10].

2.2.4 Anticoagulation during ECP in Patients with Absolute Contraindications for Heparin Use

Alternative anticoagulation is needed for patients with absolute contraindications to heparin, such as heparin-induced thrombocytopenia, risk of bleeding due to additional anticoagulation (e. g. warfarin) or heparin allergy.

Nedelcu and colleagues from the University of California, Los Angeles, developed a protocol that completely replaces heparin with ACD-A for ECP performed with the THERAKOS® device [11]. This study describes 5 patients with cutaneous T cell lymphoma (n=3), heart transplant rejection (n=1) and GVHD (n=1), all with contraindications for heparin use, undergoing a total of 94 ECP procedures. Calcium gluconate solution was administered prophylactically and as needed for symptoms of citrate toxicity. The incidence and severity of citrate toxicity and the technical data for all procedures were analyzed. All patients tolerated the procedures well without significant complications. Only minimal symptoms of citrate toxicity manifested as transient perioral tingling were observed in 24.5% (23 of 94) of all procedures. Symptoms resolved promptly following administration of additional calcium gluconate. However, in this study it was very important to calculate the flow rates during the different cycles and to be aware of citrate toxicity [11].

2.2.5 Vienna Experience on ECP with ACD-A

In 2011 we investigated the safety and efficacy of this citrate anticoagulation in 94 consecutive patients (43 male, 51 female) with acute GVHD (45% with gastrointestinal GVHD; Figure 2.5) undergoing ECP with the THERAKOS® device using ACD-A anticoagulation at a single institution (Table 2.6). Patients underwent ECP 2 to 3 times per week on a weekly basis until complete resolution of acute GVHD. Priming of the apheresis device consisted of saline containing 10.000 IU/L of heparin of which approximately 1.300 IU of heparin were infused, followed by anticoagulation with ACD-A at a ratio of 1:10 or higher (e. g. in patients with low platelet counts or additional extracorporeal treatment) during the whole procedure. Heparin instead of ACD-A priming was used to avoid possible ACD-A side effects during reinfusion after the first cycle.

A total of 1242 ECP procedures were analyzed with respect to side effects and changes in hemoglobin levels and platelet counts. Moreover, in a proportion of ECP treatments activated partial thromboplastin time was monitored (Table 2.7). Before ECP 48 (51%) patients had platelet counts below 100 G/L and 24 (26%) below 50 G/L, respectively.

ECP was tolerated well by all patients. In only 0.2 % of procedures mild citrate reactions seen as transient paraesthesia were observed but resolved without the need for calcium substitution. In no case bleeding complications were noted during or after citrate anticoagulation. During ECP, aPTT levels increased marginally. We noticed that citrate anticoagulation during ECP is a feasible and safe alternative for patients with high risk for bleeding complications, especially for those after allogeneic hematopoietic stem cell transplantation (e. g. low platelet counts, acute GVHD of the gastrointestinal tract).

Number of patients (Male/Female)	94 (43/51)
Median age years (range)	41 (18–64)
Myeloablative/Reduced Intensity Conditioning	75/19
Sibling/Unrelated Donor	24/70
HLA-identical/Mismatched donor	50/44
BM/PBSC graft	40/54
Median day of onset of acute GVHD after HCT	14 (8–43)
Median day of onset of steroids after HCT	16 (8–46)
Grade of acute GVHD at start of ECP II III IV	57 19 18
Organs involved (%) Skin alone Skin, liver Skin, gut Liver, gut Skin, liver, gut	46 (49) 15 (16) 15 (16) 4 (4) 14 (15)

BM = bone marrow, PBSC = peripheral blood stem cells, HCT = hematopoietic cell transplantation, GVHD = graft-versus-host disease.

Table 2.6. Patient Characteristics.

	Before ECP (n=1242 procedures)	After ECP (n=1242 procedures)
Median hemoglobin level mg/dL (range)	10.8 (8.6–14.0)	9.5 (8.0–12.3)
Median platelet counts G/L (range)	120 (24–326)	113 (18–255)
Median aPTT sec (range)	32.1 (25.3–44.5)	35.4 (25.4–54.7)
Median loss of hemoglobin %	–	11 (0–29)
Median loss of platelets %	–	14 (0–40)

aPPT = activated partial thromboplastin time.

Table 2.7. Laboratory Data before and after ECP.

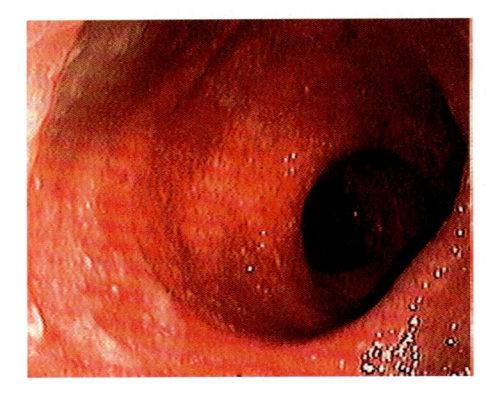

Fig. 2.5. Severe Acute Graft-versus-host Disease of the Gastrointestinal Tract as seen during Endoscopic Exam.

2.2.6 Recommendations and Conclusions

Heparin anticoagulation should be limited to certain apheresis indications (e. g. LDL-apheresis, large volume leukapheresis) and can cause major and even fatal bleeding events in up to 7% and 3% of patients, respectively depending on the amount of heparin used [1, 2]. Citrate is the preferred anticoagulant for extracorporeal circuits not only in preparative but also in therapeutic apheresis and has been shown to be safe also in ECP procedures. Symptoms of citrate toxicity are generally caused by symptomatic hypocalcemia and can be prevented through monitoring of ionized calcium and patients' symptoms [1]. Since only a small amount of citrate is used during an ECP procedure, citrate-induced symptoms are negligible. Since no bleeding events have been reported in citrate anticoagulation, this approach should be followed especially in patients with high risk for bleeding or contraindications for heparin use. Therefore, patients with bleeding risks should not be excluded from ECP.

References

[1] Lee G and Arepally GM. Anticoagulation techniques in apheresis: From heparin to citrate and beyond. J Clin Apher 2012 DOI: 10.1002/jca.21222 epub ahead.
[2] Hirsh J, Bauer KA, Donati MB, Gould M, Samma MM, Weitz JI. Parenteral anticoagulants: American College of Chest Physicians Evidence-Based Clinical Practice Guidelines (8th Edition). Chest 2008;133:141S–59S.
[3] Arepally G and Ortel TL. Heparin-induced thrombocytopenia. N Eng J Med 2006;355:809–17.
[4] Ivancic E, Knobler R, Quehenberger P, Hönigsmann H, Trautinger F. The course of anticoagulation after extracorporeal photochemotherapy. Photodermatol Photoimmunol Photomed 2005;21:150–1.
[5] Hester JP, McCullough J, Mishler JM, Szymanski IO. Dosage regimens for citrate anticoagulants. J Clin Apher 1983;1:149–57.
[6] Szymanski IO. Ionized calcium during platelet pheresis. Transfusion 1978;18:701–8.
[7] Crocco A, D'Elia D. Adverse reactions during voluntary donation of blood and/or blood components. A statistical-epidemiological study. Blood Transfus 2007;5:143–52.

[8] Rodnitzky RL, Goeken JA. Complication of plasma exchange in neurological patients. Arch Neurol 1982;39:350–4.
[9] Buchta C, Macher M, Biegelmayer C, Hoecker P, Dettke M. Reduction of adverse citrate reactions during autologous large-volume PBPC apheresis by continuous infusion of calcium-gluconate. Transfusion 2003;43:1615–21.
[10] Apsner R, Uenver B, Sunder-Plassmann G, Knobler RM. Regional anticoagulation with acid citrate dextrose-A for extracorporeal photoimmunochemotherapy. Vox Sang 2002;83:222–6.
[11] Nedelcu E, Ziman A, Fernando LP, Cook K, Bumerts P, Schiller G. Exclusive use of acid citrate dextrose for anticoagulation during extracorporeal photopheresis in patients with contraindications to heparin: an effective protocol. J Clin Apher 2008;23:66–73.

Kristina Hölig
2.3 ECP with Central Venous Access

The quality of the extracorporeal photopheresis (ECP) procedure, like other therapeutic aphereses, depends on a reliable venous access. Conveniently, ECP does not require very high blood flow rates, between 10–25 mL/min are sufficient. Therefore in most patients peripheral venous access is adequately achievable. A main goal in patient care should be to avoid central venous access, whenever possible, because each kind of central venous catheter implies its own complications.

Another point of concern is the clinical situation of the patient in general. Important factors influencing the choice of venous access are:
- The underlying disease: it affects the duration of ECP-treatment as well as the degree of immunosuppression or a possible impairment of wound healing.
- Indication for other intravenous treatments, i. e. parenteral nutrition or dialysis.
- Individual preferences of the patient.

In this respect, not every central venous catheter is appropriate for every patient and all aspects have to be considered carefully. In this chapter the pros and cons of the different options of central venous access and their suitability for ECP-treatment are discussed. There is little data on the use of central venous catheters in the literature, systematic reviews or prospective trials are missing. Therefore, recommendations can only be given from conclusions by analogy, drawn from the literature regarding patients under dialysis and plasmapheresis. Beyond that, experiences from our own ECP center and personal communications from other centers have been considered as well.

2.3.1 Arteriovenous Fistulas (AVFs) or Arteriovenous Grafts (AVGs)

AVFs or AVGs resemble the typical vascular access for hemodialysis. They allow very high blood flow rates (around 400 mL/minute) and can be used for long-term treatment periods [1]. Considering ECP-patients two completely different situations have to be taken into account:
1. Patients with an AVF already in situ.
2. Patients in need for new central venous catheters.

In the first group of patients, the AVF already available can be used for ECP, but skillful nursing and regular monitoring is crucial. This is normally the case in kidney transplant recipients, where ECP might be indicated for the treatment or prevention of organ graft rejection [2]. These patients are regularly seen by a nephrologist who can assure appropriate monitoring of the AVF. In other patients not suffering from renal disorders, an AVF might be taken into account as a reasonable alternative to a central venous catheter. In hemodialysis patients AVFs are clearly the preferred vascular access because of the lower rates of infections and thromboses, resulting in a lower morbidity and mortality [3, 4].

On the other hand, AVFs require surgical creation and a waiting period of several weeks for wound healing and maturation. For this reason most authors recommend an AVF only for patients in need of an apheresis treatment for longer than 1 year. This situation can rarely be anticipated in patients beginning ECP treatment. The specific, although infrequent complications of AVFs include steal syndrome, myocardial ischemic events and high-output cardiac failure [5]. Therefore AFVs can be contraindicated in patients with serious cardiac diseases.

From a practical point of view, it is most critical to make appropriate plans for the care of AVF in ECP-patients similar to those undergoing hemodialysis (HD). This is especially important, because treatment intervals in ECP are considerably longer than in HD patients. Vascular access blood flow monitoring every month or second month along with preventive interventions are suggested to be the standard of care [6, 7].

The staff of most photopheresis facilities is not necessarily familiar with caring for AVF like nephrologists and dialysis nurses. For all these reasons the surgical creation of an AVF for exclusive use for ECP will probably be regarded unnecessary and too risky for most patients.

2.3.2 Central Venous Catheters (CVCs)

A wide range of CVCs is available for different clinical applications. In particular, patients with acute and sometimes chronic graft-versus-host disease (GVHD) need a CVC for intravenous medication, nutrition and blood components support. It seems reasonable to also perform ECP treatment via these CVCs. Those temporary CVCs are usually inserted into the right internal or external jugular vein. If this is not possible, the same veins at the left side can be used [8]. The design of these catheters comply with the requirements of apheresis, in most cases these are three-lumen catheters. Nevertheless ECP-treatments occasionally can be performed with these accesses. Frequently, it might be necessary to increase the flow rate by connecting two lumina with a multidirectional stopcock (Figure 2.6).

Another possibility to perform aphereses in acute situations is a femoral vein catheter (FVC). This type of catheter can only be recommended for a single ECP treatment cycle in patients, where start of therapy is urgently needed and no other options of venous access are available. FVCs carry higher risks of deep venous thrombosis and infection, furthermore they limit patients' mobility [1].

Thrombosis and catheter infection are also the most important complications of temporary CVCs. Optimal nursing with strictly sterile handling and meticulous flushing is critical to prevent these problems, but will not be able to avoid them completely.

Many patients on ECP are severely immunocompromised due to their underlying disease and the immunosuppressive treatment they receive. In this patient population the use of a temporal CVC for ECP only for extended periods of time has to be discouraged.

Tunnelled catheters represent a reasonable alternative because of the lower risk of catheter dislodgement and blood stream infection [1].

Ständer and colleagues [8] systematically evaluated eight different subcutaneous right atrial catheters regarding their suitability for ECP with the UVAR XTS® photopheresis device. They found that CVCs with a length of over 90 cm reached flow rates below 7 mL/min and are therefore impractical for ECP (Figure 2.7). This problem could be partially overcome by using two lumina of the CVC simultaneously. By this means flow rates could be increased by 5–6 mL/min. The authors conclude that an acceptable flow rate can only be achieved with hemodialysis catheters. Therefore, they consider these CVCs the central venous access of choice for ECP treatment in patients with inadequate peripheral vascular access. Subcutaneous tunneled catheters should be preferred compared to short-term catheters because of the lower risk for infections.

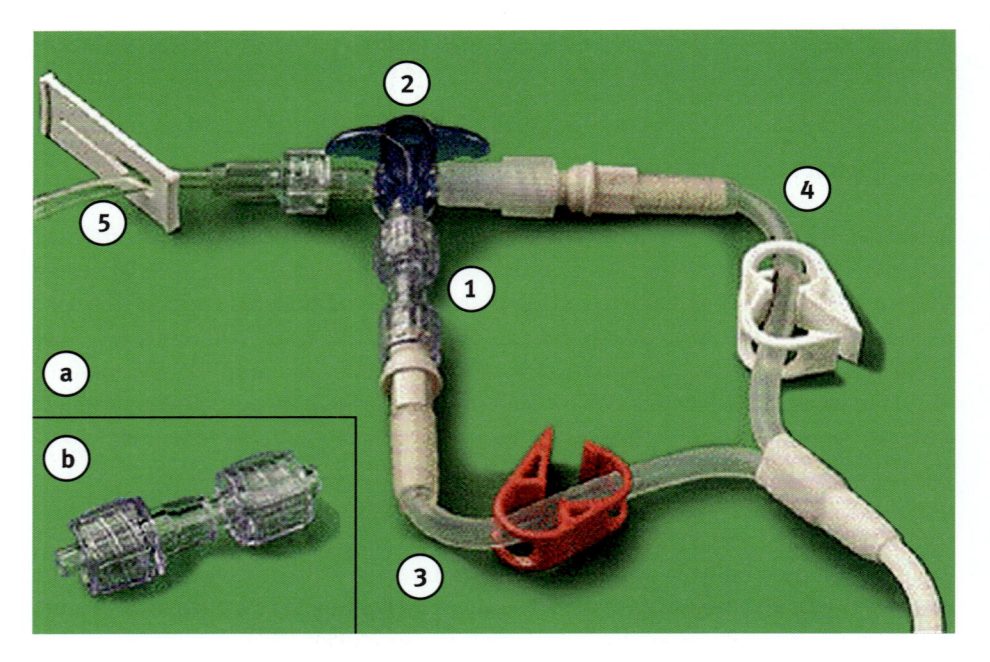

Fig. 2.6. Connection of a Dual Lumen Catheter to the UVAR XTS®.
(a) By attaching a male-male adapter (1) to a multidirectional stopcock (2) both lumina of a dual-lumen catheter (3,4) can be connected to the patient line (5) of the UVAR XTS® photopheresis system.
(b) Male-male adapter (detail); after Ständer et al. [8]. Reproduced with permission from John Wiley and Sons.

2.3 ECP with Central Venous Access — 33

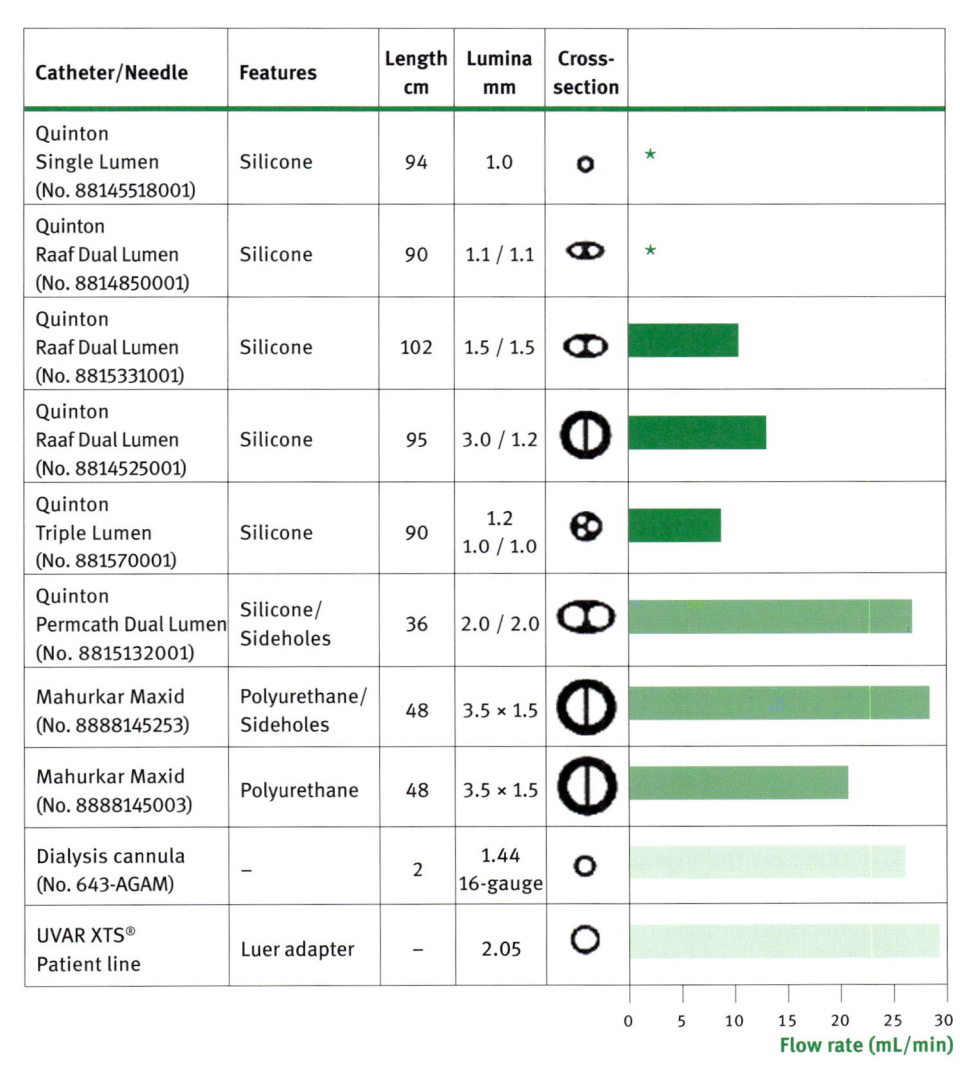

Catheter/Needle	Features	Length cm	Lumina mm	Cross-section	Flow rate
Quinton Single Lumen (No. 88145518001)	Silicone	94	1.0	○	*
Quinton Raaf Dual Lumen (No. 8814850001)	Silicone	90	1.1 / 1.1	⊂⊃	*
Quinton Raaf Dual Lumen (No. 8815331001)	Silicone	102	1.5 / 1.5	⊂⊃	▇
Quinton Raaf Dual Lumen (No. 8814525001)	Silicone	95	3.0 / 1.2	◐	▇
Quinton Triple Lumen (No. 881570001)	Silicone	90	1.2 / 1.0 / 1.0	⊗	▇
Quinton Permcath Dual Lumen (No. 8815132001)	Silicone/ Sideholes	36	2.0 / 2.0	⊂⊃	▇▇
Mahurkar Maxid (No. 8888145253)	Polyurethane/ Sideholes	48	3.5 × 1.5	◐	▇▇▇
Mahurkar Maxid (No. 8888145003)	Polyurethane	48	3.5 × 1.5	◐	▇▇▇
Dialysis cannula (No. 643-AGAM)	–	2	1.44 16-gauge	○	▇▇
UVAR XTS® Patient line	Luer adapter	–	2.05	○	▇▇

Flow rate (mL/min): 0 5 10 15 20 25 30

Fig. 2.7. In Vitro Flow Rates of Selected Implantable Central Venous Catheters which were Connected to the UVAR XTS® Photopheresis Device Outfitted with a Training ECP Kit.
Flow rates for 40% glucose solution were obtained from the control unit of the device (* = alarm: "occlusion patient"); after Ständer et al. [8]. Reproduced with permission from John Wiley and Sons.

2.3.3 Totally Implantable Central Venous Access Systems (Ports)

Port systems are devices consisting of a subcutaneously implanted chamber connected with a tunnelled catheter inserted preferentially in the subclavian or jugular vein.
Ports have the advantage of a cutaneous barrier, which effectively protects against bacterial contamination in the interval between treatments. They are, therefore, espe-

cially valuable in the outpatient setting. Many patients with hematological diseases get port systems for the application of cytostatic agents and for supportive care. Unlike temporary CVCs, these "conventional" port systems in our experience have never been suitable for therapeutic apheresis treatments like ECP. Among the various port systems very few types seem to be adapted for ECP treatment. There have not been any systematic studies published to date regarding the suitability of port systems in ECP therapy.

Our group has been using port systems for ECP treatment since 2007. The model we have exclusively applied is the Vortex® TR, SSDX-16-I (AngioDynamics® Inc, Cambridge UK), a single titanium port with a detached silicone catheter, size 9.6 F (Figure 2.8). Puncture for ECP treatment is always performed with an 18 G Huber needle SFN 1320 (PAKUMED Medical Products GmbH, Essen, Germany, Figure 2.9).

During the last 5 years 28 patients at our institution received port systems to facilitate ECP therapy. Since then about 500 ECP treatments have been performed in this group of patients, the majority with the UVAR XTS® device. Experience with the CELLEX® machine is very limited in our centre – about 15 treatments via ports have been performed by now.

Collection flow in patients with ports is in the range of 10–18 mL/min with the UVAR XTS® device; the return flow does not differ from patients with peripheral venous access (about 20–45 mL/min). Collection flow using the CELLEX® device seems to be even better, mostly > 15 mL/min. We recommend using exclusively the UVAR XTS® disposable with the small bowl for ECP-treatment in patients with port systems. With the big bowl the alarm "Occlusion patient" invariably occurs during the early return phase due to the high viscosity of the red cell sediment.

Like other central venous access devices, ports carry the risks of bacterial contamination and catheter thrombosis. To keep these risks at a minimum, optimal nursing techniques are required.

The following rules should be kept in mind when using these special port systems:
- During injections into the port high pressure has to be avoided, therefore only syringes with a minimal volume of 10 mL should be used.
- At the end of each ECP treatment, the port has to be flushed thoroughly with 20 mL of saline at the minimum.
- To avoid clotting, the port should be blocked with 5 mL of saline containing 5000 IU of heparin (in a 10 mL syringe).
- The 18G Huber needle can be left in the port for a maximum time of 48 hours.

Despite optimal care of the port systems delivery problems in our experience occur in about 40 % of ECP treatments. The collection rates drop mostly during the first two cycles of the ECP procedure. In nearly all cases this problem is encountered during the first session of a sequence, the treatment on the following day normally can be performed without any difficulties.

A variety of actions can be taken – in the order specified – to restore the flow rate of the port:
1. The patient can be positioned in the Trendelenburg's position (shock position) and is asked to breathe deeply or cough to enhance filling of intrathoracical veins.
2. The port is rinsed with saline with intermittent aspiration; simultaneously the patient should be asked to raise the arms above the head, move the head and turn around.
3. The port can be rinsed with heparinized saline.
4. The needle can be changed.
5. Solutions containing ascorbic acid can be instilled for 10–15 minutes, thereafter its aspiration is necessary.
6. Thrombolysis with urokinase can be performed as follows:
   - 5000 U/mL
   - Instillation of 1 mL (in a 10 mL syringe), clamping the line.
   - Waiting for 20 minutes, thereafter trying aspiration.
   - If no blood can be drawn, the procedure can be repeated for up to 3 times.

In our experience, steps 1–5 are sufficient to overcome most of the flow difficulties in patients with ports. Only in 2 patients thrombolysis with urokinase had to be performed and port function could be restored successfully. Generally, we would recommend controlling catheter position by X-ray before performing thrombolysis. X-ray is also necessary in all cases of pain, swelling or other discomfort during the use of the port to exclude kinking or dislocation of the catheter.

2.3.4 Summary/Conclusions

The ideal venous access for ECP is via peripheral veins; therefore, peripheral access should be always preferred. In patients who already have a temporary CVC, this catheter can be used for ECP, if the design is suitable.

If a new central venous access is needed for ECP treatment, in our experience a port currently resembles the option most feasible for adult patients. The decision for port implantation should be carefully considered in each case.

We would like to recommend the following checklist to support the decision for an ECP-port (modified after Ständer et al [8]).:
- If a patient has two previously performed ECP treatments via peripheral venous access with major access problems or treatment failure a port system is indicated. Alternatively, in patients with a history of extremely poor peripheral venous access the clinical assessment by an experienced apheresis physician is sufficient.
- The indication for ECP has to be confirmed by an interdisciplinary team of physicians including the specialists in charge of the patient's primary care.

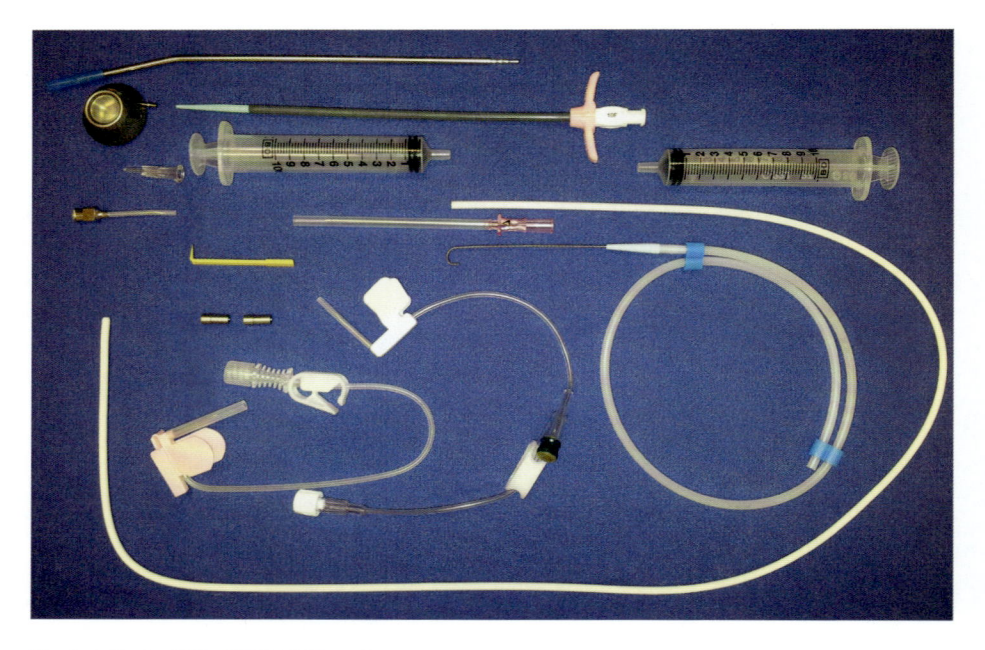

Fig. 2.8. Vortex® TR, SSDX-16-I Port System.

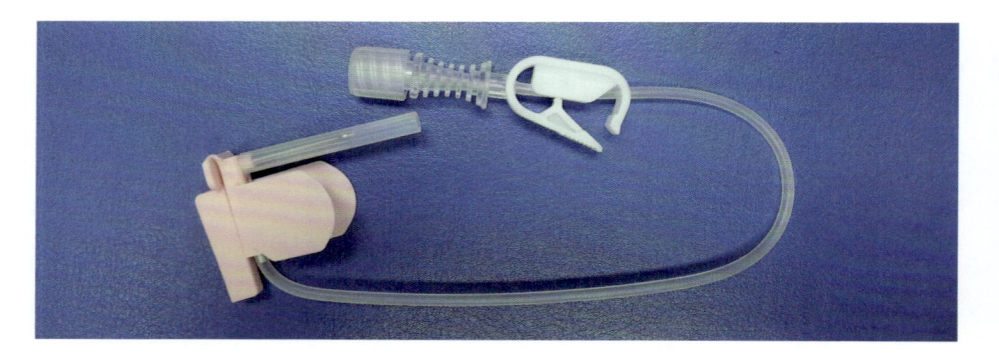

Fig. 2.9. 18 G Huber Needle SFN 1320.

- An experienced team familiar with the technique of port implantation must be available.
- Patient compliance in maintaining proper hygiene and supporting appropriate use of the port is required.
- Long-term dedicated nursing and maintenance of the port system by the apheresis staff, including the time period, when ECP-treatment might be no longer necessary, has to be available.

If all these aspects are considered carefully, port systems resemble a valuable tool to facilitate ECP treatment in patients with poor peripheral veins in the most convenient and secure way currently achievable.

References

[1] Okafor C, Kalantarinia K. Vascular access considerations for therapeutic apheresis procedures. Sem Dialysis 2012;25:140–4.
[2] Kusztal M, Kłak R, Krajewska M, Boratynska M, Patrzałek D, Klinger M. Application of extracorporeal photopheresis in kidney transplant recipients: Technical considerations and procedure tolerance. Transplant Proc 2011;43:2941–2.
[3] Dhingra RK, Young EW, Hulbert-Shearon TE, Leavey SF, Port FK. Type of vascular access and mortality in U.S. hemodialysis patients. Kidney Int 2001;60:1443–51.
[4] Clinical practice guidelines for vascular access. Vascular Access Work Group. Am J Kidney Dis 2006;48 (Suppl 1):S176–S247.
[5] Quarello F, Forneris G, Borca M, Pozzato M. Do central venous catheters have advantages over arteriovenous fistulas or grafts? J Nephrol 2006;19:265–79.
[6] Stegmayr B, Wikdahl AM. Access in therapeutic apheresis. Ther Apher Dial 2003;7:209–14.
[7] McCarley P, Wingard RL, Shyr Y, Pettus W, Hakim RM, Ikizler TA. Vascular access blood flow monitoring reduces access morbidity and costs. Kidney Int 2001;60:1164–72.
[8] Ständer H, Neugebauer F, Schneider SW, Luger TA, Schiller M. Extracorporeal photopheresis with permanent subcutaneous right atrial catheters. JDDG 2007;12: 1112–8.

Alain Bohbot, Vincent Liu, Bruno Lioure, Karin Bilger,
Annegret Laplace and Raoul Herbrecht
2.4 New Technical Developments

Introduced in 1987 in the United States of America, extracorporeal photopheresis (ECP), also called photopheresis, combines two existing therapeutic technologies: Leukapheresis and PUVA therapy.

Two concepts of photopheresis exist: The open/off-line and the closed/on-line systems. The "open" or "off-line" system requires three separate steps. The *collection* of circulating leukocytes, the *photoactivation* (which is the addition of 8-methoxypsoralen (8-MOP) to the leukocytes combined with irradiation by ultraviolet A-light), and the *reinfusion* of the treated cells to the patient. The irradiation step is the most important, because the photoactivation is presumed to induce cell damages leading to apoptosis, which is the key of the mechanism(s) of action. The second type of photopheresis system is a certified, single unit system known as "closed" or "on-line" system. This procedure is performed as a one-step, closed procedure. Currently, there are two closed photopheresis systems available: THERAKOS® UVAR XTS® Photopheresis System and the THERAKOS® CELLEX® Photopheresis System (Johnson and Johnson, New Jersey, USA and Ascot, UK).

2.4.1 Extracorporeal Photopheresis Regulatory Recommendations

Since 2003, the French Health Products Safety Agency (ANSM, Agence Nationale de Sécurité du Médicament et des produits de Santé), considers that only ECP performed with the off-line system has to comply with the cellular therapy regulatory recommendations.

What is an open or off-line system? It is any disconnected process using a cell separator in combination with a light box and a drug. For example, Caridian Spectra or Optia for white blood cell (WBC) collection (Caridian BCT, Inc., Denver, CO, USA), in combination with the Macogenic (MacoPharma, France) or PIT system (MTS GmbH, Germany) for WBC irradiation. Although the components may be individually CE-marked, they are not specifically CE-marked for photopheresis. To obtain proper CE-marking for photopheresis, a system (all components) must undergo controlled clinical trials using a drug.

In clinical use irradiated mononuclear cells retransfused after collection and treatment with 8-MOP and ultraviolet A (UVA), are considered "drugs." As a consequence, good manufacturing practice (GMP) productions have to be transferred from the clinical institutions to cell therapy facilities, which, according to GMP, are able to manufacture "drugs."

Good manufacturing practice regulations apply to all phases of cell collection, transport, processing and infusion as well as documentation, training of personnel and laboratory facilities. A number of national and international guidelines, regulations, and federal laws have to be considered [1–3].

One prerequisite for regulatory approval is the appointment of qualified personnel and place of cell processing, including a clean room facility reaching the level of air cleanliness standard class D (ISO-8 or 100000 according to US federal standard N° 209B). The aim is to avoid contamination and to ensure sterility and safety of the product.

Another major area of GMP is standard operating procedures that have to exist for all manufacturing stages, as well as for documentation, in-process controls, training, cleaning and product release. In-process control assays have to be performed. These include routine testing for sterility at different critical points, determination of cell counts and a functional test to characterize the cells in the preparation (mitogen-induced proliferation before irradiation and inhibition of mitogen-induced proliferation after irradiation).

Additional parameters to comply with GMP regulations include validation of the method used, survey of room surfaces and air, monitoring of key equipment (e. g. irradiator, UVA light energy level, lifespan of UVA lamp), and material used (e. g. bags, 8-MOP etc.).

The aim of these recommendations is first, to produce irradiated cells according to a safe and secure process, and second, to ensure traceability and avoid cross contaminations.

2.4.2 The Closed System's New Technical Developments

The THERAKOS® CELLEX® System (Figure 2.10) incorporates technical advances in the cell separation (bowl and centrifuge system) and fluid control functions (software and continuous flow). It is an integral device, performing all steps of leukocyte collection, photoactivation and reinfusion of the treated cells to the patient in one instrument. This medical device is associated with a single-use kit and with the drug, UVADEX™ 20 mcg/mL solution, which is approved by the FDA and with market authorization in many European countries including UK, France, Austria, Germany, and Italy.

How does the CELLEX® System work? During a photopheresis procedure, whole blood is withdrawn from the patient and separated by centrifugation to yield a leukocyte enriched blood fraction. In double-needle configuration, the pump draws whole blood from the patient via the collect line into the centrifuge bowl. The leukocytes are concentrated in the continuously spinning centrifuge bowl whilst red cells and plasma are simultaneously returned to the patient via the return line.

For patients with poor venous access or in case of an access loss during the procedure, the CELLEX® System offers the option of configuring the procedural kit as single-needle, resulting in discontinuous flow of whole blood to, and from, the patient. In case of single-needle configuration, the pump draws whole blood from the patient via the collect/return line into the centrifuge bowl. The leukocytes are concentrated in the spinning centrifuge bowl. Red cells and plasma are returned intermittently to the patient via the collect/return line.

In either configuration, following the leukocyte harvest, UVADEX™ 20 mcg/mL solution is injected directly into the leukocyte-enriched fraction (buffy coat) in the treatment bag. The contained leukocyte/drug product is then exposed to an automatically calculated prescribed dose of UVA light. During photoactivation, any remaining red blood cells and plasma are continuously returned to the patient, without being treated. Once photoactivation is completed, the treated cells are filtered and automatically reinfused into the patient.

In this chapter, we would like to develop the effectiveness of the leukocyte collection system, the management of the fluid balance and the system upgrade. Most of these points marked the differences in regards to the technical enhancements between the CELLEX® System and its predecessor, the UVAR XTS® System.

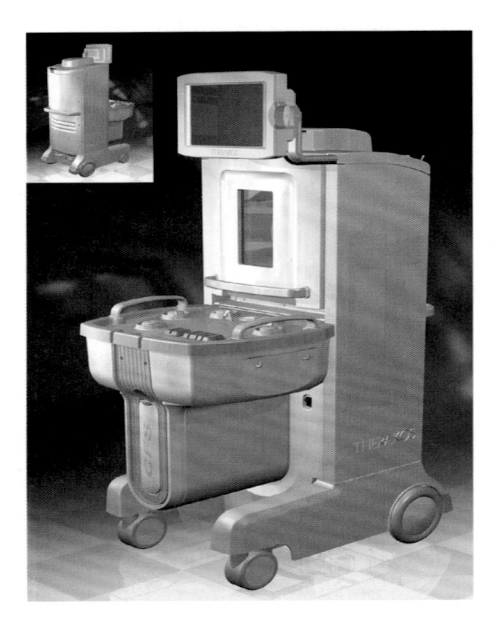

Fig. 2.10. THERAKOS® CELLEX® Photopheresis System.

2.4.2.1 Leukocyte Collection System

Medical devices used for leukocyte separation can be classified in two categories based on centrifugation speed and on collection technology. In regards to centrifugation speed, the leukocyte separation systems are based on low (between 500 to 1200 rpm) and high (between 3000 to 4800 rpm) centrifugation speeds. Medical devices using a low centrifugation speed, (e. g. Cobe Spectra or Optia), routinely used for hematopoietic stem cell collections, require for leukocyte harvest data concerning the patient, such as gender, height, body weight, hematocrit, leukocyte and platelet counts (especially for Optia). Based on these data points, the medical devices propose a treatment volume, the drawing pump flow rate and a centrifugation speed.

The second collection technology, well known in cell therapy facilities, is routinely used for bone marrow separations (e. g. Cobe 2991). By using a higher centrifuge speed, this permits separation and concentration of the cellular layers with good efficacy. The buffy coat collection is controlled by the operator who appreciates the leukocyte layer and the red cell contamination (neutrophils contaminating the buffy coat). These medical devices are operator-dependant.

The CELLEX® System is equipped with a leukocyte separation and concentration system, composed of a new custom centrifuge bowl using a high-speed centrifuge (4800 rpm). The bowl, part integral of the procedural kit, has a particular and complex internal structure. Its unique design distributes whole blood to the center of the bowl, allowing red blood cells to readily fall to the base of the bowl, while leukocytes rise to the top.

The centrifuge assembly is equipped with a bowl optic sensor that automatically identifies the red blood cells/buffy coat interface and conditions its position in the bowl. It signals the central processing unit to maintain the red cell interface at the ideal place (artificial hematocrit in the bowl) for optimal cell separation. This laser signaling is used by the system computer to establish the red cell pump speed and intermittently remove red blood cells from the base of the bowl to maintain the expanding buffy coat within the spinning centrifuge bowl. The bowl optic sensor makes the system independent from the patient's hematocrit and allows a standardization of the collection.

The collection software algorithm determines the initiation of the buffy coat phase based on the whole blood processed volume target. This value is operator selectable via the setup screen. Together, the bowl optic and hematocrit sensors (the collection and control software), select the optimal buffy coat and yield the targeted hematocrit of the leukocyte-enriched fraction. By measuring a change in light transmittance, the hematocrit sensor determines the hematocrit of the blood fraction being displaced from the centrifuge bowl during buffy coat collection. The hematocrit sensor is used to automatically stop the collection of the buffy coat.

This advantage permits an instant separation of the cellular layers and makes the system independent from the patient's hematocrit. Because of its efficacy to concentrate leukocytes, the system is effective with lower flow rates (5 or 10 mL/min) and allows the treatment of a smaller whole blood volume in comparison to the Cobe Spectra or Optia (in regard to unclear cell counts, treatment of 1.5 liters on the CELLEX® System is equivalent to 6 liters of blood treated on Cobe Spectra). Compared to the UVAR XTS® System, the CELLEX® System is more effective in terms of cellular counts and repartition (Table 2.8 and Figure 2.11). Table 2.8 summarizes a comparison of cellular counts of collected buffy coats using these two different techniques. In comparison to the UVAR XTS® System, buffy coats obtained with the CELLEX® System are more concentrated (higher cell counts) with lower volumes and good cell repartitions (low percentage of neutrophils).

Figure 2.11 shows the cellular composition of buffy coats collected from patients with chronic graft-versus-host disease (GVHD), lupus erythematosus or cutaneous T cell lymphoma (CTCL) comparing the CELLEX® with the UVAR XTS® device. This figure demonstrates better cellular repartitions for buffy coats collected with the CELLEX® (higher percentage of lymphocytes and lower percentage of neutrophils).

Both double-needle and single-needle configurations utilize the new continuous flow centrifuge, which continuously concentrates the leukocytes prior to a single harvest of the buffy coat. The continuous flow centrifuge provides an automated, more consistent buffy coat cut fraction and reduces the overall leukocyte collection time (on average less than 2 hours for a procedure with CELLEX® System versus 3.5 hours using the UVAR XTS® System, and more than 5 hours for the open system). This allows greater comfort to the patient and to the nurses who will have the option of planning more photopheresis treatments in one day on the same instrument (Figure 2.12).

The CELLEX® System technology allows a full automation of the leukocyte collection. Because of a total independence of the system from the patient's parameters (such as gender, body weight, size, hematocrit, leukocyte count, etc.), it allows to standardize the leukocyte harvest in all the patients (good or poor venous access like high or lower cell counts). Biologically, the patients treated are very different as demonstrated by the diversity of the clinical indications treated by the CELLEX® System. The CELLEX® System easily allows to treat an acute GVHD patient with low leukocyte counts (2 or 3×10^9/L), as well as a Crohn's disease patient given steroids (high leukocyte counts including high percentage of neutrophils).

	CELLEX® (n = 109)	UVAR XTS® (n = 540)
Buffy Coat volumes (mL)	215.33 ± 29.25	272.48 ± 32.93
Leukocytes (x10^9/L)	21.14 ± 9.74	7.22 ± 18.51
Hematocrit (%)	2.15 ± 0.96	1.23 ± 1.96

Table 2.8. Cellular Counts of Collected Buffy Coats Comparing CELLEX® and UVAR XTS®.
Buffy coats collected from patients with chronic graft-versus-host disease, lupus erythematosus and cutaneous T cell lymphoma were analysed. Absolute mean values and SD were calculated from 109 procedures with CELLEX® and 540 procedures with UVAR XTS®. Treatment volume was 1531.20 ± 121.13 mL and all patients received ECP in double-needle mode when using the CELLEX®.

2.4.2.2 Fluid Balance Management

The fluid balance management on the CELLEX® System has been improved in three different ways: Procedural kit, instrument and software improvements. Many times any three of these components rely on each other to ensure system reliability. The CELLEX® System offers the option of configuring the disposable kit for double-needle or single-needle use. The double-needle configuration provides **continuous flow**, re-

2.4 New Technical Developments — 43

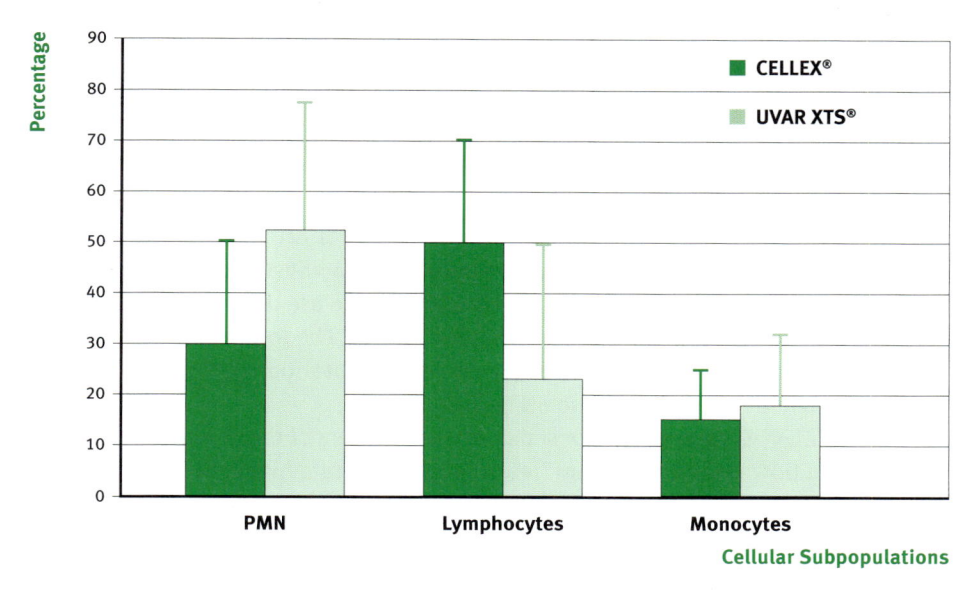

Fig. 2.11. Cellular Composition of Buffy Coats Comparing CELLEX® and UVAR XTS®.
Cells were collected from patients with chronic graft-versus-host disease, lupus erythematodes and cutaneous T cell lymphoma using either CELLEX® (n=109 procedures) or UVAR XTS® (n=540 procedures). This figure demonstrates better cellular repartitions for buffy coats collected with the CELLEX® device (higher percentage of lymphocytes and lower percentage of neutrophils). PMN are peripheral blood mononuclear cells.

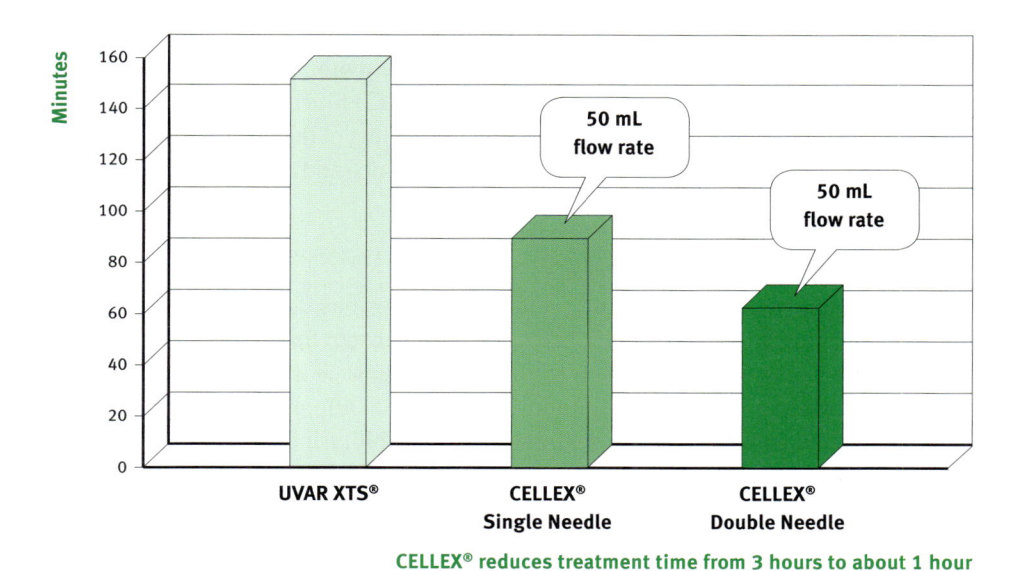

CELLEX® reduces treatment time from 3 hours to about 1 hour

Fig. 2.12. Substantially Reduced Treatment Times Using CELLEX® Compared to UVAR XTS®.
(Source Therakos Inc.).

sulting in a lower extracorporeal volume. Single-needle configuration results in **discontinuous flow,** which requires a higher extracorporeal volume.

A minimum amount of whole blood must be processed to prime the centrifuge bowl and establish the proper red blood cell/plasma interface (140 mL). This volume, called the kit extracorporeal volume (ECV), increases in inverse proportion to the patient's hematocrit (i.e. a lower hematocrit leads to a higher ECV). For comparison, at a 40% hematocrit, the UVAR XTS® System Procedural Kit XT 125 has an ECV of approximately 400 mL, while the ECV for the UVAR XTS® System Procedural Kit XT 225 mL bowl is approximately 550 mL. The double-needle use of the CELLEX® System and the structure of the kit allow the reduction of ECV. The total volume within the disposable tubing set path using double-needle configuration is 180 mL, while it is 236 mL in single-needle configuration (Figure 2.13).

The CELLEX® System allows for separate management of the drawing and return pumps. Good flow rate management (return pump flow rate higher than the drawing pump one) makes it possible to reduce extracorporeal volumes (lower volume accumulated in the return bag). The approximate residual blood volume in the procedural kit is 20 mL for the CELLEX® System and is 50 mL for the UVAR XTS® System. With less ECV and less residual blood loss at the end of a treatment, the new system is tolerated by a broader range of patients such as those with low body weight (children under 20 kg), those with cardiac or pulmonary insufficiencies and hemodynamically unstable patients.

The CELLEX® System has been enhanced by reducing treatment times, extracorporeal and residual volumes, but also by modifying anticoagulant dosing. Post-prime, the software minimizes the anticoagulant dose in the tubing circuit. It significantly reduces the anticoagulant concentration within the patient return tubing circuit at the onset of treatment. A central processing unit equipped with a LCD touch screen allows the operator to manage all the parameters necessary for handling of the device. This interface displays the treatment status, treatment data, fluid balance and any alarm information.

2.4.2.3 CELLEX® System Improvements

Working closely with clinicians and patients, Therakos has developed the CELLEX® System delivering a technology that takes a significant step forward in the flexibility of photopheresis therapy. Since its introduction into Europe in the summer of 2008, this medical device has been continuously upgraded. Different modifications have been introduced, in order to improve the system's reliability, intelligence, and to eliminate software bugs in order to deliver reproducible results.

The system has been improved by reducing alarms such as red blood cells alarms, system and patient pressure alarms and prime 10 alarms. It provides increased system reliability and reduces the need to manually intervene throughout the treatment. For system and patient pressure alarms, the added system intelligence is able to create recognition of system pressure spikes and adapt without alarming. The system's im-

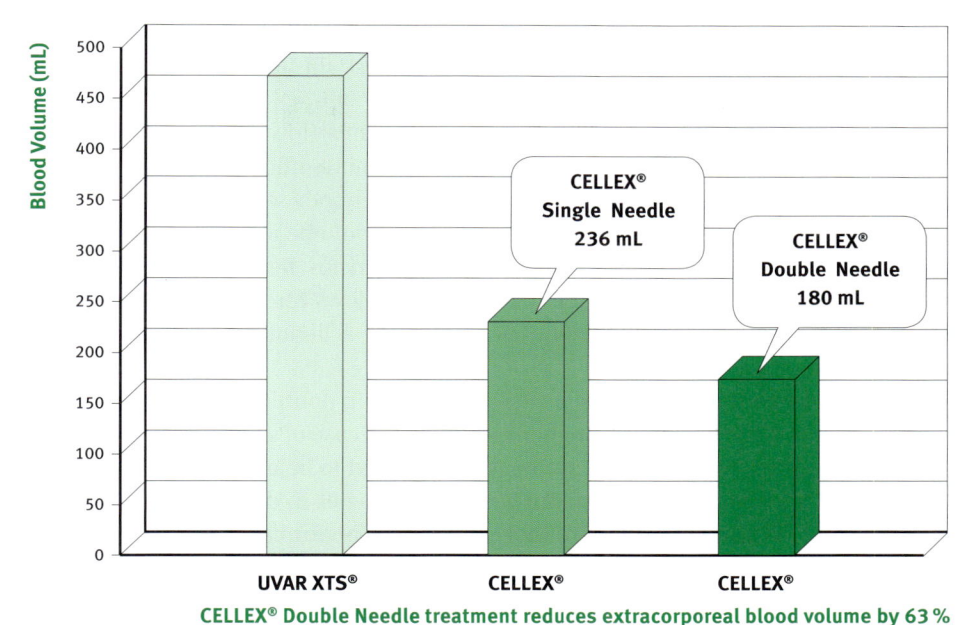

Fig. 2.13. Lower Extracorporeal Blood Volume Using CELLEX® Compared to UVAR XTS®. (Source Therakos Inc.).

provements have been implemented to significantly reduce the possibility of unexpectedly entering buffy coat mode and to enhance the system's ability to recognize blood interface changes more accurately.

The software amendments now broaden re-infusion parameters and minimizes the anticoagulant dose in tubing circuit post prime. It improves the system's safety and the ability to treat additional low body weight patients by creating the flexibility of returning treated buffy coat cells at lower flow rates. It provides the ability to return the buffy coat product from 1 mL/min to 5 mL/min in 1 mL increments. It allows complete treatments, while reducing the total anticoagulant dose given to a patient. Since 2010, we have been using the instrument in routine with ACD-A as a source of anticoagulant (more than 1500 procedures). ACD-A is the most commonly used anticoagulant within the framework of therapeutic hemapheresis. It enables the treatment of patients with very high platelet counts and avoids platelets clumps from the bowl and the tubing set.

2.4.3 Conclusions

Introduced into Europe by Therakos Inc. in the summer of 2008, the CELLEX® System is the successor to UVAR XTS®, which was launched in 1998. The CELLEX® System is an integrated system, all its components are approved and validated to work as a complete, closed treatment unit. It delivers consistent treatment, and one operator can perform the entire treatment. The CELLEX® System built-in quality systems alleviate the need for additional outside safety and quality controls.

Due to the CELLEX® System hemodynamic features (lower extracorporeal volumes), the system performs photopheresis therapy more efficiently and allows the treatment of a wider range of patients, including lower body weight patients and hemodynamically unstable ones. Lower residual blood volume allows for treatment of patients with anemia, cardiac or pulmonary insufficiencies. Reduced treatment time, enhanced patient comfort and added convenience allows for increased operational efficiency, higher patient throughput, more efficient scheduling and improved resource management.

This instrument is designed to be used in routine in double-needle mode and offers the possibility to be used in single-needle mode in case of venous access loss during the procedure. The collection system was designed to be effective, but also fully automatic. This device profits from the latest technologies in the field of traceability. Each kit comes with a magnetic card that captures the performance of the instrument during a procedure. This technology makes the CELLEX® System very accessible to any user. It is not just for an elite of specialists authorized within the framework of therapeutic hemapheresis.

The CELLEX® System is perfectible, and in the coming months, this medical device will offer new technical developments. Similar to the UVAR XTS® System, the CELLEX® System has demonstrated excellent tolerance by patients with no serious side effects. These features make this medical device a success.

Acknowledgments

We are grateful to Dr Vanita Sharma (Therakos Inc.) for critically reading the manuscript.

References

[1] Directive 2004/23/EC of the European Parliament and of the Council of 31 March 2004 on setting standards of quality and safety for the donation, testing, processing, preservation, storage and distribution of human tissues and cells.
[2] Directive 2006/86/EC implementing Directive 2004/23/EC of the European Parliament and of the Council as regards traceability, requirements, notification and serious adverse reactions and events and certain technical requirements for the coding, processing, preservation, storage and distribution of human tissues and cells.
[3] Directive 2006/17/EC implementing Directive 2004/23/EC of the European Parliament and of the Council as regards certain technical requirements for the donation, procurement and testing of human tissues and cells. Text with EEA relevance.

Section 3: Mechanisms of Action of ECP

3 Mechanisms of Action of ECP

Erin Gatza and James L.M. Ferrara

3.1 Preclinical GVHD Model

3.1.1 Introduction

Graft-versus-host disease (GVHD) occurs when donor T cells respond to foreign histocompatibility antigens presented by host antigen presenting cells [1, 2] and results in significant morbidity and mortality. Steroids, the first line therapy for treating GVHD, fail in 50% of patients and are broadly immunosuppressive, increasing the risk of relapse, infection, and other toxicities [3–5]. Strategies to mitigate GVHD while preserving immune function are important to improve outcomes after allogeneic marrow and stem cell transplantation (BMT). Extracorporeal photopheresis (ECP) has demonstrated efficacy in treating both acute and chronic GVHD, even in some patients who are refractory to conventional immunosuppressive therapy, with few reported side effects [3, 6–12].

Although the definitive mechanism of ECP in immune modulation has not yet been elucidated, a number of immunological alterations are induced by ECP, including expansion of regulatory T cells (Tregs) [13, 14], modulation of cytokine production and maturation of dendritic cells (DCs) [15–17].

We developed a novel method for incorporating ECP treatment into well established and clinically relevant murine models of GVHD to examine the effects of ECP on established, progressive disease. The infusion of ECP treated cells reduced established severe GVHD, suppressed allogeneic responses of donor effector T cells that had never been exposed to psoralen and ultraviolet A irradiation (PUVA), and increased the number of Foxp3⁺ T regulatory cells derived from the graft. This increase in Tregs was required to reduce GVHD and mortality after allogeneic BMT.

3.1.2 Results

3.1.2.1 Infusion of Cells Treated with ECP Reduces GVHD

We tested the hypothesis that ECP would modulate the function of lymphocytes that had not been directly exposed to ECP in an allogeneic murine HCT model of GVHD where donor and recipient are identical at the major histocompatibility complex (MHC) but mismatched at multiple minor histocompatibility antigens (miHAs) (B6→C3H.SW) and GVHD is mediated by donor CD8⁺ T cells [1]. Lethally irradiated (11 Gy of total body irradiation) recipient C3H.SW mice were transplanted with bone marrow (BM) and T cells from either syngeneic (C3H.SW) or congenic allogeneic (B6-Ly5.2) donors. Thirty million splenocytes were isolated from a second cohort of B6→C3H.SW BMT recipients, incubated ex vivo with 8-MOP (UVADEX®) followed by exposure to UVA light [18], and infused intravenously into the first cohort of BMT recipients 7 days after BMT (Figure 3.1), when clinical disease was already evident. Four weekly infusions of ECP treated splenocytes significantly improved both survival and GVHD clinical scores (Figure 3.2a), reduced histopathologic damage in GVHD target organs (Figure 3.2b) and dramatically improved immune reconstitution 56 days post-BMT (Figure 3.2c). Importantly, complete (>99.8%) engraftment with donor cells was confirmed in all recipients. We confirmed these results in a second, haploidentical model (B6-Ly5.2→B6D2F1) where GVHD is driven by CD4⁺ T cells [19] (Figure 3.2d).

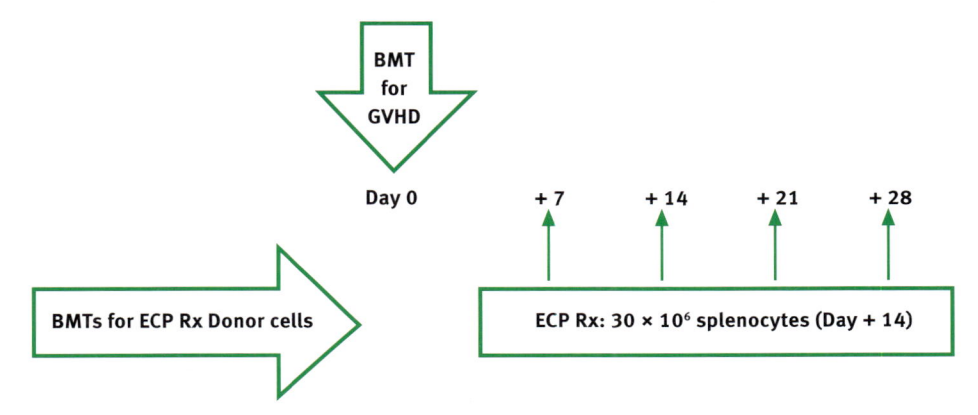

Fig. 3.1. ECP Treatment Schema.
Mice to receive treatment infusions were transplanted on day 0 as described in [18]. 30x10⁶ splenocytes from a second cohort of allogeneic BMT recipients (identically transplanted, 14 days earlier) were isolated, exposed to 200 ng/mL 8-MOP and 2 J/cm² UVA ex vivo and infused i.v. into the first cohort of BMT recipients 7, 14, 21 and 28 days after transplant.

3.1.2.2 Cells Treated with ECP Modulate Allogeneic T Cell Responses and Increase Foxp3⁺ T Regulatory Cells

Splenocytes from the BMT cohorts that were exposed to PUVA were all (>98%) Annexin-V⁺ within 24 hours of exposure. Although no ECP-treated cells were detectable in lymphoid organs 72 hours after infusion, at 96 hours they had caused a three-fold decrease in CD8⁺interferon (IFN)-γ⁺ donor effector splenocytes that had never been directly exposed to PUVA (Figure 3.3a). ECP-treated splenocytes from B6→B6D2F1 mice also suppressed allogeneic responses of naïve B6 T cells in vitro, where their addition reduced CD8⁺IFN-γ⁺ responders and T cell proliferation in response to B6D2F1 bone marrow-derived dendritic cells by 50% (Figure 3.3b).

Donor CD4⁺Foxp3⁺ cells were increased in mixed lymphocyte reaction (MLR) cultures containing ECP treated splenocytes (Figure 3.3c), resulting in an average 1.8-fold increase in donor CD4⁺Foxp3⁺ Treg numbers per well. B6-Ly5.2 responders from primary MLR cultures containing ECP treated splenocytes were refractory to secondary stimulation with fresh B6D2F1 DC and their bulk transfer from the first MLR suppressed

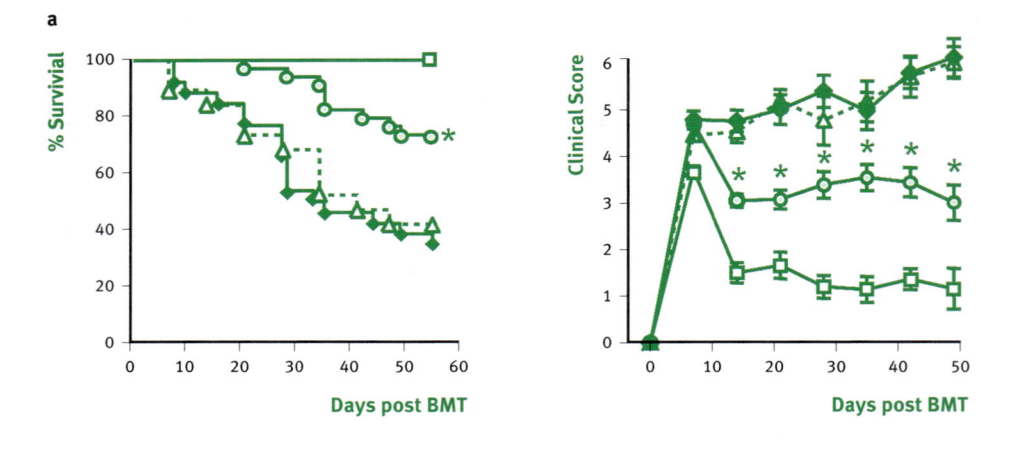

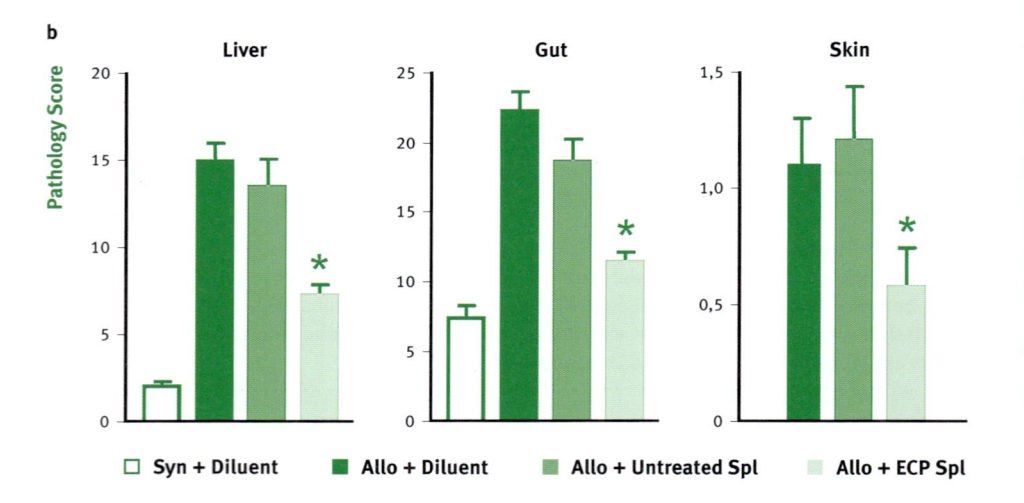

Fig. 3.2. ECP-Treated Cells Reduce GVHD and Mortality After Allogeneic BMT.
(a) Survival and clinical GVHD scores after BMT. C3H.SW mice received syngeneic (C3H.SW; open square, n=15) or allogeneic (B6-Ly5.2) BMT followed by four weekly infusions of diluent (♦, n=26) or of B6→C3H.SW splenocytes that were untreated (Δ, n=19) or treated with ECP (green circle, n=34); green circle vs Δ or ♦, *p<0.004. (b) Histopathology scores 56 days post-BMT (n=8-20 per group); Allo + untreated Spl vs Allo + ECP Spl, *p<0.03. (c) Spleen reconstitution with donor lymphocytes (B6-Ly5.2) 56 days post-BMT (n=6–8 per group); Allo + ECP Spl vs Allo + Diluent, *p<0.02.
(d) Survival and clinical GVHD scores after haploidentical BMT. B6D2F1 mice received syngeneic (B6D2F1; open square, n=6) or allogeneic (B6-Ly5.2) BMT followed by four weekly infusions of diluent (♦, n=18) or of B6→B6D2F1 splenocytes that were treated with ECP (green circle, n=13); green circle vs ♦, *p<0.02. Data are means ± SD pooled from at least 2 independent experiments.

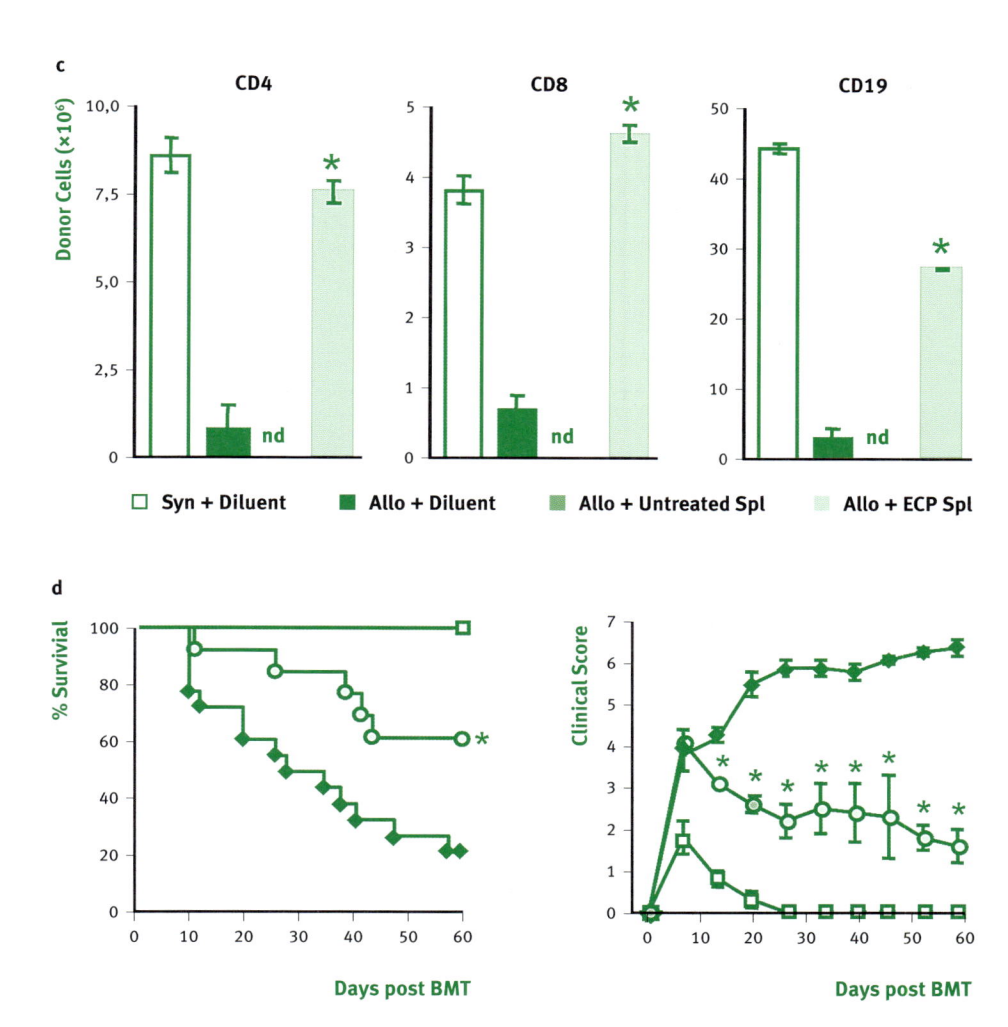

allogeneic proliferation of fresh responders more than 200-fold (Figure 3.3d). Similarly, one infusion of ECP treated cells caused the number of donor CD4⁺CD25⁺Foxp3⁺ splenocytes in transplanted mice to nearly double within four days (Figure 4a). Tregs remained elevated in the spleen, mesenteric lymph nodes (MLN) and the thymus for at least 49 days after transplant (Figure 3.4a). The increase in Tregs 11 days after transplant was due to a significant increase in the percent of CD4⁺CD25⁺Foxp3⁺ cells originating from mature T cells in the BMT inoculum, whereas the increases at later time points were also due to increased donor cell reconstitution at these sites, with Tregs deriving from the bone marrow graft and differentiating in the thymus (Figure 3.4b).

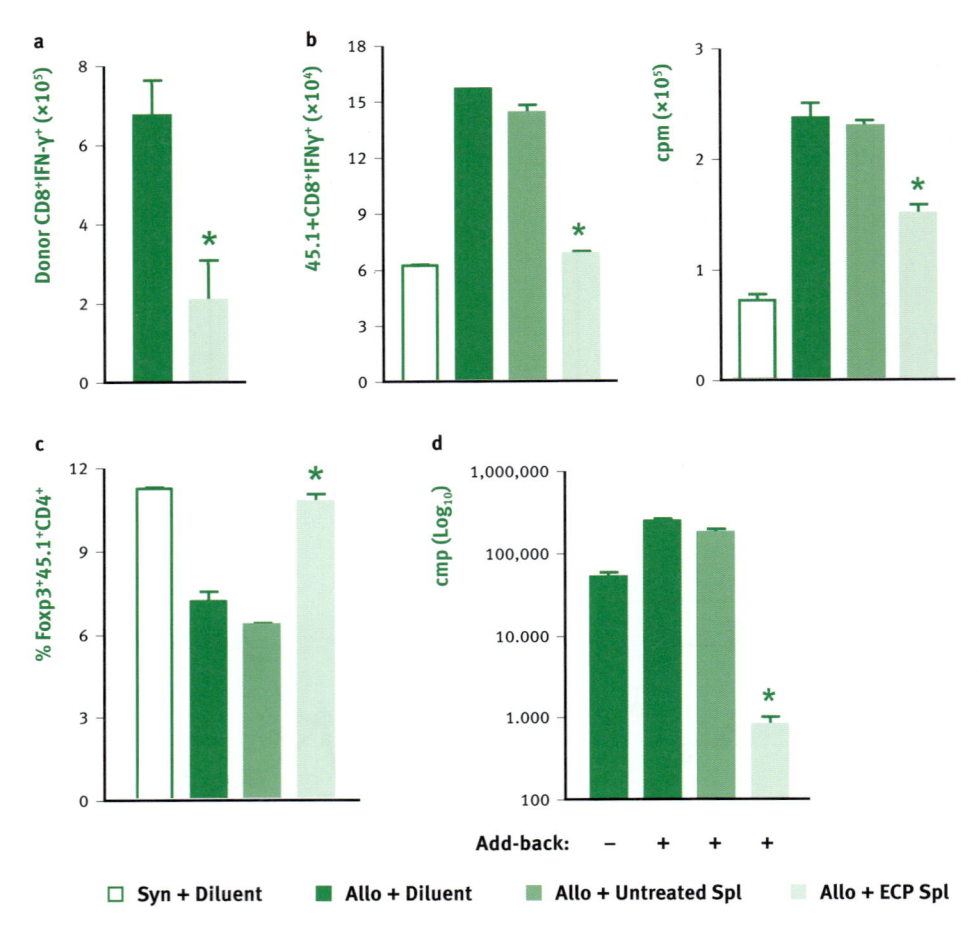

Fig. 3.3. ECP-Treated Splenocytes Modulate Allogeneic T Cell Responses and Increase Foxp3 Expression.
(a) C3H.SW recipient mice received bone marrow and T cells from syngeneic (C3H.SW; white bar) or allogeneic (B6-Ly5.2; dark green and light green bars) donors on day 0 followed by infusion of B6→C3H.SW ECP-treated cells (light green bar) on day 7. Numbers of donor CD8⁺IFN-γ⁺ cells per allogeneic recipient spleen 96 hours after infusion of ECP-treated cells (light green bar) vs diluent (dark green bar), *p<0.05. Data are means ± SD pooled from 3 independent experiments (n=9-20 per group).
(b, c) B6-Ly5.2 responder T cells were incubated at a 10:1 ratio with syngeneic B6 (white bar) or allogeneic B6D2F1 (dark green bar) stimulator DC for 60 hours in the presence of untreated (medium green bar) or ECP-treated (light green bar) B6→B6D2F1 splenocytes at a 1:1 ratio with responders.
(b) Numbers of responder CD8⁺IFN-γ⁺ cells per well (left) and proliferation of bulk responder cells (right); medium green light green bar vs dark green or medium green bar, *p<0.05.
(c) Percent of CD4⁺Foxp3⁺cells; medium green light green bar vs dark green or medium green bar, *p<0.05. (d) Proliferation of fresh MLR cultures containing 10 B6-Ly5.2 responder T cells per B6D2F1 stimulator DC after cells harvested from (b, c) were added at a 1:1 ratio with responders. – indicates nothing added; +, cells added from primary cultures as colored in panels (b) and (c); medium green light green bar vs dark green or medium green bar, *p<0.05. Syngeneic control groups had low background proliferation (< 2.0x10³ cpm) which was un-affected by addition of cells from (b, c) (data not shown). Data are means ± SD pooled from at least 2 independent experiments (n=6–9 wells per group).

3.1.2.3 Regulatory T Cells are Required for Reversal of GVHD by ECP Treatment

We incapacitated Tregs in vivo using anti-CD25 (PC61) [20] before and after the infusion of ECP treated splenocytes. PC61 infusion completely prevented the increases in Foxp3+ cells (Figure 3.5a) observed after infusion of ECP treated cells. Anti-CD25 also abolished the ability of cells treated with ECP to reverse GVHD (Figures 3.5b and 3.5c), confirming the requirement of Tregs for disease reversal.

3.1.3 Discussion

We modeled ECP treatment of GVHD using two well-defined murine models of GVHD, one to minor histocompatibility antigens (B6→C3H.SW) mediated by CD8+ T cells and the other (B6→B6D2F1) mediated primarily by CD4+ T cells. Our system used splenocytes obtained on day 14 from cohorts of mice with ongoing GVHD to model the cells from a patient undergoing apheresis. We assumed that the mouse spleen is representative of peripheral blood as a cell source early after transplant and the dose of 30 million cells was approximately 10 % of viable donor leukocytes on day 14.

Several studies suggest that GVHD can be considered an imbalance of effector T cells and Tregs [21–23] and increases in Tregs in patients with GVHD who responded to ECP treatment have been reported [13, 24, 25]. In our study, ECP induced profound and stable increases in peripheral CD4+CD25+Foxp3+ Treg cells early after transplantation, and functionally changed the response of effector T cells, thus reducing GVHD. Mice receiving ECP treated cells demonstrated improved immune reconstitution, which is consistent with reduced GVHD and with the relative immunocompetence of patients who receive ECP therapy compared to immunosuppressive therapy [26, 27].

Our studies do not address the role of cytokines or dendritic cells in determining the clinical response following ECP treatment. Indeed, apoptotic cells resulting from PUVA exposure have now been shown to exert modulatory effects on antigen presenting cell function [16, 17, 28–30]. Recent studies using similar murine models of allogeneic BMT and ECP treatment methodology have confirmed and extended our findings to show that ECP-treated splenocytes infused prior to donor lymphocyte infusions (DLI) in thymectomized T cell depleted BMT recipients effectively prevented GVHD and that interleukin (IL)-10 produced by BM-derived non-T cells was required for the attenuation [28]. Interestingly, co-culture of myeloid DCs with ECP-treated splenocytes in the presence of low concentrations of LPS resulted in a pronounced increase in IL-10 production and a reduced ability of the DCs to induce CD8+ immune responses in vivo, which was lost on stimulation with higher LPS concentrations [28]. Thus, the immune response invoked by ECP treatment is likely governed by the state of the antigen presenting cells and the maturation signals present in the patient at the time of therapy.

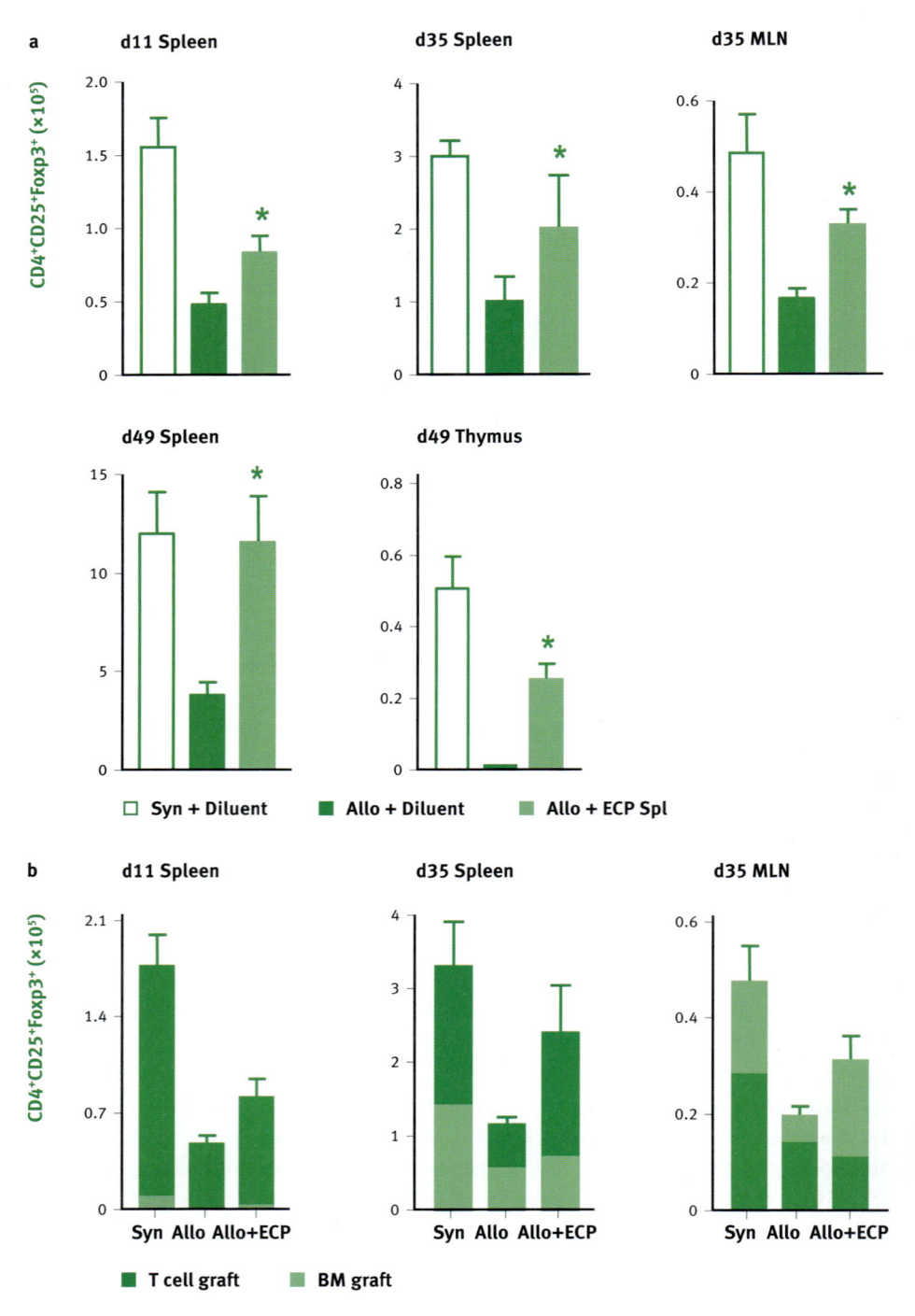

Fig. 3.4. Infusion of ECP-treated Splenocytes Increases Donor Treg After Allogeneic BMT.

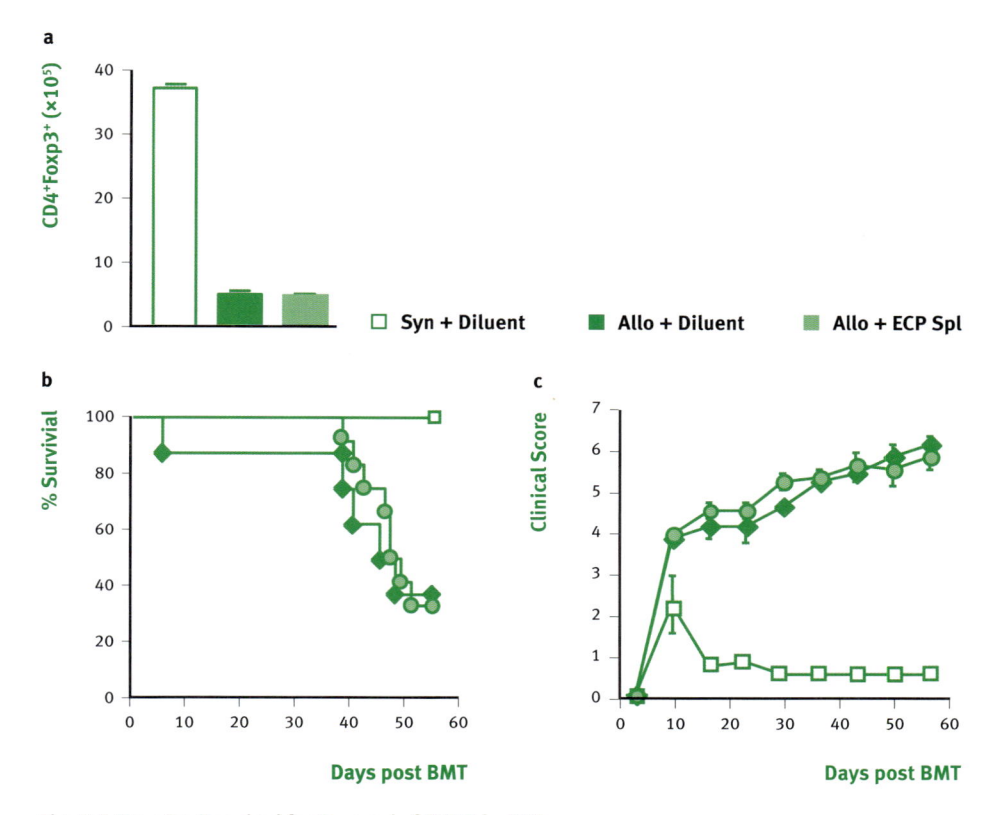

Fig. 3.5. Treg Are Required for Reversal of GVHD by ECP.
(a–c) C3H.SW recipient mice received syngeneic (C3H.SW; open square, n=3) or allogeneic (B6-Ly5.2) BMT and four weekly infusions of ECP-treated B6→C3H.SW splenocytes (green circle, n=12) or diluent (♦, n=8). All BMT recipients were injected intraperitonealy. with 0.5 mg CD25 depleting mAb (PC61) on day 1 and 0.1mg on days 8, 15, 22 and 29 post-BMT. (a) Number of CD4$^+$Foxp3$^+$ Tregs 56 days post-BMT (n=3–4 per group). Bars represent means ± SD. (b) Survival. (c) Clinical GVHD scores.

Fig. 3.4. Infusion of ECP-treated Splenocytes Increases Donor Treg After Allogeneic BMT.
B6 and C3H.SW (CD45.2$^+$Thy1.2$^+$) recipient mice received T cell depleted B6-Ly5.2 (CD45.1$^+$Thy1.2$^+$) bone marrow and B6-Thy1.1 (CD45.2$^+$Thy1.1$^+$) T cells followed by infusion of ECP-treated B6→C3H. SW splenocytes. CD4$^+$Foxp3$^+$ or CD4$^+$CD25$^+$Foxp3$^+$ cells were gated on whole cell scatter followed by segregation into CD45.1$^+$Thy1.1$^-$ BM or CD45.1$^-$Thy1.1$^+$ T cell inoculum-derived cells. (a) Total numbers of CD4$^+$CD25$^+$Foxp3$^+$ cells after infusion of ECP-treated cells from second BMT cohort; grey bar vs black bar, *p<0.04. At day 11, mice had received 1 infusion of ECP-treated cells, and at days 35 and 49 they had received 4 infusions. (b) Numbers of donor CD4$^+$CD25$^+$Foxp3$^+$ cells from the bone marrow (BM) and T cell grafts in the spleen and mesenteric lymph nodes (MLN) 11 and 35 days post-BMT. Allo+Diluent vs Allo+ECP in the spleen, dark green bars, p<0.03; Allo+Diluent vs Allo+ECP in the MLN, light green bars, p=0.04. Bars represent means ± SD. Data pooled from 3–4 independent experiments (n=12–20/group).

Previous studies have suggested that the efficacy of ECP is dependent on the presence of particular cell types in ECP-treated cell populations. We compared the use of donor-type ECP-treated splenocytes from transplanted cohorts with ongoing GVHD (B6-Ly5.2→C3H.SW) to naïve B6-Ly5.2 donors. Despite very different splenic compositions (Figure 3.6), the two donor populations were equally effective in reducing ongoing GVHD and associated mortality. Capitini et al have recently confirmed these findings and additionally showed that equivalent improvement in GVHD could be achieved using MHC-matched donor-type, recipient-type or third-party splenocytes, MHC-mismatched splenocytes or splenocytes depleted of T or B cells [28]. These data warrant further exploration as the use of healthy donors to generate ECP treatment cells may enable additional approaches to the treatment of GVHD in patients who are unable to undergo the procedure.

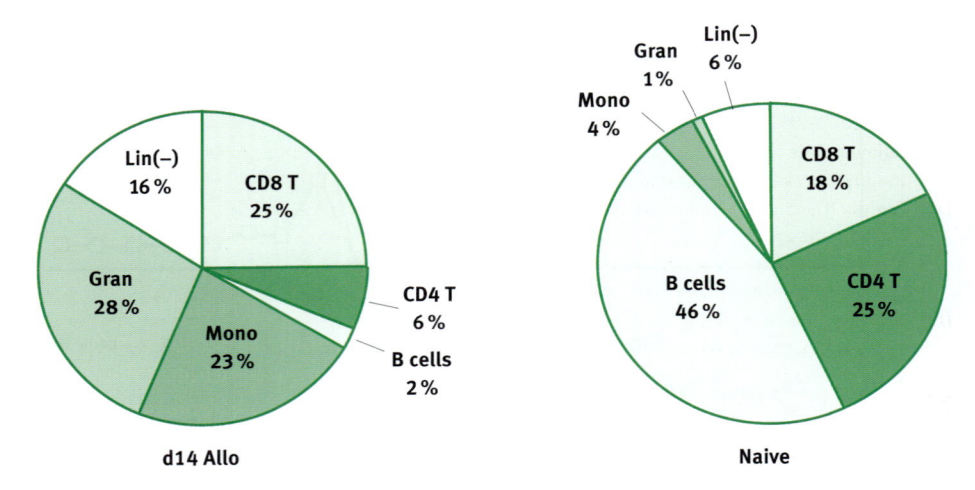

Fig. 3.6. Comparison of Splenic Leukocytes Obtained From Transplanted and Naïve Donor Cohorts as a Cell Source for ECP Treatment.
Splenocytes from cohorts of B6-Ly5.2→C3H.SW BMT recipients (transplanted 14 days earlier) and naive, age-matched B6-Ly5.2 littermates were isolated, exposed to 8-MOP and UVA ex vivo and infused i.v. into B6→C3H.SW BMT recipients as ECP treatment. Leukocyte populations determined by flow cytometry prior to infusion were defined as: CD8 T cell, CD45.1$^+$CD8$^+$; CD4 T cell, CD45.1$^+$CD4$^+$; B cell, CD45.1$^+$CD19$^+$; Monocyte (Mono), CD45.1$^+$CD11b$^+$CD49d$^+$; Granulocyte (Gran), CD45.1$^+$CD11b$^+$Ly6C/G$^+$; Lin(−), viable scatter without lineage marker expression. Data are combined from 6 independent cohorts of donor spleens per group.

Acknowledgements

This research was originally published in *Blood*. Gatza E, Rogers C, Clouthier SC, Lowler KP, Tawara I, Liu C, Reddy P and Ferrara JLM. Extracorporeal photopheresis reverses experimental graft-versus-host disease through regulatory T cells. *Blood*. 2008; 112:1515–1521. © the American Society of Hematology.

References

[1] Shlomchik WD, Couzens MS, Tang CB, et al. Prevention of graft versus host disease by inactivation of host antigen-presenting cells. Science 1999;285:412–5.

[2] Teshima T, Ordemann R, Reddy P, et al. Acute graft-versus-host disease does not require alloantigen expression on host epithelium. Nat Med 2002;8:575–81.

[3] Marshall SR. Technology insight: ECP for the treatment of GvHD--can we offer selective immune control without generalized immunosuppression? Nat Clin Pract Oncol 2006;3:302–14.

[4] Holler E. Risk assessment in haematopoietic stem cell transplantation: GvHD prevention and treatment. Best Pract Res Clin Haematol 2007;20:281–94.

[5] Messina C, Faraci M, de Fazio V, Dini G, Calo MP, Calore E. Prevention and treatment of acute GvHD. Bone Marrow Transplant 2008;41 Suppl 2:S65–70.

[6] Dall'Amico R, Messina C. Extracorporeal photochemotherapy for the treatment of graft-versus-host disease. Ther Apher 2002;6:296–304.

[7] Flowers ME, Apperley JF, van Besien K, et al. A multicenter prospective phase 2 randomized study of extracorporeal photopheresis for treatment of chronic graft-versus-host disease. Blood 2008;112:2667–74.

[8] Greinix HT, Knobler RM, Worel N, et al. The effect of intensified extracorporeal photochemotherapy on long-term survival in patients with severe acute graft-versus-host disease. Haematologica 2006;91:405–8.

[9] Kaloyannidis P, Mallouri D. The role of the extracorporeal photopheresis in the management of the graft-versus-host disease. Transfus Apher Sci 2012;46:211–9.

[10] Greinix HT, van Besien K, Elmaagacli AH, et al. Progressive improvement in cutaneous and extracutaneous chronic graft-versus-host disease after a 24-week course of extracorporeal photopheresis-results of a crossover randomized study. Biol Blood Marrow Transplant 2011;17:1775–82.

[11] Gonzalez Vicent M, Ramirez M, Sevilla J, Abad L, Diaz MA. Analysis of clinical outcome and survival in pediatric patients undergoing extracorporeal photopheresis for the treatment of steroid-refractory GVHD. J Pediatr Hematol Oncol 2010;32:589–93.

[12] Perfetti P, Carlier P, Strada P, et al. Extracorporeal photopheresis for the treatment of steroid refractory acute GVHD. Bone Marrow Transplant 2008;42:609–17.

[13] Biagi E, Di Biaso I, Leoni V, et al. Extracorporeal photochemotherapy is accompanied by increasing levels of circulating CD4+CD25+GITR+Foxp3+CD62L+ functional regulatory T-cells in patients with graft-versus-host disease. Transplantation 2007;84:31–9.

[14] Maeda A, Schwarz A, Kernebeck K, et al. Intravenous infusion of syngeneic apoptotic cells by photopheresis induces antigen-specific regulatory T cells. J Immunol 2005;174:5968–76.

[15] Di Renzo M, Rubegni P, Pasqui AL, et al. Extracorporeal photopheresis affects interleukin (IL)-10 and IL-12 production by monocytes in patients with chronic graft-versus-host disease. Br J Dermatol 2005;153:59–65.

[16] Spisek R, Gasova Z, Bartunkova J. Maturation state of dendritic cells during the extracorporeal photopheresis and its relevance for the treatment of chronic graft-versus-host disease. Transfusion 2006;46:55–65.

[17] Di Renzo M, Sbano P, De Aloe G, et al. Extracorporeal photopheresis affects co-stimulatory molecule expression and interleukin-10 production by dendritic cells in graft-versus-host disease patients. Clin Exp Immunol 2008;151:407–13.

[18] Gatza E, Rogers CE, Clouthier SG, et al. Extracorporeal photopheresis reverses experimental graft-versus-host disease through regulatory T cells. Blood 2008;112:1515–21.

[19] Reddy P, Negrin R, Hill GR. Mouse models of bone marrow transplantation. Biol Blood Marrow Transplant 2008;14:129–35.

[20] Kohm AP, McMahon JS, Podojil JR, et al. Cutting Edge: Anti-CD25 monoclonal antibody injection results in the functional inactivation, not depletion, of CD4+CD25+ T regulatory cells. J Immunol 2006;176:3301–5.
[21] Nguyen VH, Zeiser R, Negrin RS. Role of naturally arising regulatory T cells in hematopoietic cell transplantation. Biol Blood Marrow Transplant 2006;12:995–1009.
[22] Rezvani K, Mielke S, Ahmadzadeh M, et al. High donor FOXP3-positive regulatory T-cell (Treg) content is associated with a low risk of GVHD following HLA-matched allogeneic SCT. Blood 2006;108:1291–7.
[23] Edinger M, Hoffmann P, Ermann J, et al. CD4+CD25+ regulatory T cells preserve graft-versus-tumor activity while inhibiting graft-versus-host disease after bone marrow transplantation. Nat Med 2003;9:1144–50.
[24] Quaglino P, Comessatti A, Ponti R, et al. Reciprocal modulation of circulating CD4+CD25+bright T cells induced by extracorporeal photochemotherapy in cutaneous T-cell lymphoma and chronic graft-versus-host-disease patients. Int J Immunopathol Pharmacol 2009;22:353–62.
[25] Di Biaso I, Di Maio L, Bugarin C, et al. Regulatory T cells and extracorporeal photochemotherapy: correlation with clinical response and decreased frequency of proinflammatory T cells. Transplantation 2009;87:1422–5.
[26] Lim HW, Edelson RL. Photopheresis for the treatment of cutaneous T-cell lymphoma. Hematol Oncol Clin North Am 1995;9:1117–26.
[27] Suchin KR, Cassin M, Washko R, et al. Extracorporeal photochemotherapy does not suppress T- or B-cell responses to novel or recall antigens. J Am Acad Dermatol 1999;41:980–6.
[28] Capitini CM, Davis JP, Larabee SM, Herby S, Nasholm NM, Fry TJ. Extracorporeal photopheresis attenuates murine graft-versus-host disease via bone marrow-derived interleukin-10 and preserves responses to dendritic cell vaccination. Biol Blood Marrow Transplant 2011;17:790–9.
[29] Fry TJ, Shand JL, Milliron M, Tasian SK, Mackall CL. Antigen loading of DCs with irradiated apoptotic tumor cells induces improved anti-tumor immunity compared to other approaches. Cancer Immunol Immunother 2009;58:1257–64.
[30] Morelli AE, Larregina AT. Apoptotic cell-based therapies against transplant rejection: role of recipient's dendritic cells. Apoptosis 2010;15:1083–97.

Thomas Schwarz
3.2 Preclinical Hypersensitivity Models

3.2.1 Introduction

Extracorporeal photopheresis (ECP) is based on the reinfusion of autologous leukocytes exposed extracorporeally to 8-methoxypsoralen (8-MOP) and ultraviolet-A (UVA) radiation [1]. It has been approved for the treatment of cutaneous T cell lymphoma [2], in particular of Sezary syndrome [3]. Because of its safety and efficacy, ECP has been subsequently investigated in a variety of diseases with suspected involvement of T cells including organ transplant rejection, graft-versus-host-disease (GVHD) and some autoimmune disorders. Accordingly, ECP prevented chronic [4] and reduced acute rejection of cardiac transplants [5]. In patients with GVHD ECP reduced alloreactive T-cell responses [6] and exerted beneficial effects in acute and chronic GVHD [7, 8]. Success has also been observed occasionally in other autoimmune diseases [9–11].

Although ECP has been in use for more than 25 years, the mode of action is still unclear. The beneficial effects of ECP in GVHD, in preventing the rejection of solid organ transplants and in various autoimmune diseases gave rise to the speculation that ECP may act via immunosuppression [12]. However, in contrast to conventional immunosuppressive drugs, ECP does not induce a generalized immune suppression since patients undergoing long term ECP do not suffer from a higher risk of infections or malignancies [13] and respond normally to both novel and recall antigens [14]. Accordingly this line, it has been suggested that ECP may induce antigen-specific immunomodulation, possibly via regulatory T cells (Treg) [15].

Regulatory T cells comprise a heterogeneous group of T lymphocytes, which actively inhibit immune responses [16]. They have been recognized to play an important role in the prevention of autoimmunity, GVHD, and transplant rejection [17–19]. Clinically, there is great enthusiasm about the potential to develop strategies that can enhance Treg number or activity for therapeutic use in immune-mediated diseases. The best characterized subtype of Treg are those expressing CD4 and CD25 [20]. UV radiation (UVR), in particular the mid wave range (UVB, 290–320 nm), has been long recognized to exhibit the capacity to induce immunotolerance [21]. This appears to be at least in part mediated via antigen-specific Treg which meanwhile are pretty well characterized [22].

3.2.2 The Experimental Model

To clarify whether ECP induces Treg, in 2004 we set up an experimental *in vivo* model [15]. We utilized the model of hapten-mediated contact hypersensitivity (CHS) in mice. In this system UVR-induced Treg had been successfully characterized phenotypically and functionally. It harbors the advantages to check for antigen specificity and to prove the induction of Treg on a functional level by adoptive transfer experiments. We utilized the contact allergen dinitrofluorobenzene (DNFB) as a hapten. Topical painting of 0.5% DNFB on razor shaved skin results in almost 100% sensitization. Once sensitized, mice react with a pronounced ear swelling response to 0.3% DNFB painted on one ear. The reaction is not toxic and antigen-specific. To simulate the ECP procedure, we obtained leukocytes from spleens and lymph nodes from DNFB-sensitized mice and exposed these cells *in vitro* to UVA in the presence of 8-MOP (PUVA). 24 hours later cells were injected intravenously (i. v.) into naïve mice. Recipients were then sensitized against DNFB and showed a reduced sensitization response to DNFB. Reactions to other unrelated haptens like oxazolone were not affected, indicating that the infusion of PUVA-exposed leukocytes from DNFB-sensitized donors inhibits the induction of CHS against DNFB but not against other antigens. To further elucidate whether this suppression is due to the induction of Treg in the recipients, T cells were obtained from these mice and were injected into another group of naive mice. Upon sensitization, these recipients turned out not to react to DNFB, indicating that injection of PUVA-treated leukocytes might induce Treg and thus, indicated this model as suitable for our purposes (Figure 3.7).

3.2.3 Characterization of ECP/PUVA-Induced Treg

Depletion studies utilizing specific antibodies revealed that PUVA-induced Treg express CD4 and CD25 and thus, belong to the $CD4^+CD25^+$ Treg subtype. In addition, they release *in vitro* upon antigen specific stimulation by dendritic cells interleukin (IL)-10 and transforming growth factor-ß [15].

The crucial cells for inducing Treg in the i.v. infused PUVA-treated leukocytes are not as initially presumed T cells but dendritic cells since the suppressive effect was lost upon depletion of $CD11c^+$ cells but not of $CD3^+$ cells before transfer. The vast majority of cells upon infusion migrate into the spleen and the lymph nodes. Interestingly, all cells upon *in vitro* PUVA undergo apoptosis but with different kinetics. Whereas the vast majority of T cells are dead after 24 hours, dendritic cells undergo cell death with a delay of 72 to 96 hours. This gives rise to the speculation that damaged but still alive dendritic cells are infused. Since some of them are loaded with the hapten they may present the antigen in the lymph nodes to T cells but because of their damage in a non-professional fashion and thus, do not induce T effector cells but Treg. A similar phenomenon appears to be responsible for the induction of UVR-Treg [23].

3.2.4 Interleukin-10 is a Crucial Mediator

IL-10 appears to be important for the induction of Treg since injection of PUVA-treated leukocytes obtained from IL-10 knock-out mice did not induce Treg. Injection of PUVA-treated leukocytes into sensitized mice inhibited the elicitation of CHS, indicat-

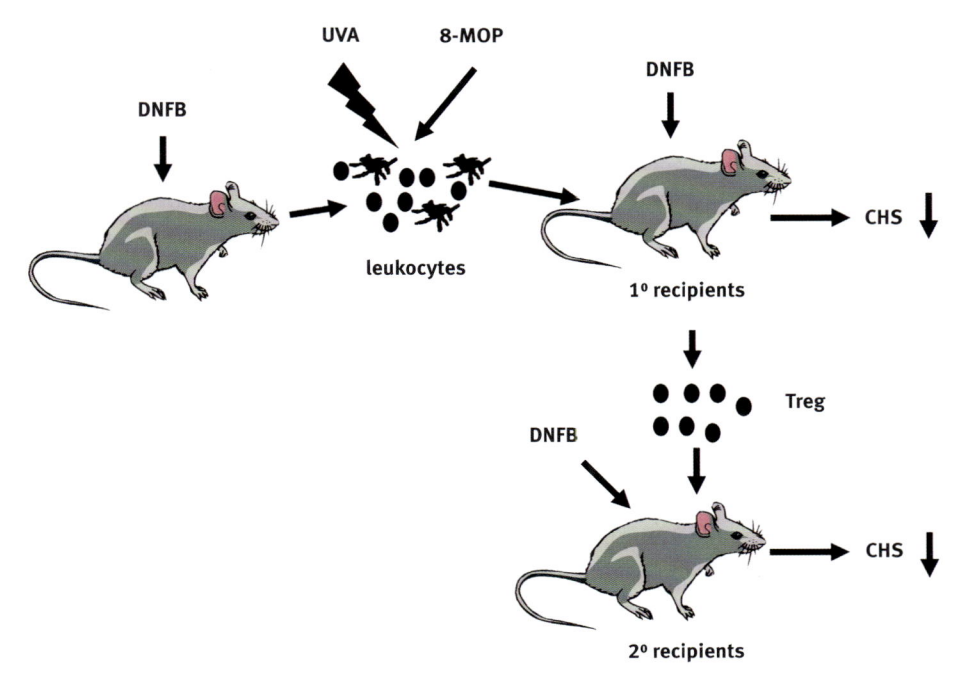

Fig. 3.7. Scheme of Experimental *in vivo* Model for ECP Utilizing Contact Hypersensitivity as an Immunologic Model.
Spleen and lymph node cells (leukocytes) were obtained from mice which were sensitized with dinitrofluorobenzene (DNFB). Cells were exposed extracorporeally to 8-methoxypsoralen (8-MOP) and UVA radiation. Treated cells were injected intravenously (i.v.) into naïve syngeneic recipients (1° recipients). Five days after injection, recipients were sensitized against DNFB and ear challenge performed 5 days later. Lymph node cells were obtained from the recipient mice and transferred i.v. into a second generation of syngeneic naïve mice (2° recipients). 24 hours after transfer, mice were sensitized against DNFB and ear challenge performed 5 days later. Both in the 1° and 2° generation recipients CHS against DNFB was suppressed. (Taken and adapted from Maeda et al., J Immunol 2005;174:5968–76).

ing that this ECP model does not only prevent the induction but also inhibits the effector phase of CHS [24]. Interestingly, injection of PUVA-induced Treg into sensitized mice did not inhibit the effector phase, indicating that this effect cannot be due to the activity of Treg. Utilizing IL-10 knock-out mice we could show that the injection of PUVA-treated leukocytes induces the release of IL-10 in the recipients which could explain the inhibition of the elicitation phase of CHS [25]. Together these data indicate that the inhibition of CHS does not require Treg but may be mediated via enhanced IL-10. In parallel, Treg are induced as demonstrated by the adoptive transfer experiments and these cells could be important in maintaining or inhibiting induction of immune responses and explain the antigen specificity. This explains why both the sensitization and the effector phases are blocked.

3.2.5 Other Models and Data Indicating a Role of Treg in ECP

Soon after the description of the induction of Treg by ECP in the CHS model, similar studies were performed in other models. Gatza et al. investigated the effect of experimental ECP in a murine model of acute GVHD [26]. They demonstrate that the transfer of cells treated with ECP reverses established GVHD by increasing donor Treg and indirectly by reducing the number of donor effector lymphocytes that themselves had never been exposed to PUVA.

There are also indications that ECP in a clinical setting might induce Treg in humans. However, the limitation of these studies is the fact that such indicative functional studies with adoptive transfer experiments as in mice cannot be done in humans. Most of these studies confine themselves to a measurement in the alteration of numbers of Treg before and after ECP and *in vitro* analyses with *ex vivo* obtained leukocytes.

Since acute GVHD in patients with allogeneic grafts can be associated with a low number of Treg [27–29], several groups studied the effect of ECP on the number of Treg in patients undergoing ECP. In the majority of both CTCL and GVHD patients an increase in Treg and an enhanced suppressive activity could be observed [30–35]. This could explain at least partially the beneficial effect of ECP in GVHD and autoimmune diseases. How this relates to the positive effect in CTCL remains elusive. However, reduced numbers of Treg have been observed also in patients with Sézary syndrome [36, 37]. In addition their suppressive function appears to be impaired [38]. This gives rise to the speculation whether Treg exert the capacity to suppress CD4-positive tumor cells in Sézary syndrome. Whether this is the case, however, remains to be determined.

3.2.6 Conclusion

Although we are still far away from understanding the mode of action of ECP, the experimental murine models gave an idea and fostered the concept of Treg induced by ECP. The same applies for the human situation, however most of these studies simply describe a change in the number of Treg upon ECP and do not provide in depth functional data. In addition, these models may represent a nice tool to optimize the ECP regimen, e. g. to determine the optimal UVA dose, number of cells infused, frequency of infusion etc. This appears to be important because, since its original description 25 years ago, the regimen has remained almost unmodified as, probably by coincidence, it was working from the start. This, however, does not exclude chances for improvement.

References

[1] Knobler R. Extracorporeal photochemotherapy--present and future. Vox Sang 2000; 78 (Suppl 2): 197–201.
[2] Edelson R, Berger C, Gasparro F et al. Treatment of cutaneous T-cell lymphoma by extracorporeal photochemotherapy. Preliminary results. N Engl J Med 1987;316:297–303.
[3] Heald P, Rook A, Perez M, et al. Treatment of erythrodermic cutaneous T-cell lymphoma with extracorporeal photochemotherapy. J Am Acad Dermatol 1992;27:427–33.
[4] Maccherin M, Diciolla F, Laghi Pasini F, et al. Photopheresis immunomodulation after heart transplantation. Transplant Proc 2001;33:1591–4.
[5] Barr ML, Meise BM, Eisen HJ, et al. Photopheresis for the prevention of rejection in cardiac transplantation. Photopheresis Transplantation Study Group. N Engl J Med 1998;339:1744–51.
[6] Gorgun G, Miller KB, Foss FM. Immunologic mechanisms of extracorporeal photochemotherapy in chronic graft-versus-host disease. Blood 2002;100:941–7.
[7] Greinix HT, Volc-Platzer B, Kalhs P, et al. Extracorporeal photochemotherapy in the treatment of severe steroid-refractory acute graft-versus-host disease: a pilot study. Blood 2000;96:2426–31.
[8] Greinix HT, Volc-Platzer B, Rabitsch W, et al. Successful use of extracorporeal photochemotherapy in the treatment of severe acute and chronic graft-versus-host disease. Blood 1998;92:3098–104.
[9] Reinisch W, Nahavandi H, Santella R, et al. Extracorporeal photochemotherapy in patients with steroid-dependent Crohn's disease: a prospective pilot study. Aliment Pharmacol Ther 2001;15:1313–22.
[10] Malawista SE, Trock D, Edelson RL. Photopheresis for rheumatoid arthritis. Ann NY Acad Sci 1991;636:217–26.
[11] Ludvigsson J, Samuelsson U, Ernerudh J, Johansson C, Stenhammar L, Berlin G. Photopheresis at onset of type 1 diabetes: a randomised, double blind, placebo controlled trial. Arch Dis Child 2001;85:149–54.
[12] Oliven A, Shechter Y. Extracorporeal photopheresis: a review. Blood Rev 2001;15:103–8.
[13] Lim HW, Edelson RL. Photopheresis for the treatment of cutaneous T-cell lymphoma. Hematol Oncol Clin North Am 1995;9:1117–26.
[14] Suchin KR, Cassin M, Washko R, et al. Extracorporeal photochemotherapy does not suppress T- or B-cell responses to novel or recall antigens. J Am Acad Dermatol 1999;41:980–6.
[15] Maeda A, Schwarz A, Kernebeck K, et al. Intravenous infusion of syngeneic apoptotic cells by photopheresis induces antigen-specific regulatory T cells. J Immunol 2005;174:5968–76.
[16] Beissert S, Schwarz A, Schwarz T. Regulatory T cells. J Invest Dermatol 2006;126:15–24.
[17] Chatenoud L, Salomon B, Bluestone JA. Suppressor T cells--they're back and critical for regulation of autoimmunity! Immunol Rev 2001;2182:149–63.
[18] Zheng SG, Wang JH, Koss MN, et al. CD4+ and CD8+ regulatory T cells generated ex vivo with IL-2 and TGF-beta suppress a stimulatory graft-versus-host disease with a lupus-like syndrome. J Immunol 2004;172:1531–9.
[19] Wood KJ, Sakaguchi S. Regulatory T cells in transplantation tolerance. Nat Rev Immunol 2003;3:199–210.
[20] Shevach EM, DiPaolo RA, Andersson J, et al. The lifestyle of naturally occurring CD4+ CD25+ Foxp3+ regulatory T cells. Immunol Rev 2006;212:60–73.
[21] Schwarz T. The dark and the sunny sides of UVR-induced immunosuppression: photoimmunology revisited. J Invest Dermatol 2010;130:49–54.
[22] Schwarz T. 25 years of UV-induced immunosuppression mediated by T cells-from disregarded T suppressor cells to highly respected regulatory T cells. Photochem Photobiol 2008;84:10–8.
[23] Schwarz A, Maeda A, Kernebeck K, et al. Prevention of UV radiation-induced immunosuppression by IL-12 is dependent on DNA repair. J Exp Med 2005;201:173–9.

[24] Maeda A, Schwarz A, Bullinger A, et al. Experimental extracorporeal photopheresis inhibits the sensitization and effector phases of contact hypersensitivity via two mechanisms: generation of IL-10 and induction of regulatory T cells. J Immunol 2008;181:5956–62.
[25] Schwarz A, Grabbe S, Riemann H. et al. In vivo effects of interleukin-10 on contact hypersensitivity and delayed-type hypersensitivity reactions. J Invest Dermatol 1994;103:211–6.
[26] Gatza E, Rogers CE, Clouthier SG, et al. Extracorporeal photopheresis reverses experimental graft-versus-host disease through regulatory T cells. Blood 2008;112:1515–21.
[27] Rezvani K, Mielke S, Ahmadzadeh M, et al. High donor FOXP3-positive regulatory T-cell (Treg) content is associated with a low risk of GVHD following HLA-matched allogeneic SCT. Blood 2006;108:1291–7.
[28] Wolf D, Wolf AM, Fong D, et al. Regulatory T-cells in the graft and the risk of acute graft-versus-host disease after allogeneic stem cell transplantation. Transplantation 2007;83:1107–13.
[29] Zhai Z, Sun Z, Li Q, et al. Correlation of the CD4+CD25high T-regulatory cells in recipients and their corresponding donors to acute GVHD. Transpl Int 2007;20:440–6.
[30] Quaglino P, Comessatti A, Ponti R, et al. Reciprocal modulation of circulating CD4+CD25+bright T cells induced by extracorporeal photochemotherapy in cutaneous T-cell lymphoma and chronic graft-versus-host-disease patients. Int J Immunopathol Pharmacol 2009;22:353–62.
[31] Rao V, Saunes M, Jørstad S, Moen T. Cutaneous T cell lymphoma and graft-versus-host disease: a comparison of in vivo effects of extracorporeal photochemotherapy on Foxp3+ regulatory T cells. Clin Immunol. 2009;133:303–13.
[32] Di Biaso I, Di Maio L, Bugarin C, et al. Regulatory T cells and extracorporeal photochemotherapy: correlation with clinical response and decreased frequency of proinflammatory T cells. Transplantation. 2009;87:1422–5.
[33] Schmitt S, Johnson TS, Karakhanova S, et al. Extracorporeal photopheresis augments function of CD4+CD25+FoxP3+ regulatory T cells by triggering adenosine production. Transplantation 2009;88:411–6.
[34] Tsirigotis P, Kapsimalli V, Baltadakis I, et al. Extracorporeal photopheresis in refractory chronic graft-versus-host disease: The influence on peripheral blood T cell subpopulations. A study by the Hellenic Association of Hematology. Transfus Apher Sci 2012;46:181–8.
[35] Biagi E, Di Biaso I, Leoni V, et al. Extracorporeal photochemotherapy is accompanied by increasing levels of circulating CD4+CD25+GITR+Foxp3+CD62L+ functional regulatory T-cells in patients with graft-versus-host disease. Transplantation 2007;84:31–9.
[36] Heid JB, Schmidt A, Oberle N, et al. FOXP3+CD25- tumor cells with regulatory function in Sézary syndrome. J Invest Dermatol. 2009;129:2875–85.
[37] Klemke CD, Fritzsching B, Franz B, et al. Paucity of FOXP3+ cells in skin and peripheral blood distinguishes Sézary syndrome from other cutaneous T-cell lymphomas. Leukemia 2006;20:1123–9.
[38] Tiemessen MM, Mitchell TJ, Hendry L, et al. Lack of suppressive CD4+CD25+FOXP3+ T cells in advanced stages of primary cutaneous T-cell lymphoma. J Invest Dermatol 2006;126:2217–23.

Robert M. Whittle and Peter C. Taylor
3.3 Mechanism of Action of ECP – Clinical Evidence

3.3.1 Introduction

Despite being in clinical use for over a quarter of a century the precise mechanisms underlying the immunomodulatory effects on the diseases in which extracorporeal photopheresis (ECP) has shown efficacy remain somewhat enigmatic. What is clear is that whilst traditional therapies act to restrain the effector arm of the immune response in inflammatory conditions such as graft-versus-host disease (GVHD) in a broad manner, ECP provides the possibility of targeting immune tolerance without either substantive suppression of graft versus leukemia effect or generalized immunosuppression associated with increased infection risk [1]. The contrasting promotion of induction of active anti-tumour responses in the ECP treatment of the cutaneous T cell lymphomas (CTCL) precludes a single all-encompassing model to explain the action of photopheresis. In light of this divergence in action, two main hypotheses have been forwarded to explain this apparent mechanistic dichotomy. It is proposed that in the treatment of GVHD and other pro-inflammatory conditions ECP induces immune tolerance. Although the clinical evidence is indirect, it is supported by elegant animal studies. For the treatment of cutaneous T cell lymphomas the cellular vaccination hypothesis has strong evidence and is rooted in the earliest clinical observations of extracorporeal photopheresis treatment.

3.3.2 Cellular Vaccination Hypothesis

The initial application of extracorporeal photopheresis in the treatment of cutaneous T cell lymphoma was the culmination of in-vitro and in-vivo scientific observations promising the potential for photopheresis to provoke the human immune system to produce active immunization against disease causing T lymphocytes. The interest in a possible "vaccination" response was in part based upon the observations that in animal models of autoimmune encephalomyelitis and arthritis induction of an apparent anti-clonotypic response could be generated by infusion of pathogenic T cells [2–4]. Additionally, the sensitivity of T cells to the combined effects of 8-methoxypsoralen (8-MOP) and ultraviolet-A (UVA) had been established in Richard Edelson's laboratory in the same period, and the possibility that UVA and 8-MOP treated cells may provide a highly appropriate vaccination vehicle gathered pace [5]. The subsequent report of the clinical success of ECP treatment for CTCL in 1987 offered further support [6]. The cellular vaccination theory was developed by the Edelson group following observations that anti-clonal activity was attributed to the generation of clone-specific suppressor T cells [4, 7]. This anti-idiotypic response to T cell receptor

(TCR) antigens was proposed to be generated when the CTCL tumour T cells, treated by ECP and undergoing apoptosis, were ingested by antigen presenting cells and the peptide components of the CTCL TCR clone were presented to competent patient non-malignant T cells. It has been suggested that 8-MOP targets proteins, presumably including tumour antigens, for degradation and possible translocation into the major histocompatibility (MHC) class I pathway [8]. Increased display of MHC molecules in photoactivated 8-MOP treated lymphocytes would serve to enhance the presentation of these peptide targets. Strong evidence exists that the processing of engulfed apoptotic cells yields T cell epitopes and that preferential recognition of TCR hypervariable regions by anti-idiotypic clonal T cells is induced by T cell vaccination [9, 10].

The observed alterations in T cell clonality associated with clinical improvement in ECP-treated CTCL patients are relevant here. Therapeutic response is seemingly most potent in patients with evidence of T cell clonality in the circulation. Intriguingly the clones largely disappear in response to treatment [11]. Systemic sclerosis (SS) patients with a T cell clonal profile are also more responsive to ECP treatment than those without a T cell clone [12, 13]. Animal models of ECP where an anti-clonotypic response may be responsible for disease control lend weight to these observations [14–16].

Indirect evidence of anti-clonal response in treatment of GVHD may be claimed from the attenuation of effector T cells by ECP and the disease response to therapy correlating with the regression of amplified clonal T cell populations incriminated in driving the inflammatory process [12]. Additional indirect evidence may be derived from the animal models of GVHD treated with Psoralen and Ultraviolet Light A (PUVA) which demonstrated that greater MHC disparity between donor and recipient animals led to more complete and higher rates of response [7].

3.3.3 Apoptosis of ECP-Treated Lymphocytes

Combination of 8-MOP and UVA irradiation causes the majority of lymphocytes to apoptose within 48 hours [17, 18]. Lymphocytes demonstrate distinctive apoptotic morphology and DNA laddering [19, 20]. We demonstrated that these apoptotic lymphocytes then externalise phosphatidylserine, which is a key target recognition site for phagocytosis of the cell by antigen presenting cells [21]. Annexin V, a hallmark of early apoptosis is expressed almost immediately on a proportion of lymphocytes after treatment with ECP and positivity increases to over 75% 48 hours after exposure as shown in Figure 3.8 [17, 22, 23].

Whilst early apoptotic processes occur within the first 24 hours post-treatment including the depolarisation of the mitochondrial membrane and alteration of pro-apoptotic protein expression a second later apoptotic wave appears to account for the final cell death [22, 24]. Upregulation of Fas (CD95) and Fas-ligand have been reported which leaves the cell susceptible to the Fas pathway induction of intracellular caspases, a family of apoptotic proteases. The caspases, which have been detected in ECP-treated cells, ultimately dissemble the cell (Figure 3.9) [25].

It is assumed that the re-infused apoptotic lymphocytes are removed by the host antigen presenting cell population in locations such as the spleen, liver and other lymphoid tissues. Recent experiments in which 8-MOP/UVA treated peripheral blood leukocytes were radio-labelled demonstrated that peripheral blood mononuclear cells (PBMC) and neutrophils have different kinetic patterns after intravenous re-injection. The most prominent difference was immediate retention of PBMC but not of neutrophils in the lungs. After 24 hours more than 80% of both cell populations could be detected in liver and spleen [26]. The uptake of circulating apoptotic cells by splenic dendritic cells (DC) is a previously reported phenomenon [27], and ECP-treated, apoptotic lymphocytes are phagocytosed readily by monocytes [17, 24].

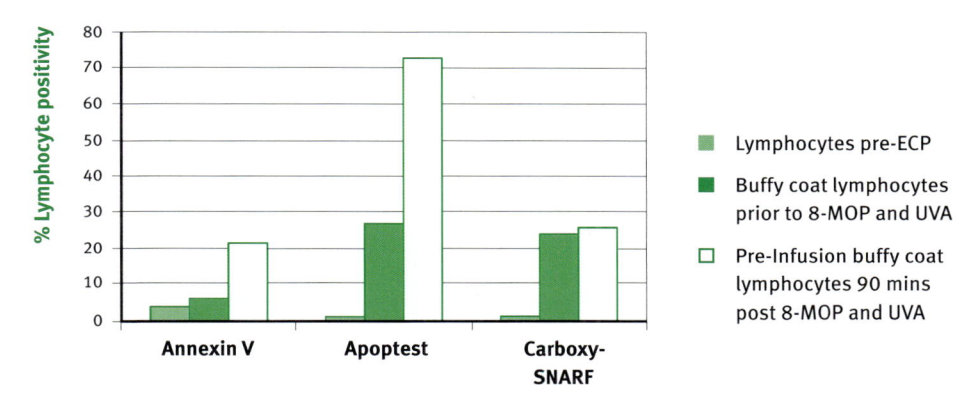

Fig. 3.8. Mean Levels of Lymphocyte Apoptosis After ECP Treatment as Measured by Different Methods. ECP induces rapid apoptotic processes in lymphocytes of GVHD and CTCL patients. Levels of apoptotic markers as measured by Annexin V expression, chromatin texture change (ApoptestTM) and changes in intracellular pH (Caboxy –SNARF-1-AM) increase significantly when lymphocytes are exposed to 8-MOP and UVA light [18].

3.3.4 Direct Effect of ECP on Effector Cells

Activated lymphocytes, which presumably include effector cell populations in pro-inflammatory conditions, appear particularly susceptible to rapid apoptosis [28]. Apoptosis induction in treated lymphocytes renders them unable to proliferate in-vitro, eliminating clonal expansion [29, 30]. Such apoptotic lymphocytes are also destined to be phagocytosed by macrophages [31]. However, the apoptosis, inactivation and removal of lymphocytes exposed to 8-MOP and UVA in the treatment cannot fully explain the efficacy of ECP as only a small proportion of the circulating T cells

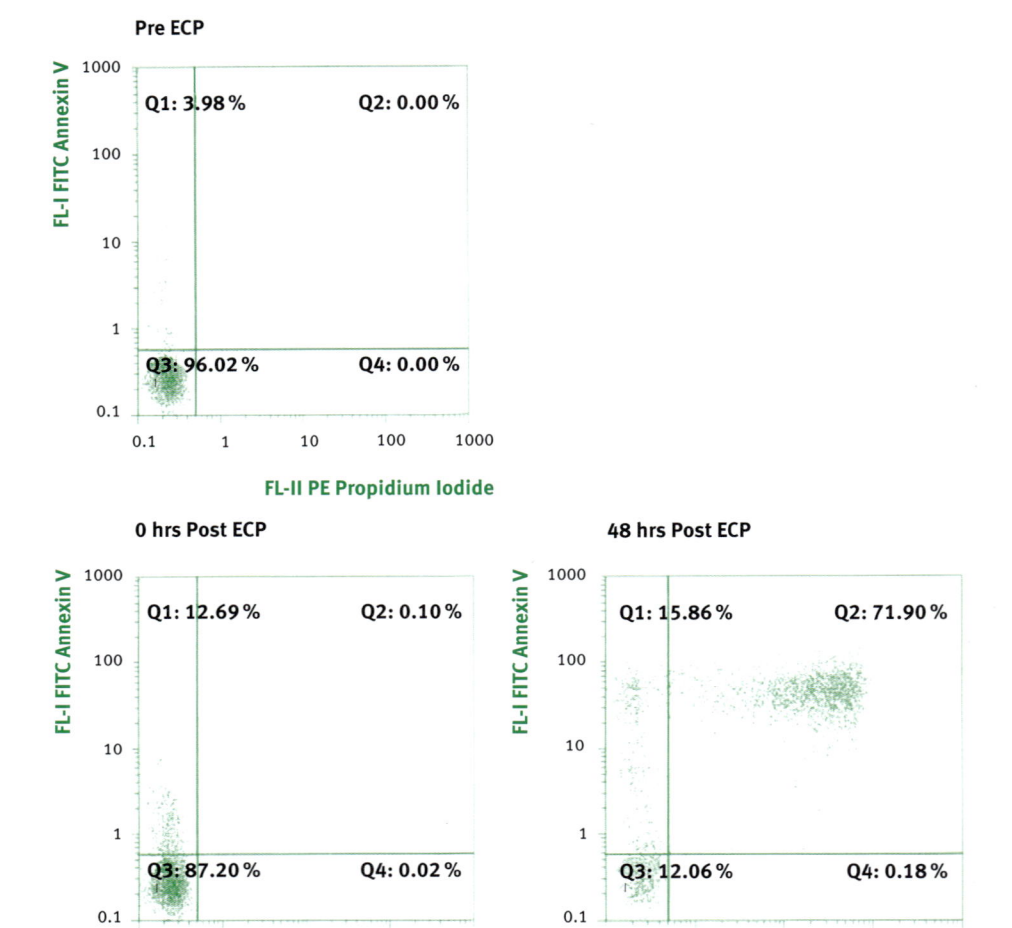

Fig. 3.9. Flow cytometric representation of Annexin V/ Propidium iodide (PI) expression pre ECP, immediately post ECP and in the 'late apoptosis' population 48 hours post ECP.
Compared to untreated lymphocytes, the number of Annexin V positive lymphocytes is significantly raised immediately post ECP. At 48 hours post ECP the majority of lymphocytes demonstrate both Annexin V and PI positivity, a phenotype consistent with secondary necrosis and late apoptotic processes [22].

are treated. Proportional estimates may vary on the procedure but figures between 5–15% of circulating lymphocytes are commonly treated [32]. Moreover, the majority of pathogenic T cells in either CTCL or GVHD, are likely to be located either at the site of inflammation or in the lymphoid tissues and are not subject to the therapy.

3.3.5 ECP Modulation of Peripheral Blood Monocytes and Dendritic Cells

Whilst the widespread and rapid kinetics of apoptosis in treated lymphocytes are consistently reported in the literature, the kinetics of apoptosis in monocytes are more controversial and subsequently their potential contribution to the overall immunomodulation generated by ECP remains open to debate.

Studies have demonstrated a resistance to apoptosis induction by ECP with ECP-exposed monocytes showing significant survival (approx 25%) up to 6 days post-treatment [17, 33, 34]. Contrastingly, other investigators have reported relatively rapid apoptotic kinetics in treated monocytes with over 80% of cells exhibiting apoptotic features within 48 hours of ECP [35, 36]. The contrast in the findings of the different studies is important as the concept of a dynamic, active role of ECP-treated monocytes in immunomodulation is linked to their survival in vivo; rapid apoptosis may argue for their role being somewhat restricted to acting as an apoptotic cell load to be ingested by untreated antigen presenting cells (APCs) whilst longer-term survival could allow a significant window of opportunity for ECP-treated monocytes to contribute directly. Evidence has emerged of monocytes undergoing pro-tolerogenic changes following ECP treatment.

Induction of monocyte differentiation to immature forms of dendritic cells by photopheresis, have been reported by a series of studies [35, 37]. Other recent experiments suggest that surviving monocytes differentiate into functional DC only with the addition of differentiation inducing cytokines [34]. Resistance to apoptosis of re-infused monocytes may in part be dependant on specific protectant cytokine bioavailability such as interleukin-12 (IL-12) [38], or granulocyte macrophage colony stimulating factor (GM-CSF) [17].

Evidence that ingestion of apoptotic cells by APCs has profound effects on immune regulation was clearly applicable to ECP treatment [39–41]. Key to this observation is the role of immature dendritic cells in promoting peripheral tolerance as a function of their specific phenotype [42, 43]. Additionally uptake of apoptotic cells is thought to inhibit pro-inflammatory cytokine production by APCs [44]. Since the specific characteristics and relative maturity of monocyte-derived dendritic cells is known to have a profound influence on the induction of alloreactivity, inflammation and immune tolerance [45], the fate of ECP treated APCs has logically received attention.

A study by Alcindor and colleagues suggested a modulation of circulating DC populations in ECP-treated patients with reduction in CD80+ CD123+ mature dendritic cells in circulation [46]. It should be noted that this and similar studies examining the phenotype of circulating DC populations cannot provide direct evidence of the effect of ECP/PUVA on these cell types.

However, the data from in-vitro studies for the direct ECP-effect on treated cells, is variable. A profoundly immature DC phenotype was reported to be prevalent in ECP-treated cell populations by Spisek et al in a group of 3 chronic GVHD patients [47]. These immature DCs retained their ability for activation, were highly phagocytic, could not generate allogeneic T cell proliferation and increased production of the anti-inflammatory cytokine, interleukin-10 (IL-10), which is ordinarily deficient in chronic GVHD [48]. Di Renzo and co-workers reported that cytokine-induced immature dendritic cells from GVHD patients produced enhanced amounts of IL-10 [49]. Evidence for 8-MOP/UVA induction of immature dendritic cells was also presented by the Pisa group but in these experiments additional cytokines were required and the presence of apoptotic cells was insufficient to promote monocyte-DC maturation. Interestingly, DCs that were matured in the presence of PUVA treated cells were of a tolerogenic phenotype, highly phagocytic and exhibited a lower ability to induce T cell proliferation [50].

It can be argued that the exposure of untreated antigen presenting cells to ECP/PUVA-treated cells most closely resembles the in-vivo scenario post-reinfusion. In light of this, the illustration of increased mRNA production of IL-10 and interleukin-1 (IL-1) receptor antagonist (IL-1Ra) by untreated PBMC exposed to ECP-treated lymphocytes by Craciun is significant [51]. We also demonstrated that LPS-stimulated monocytes exposed to ECP-treated monocytes produce reduced relative quantities of the pro-inflammatory cytokines IL-1 α, IL-1 β, and interleukin-6 (IL-6) in chronic GVHD patients [52]. This reduction in pro-inflammatory cytokines was also in evidence when the untreated monocytes were exposed to ECP-treated lymphocytes [53]. Subsequently dendritic cells isolated directly post-ECP from the blood of GVHD patients revealed impaired IL-1 β, tumor necrosis factor (TNF)-α and IL-12 and an inability to drive Th1 cells responses [54]. A skewing of T-cell responses away from pro-inflammatory Th1 response by PUVA-treated APCs was recently reported by Holtick and co-workers who illustrated that the signature chemokine receptor expression of Th2 cells (CCR4 and CCR10) was upregulated when co-cultured with PUVA-treated dendritic cells (Figure 3.10) [35].

In summary it appears that for GVHD patients, the exposure of APC populations to ECP-treated cells leads to production of anti-inflammatory cytokines, reduction in pro-inflammatory cytokines and the maintenance of an immature, tolerogenic phenotype. ECP-treated APCs that may survive for a period after re-infusion also show diminished immunostimulatory capacity and a promotion of anti-inflammatory status.

3.3.6 Distal Effects on Untreated Lymphocytes in GVHD

In addition to the observations that lymphocytes treated by ECP demonstrated apoptosis and reduced proliferative responses to mitogen, a number of reports indicate evidence of global immune modulation in treated patients following ECP. In consideration that less than 1 % of the total lymphoid mass is exposed to the treatment at any time [55], (5–15 % of circulating lymphocytes) this is highly significant. These global changes are largely consistent with the pro-tolerogenic, anti-inflammatory augmentation suggested by the antigen presenting cell behavioral experimental data. ECP-treated GVHD patients may demonstrate a normalization of CD4/CD8 T cell ratios

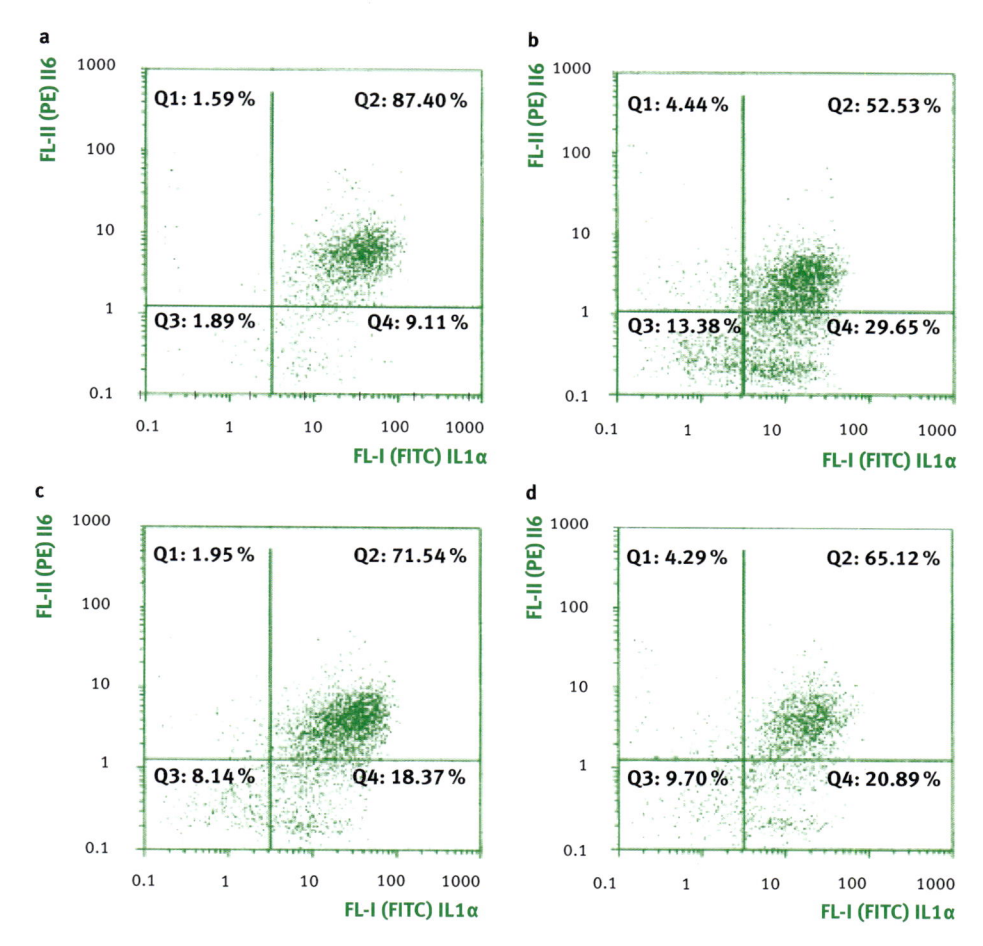

Fig. 3.10. Extracorporeal Photopheresis Suppresses IL1α and IL6 Production in ECP-treated and Untreated Monocytes.
Data represented are **(a)** pre ECP lymphocytes incubated with pre ECP monocytes (control); **(b)** post ECP lymphocytes co-cultured with post ECP monocytes (control) **c**; post ECP lymphocytes co-cultured with pre ECP monocytes and **d**; pre ECP lymphocytes co-cultured with post ECP monocytes. Co-culture mixture experiments demonstrate that ECP directly reduces the mean fluorescence intensity (MFI) of treated monocytes positive for interleukin 1 (IL1)α Q2 + Q4 and interleukin 6 (IL6) Q1 + Q2 and exposure to ECP-treated lymphocytes also indirectly reduces IL1α and IL6 production in untreated monocytes. Whilst the largest reduction in pro-inflammatory cytokines is demonstrated when both populations are ECP-treated, the exposure of untreated monocytes to ECP-treated lymphocytes generates a significant reduction in monocyte cytokine production [52].

[46, 56, 57], although this is not a universal finding in all reports [58]. It should be noted that the observed increase in circulating lymphocyte numbers may in part be as a result of decreasing cyclosporine and steroid dose in responding patients [57]. More subtle alterations in T cell phenotype have also been observed in ECP treated chronic GVHD patients with a report of increase in central memory CD8+ T cells and a decrease in central memory CD4+ T cells in patients with chronic GVHD [59]. This study also demonstrated that the balance of memory T cells normalizes after ECP treatment in tandem with improvement of clinical symptoms.

Modulation in the functional capacity of circulating T lymphocytes in patients undergoing ECP treatment is also evident. However, the findings in different diseases and studies vary. In chronic GVHD patients, a shift from a Th2 to a Th1-related IFN-γ producing cytokine profile and reduction in Th2 cytokines (interleukin-4, IL-4) was reported by several studies [58, 60]. Contrastingly, data from Gorgun and co-workers suggested a reduction in IFN-γ producing T cells in 10 chronic GVHD ECP patients with a switch to a Th2, (IL-4, IL-10) producing phenotype [61]. This latter study is consistent with the Th2 skewing of normal healthy volunteer lymphocytes when exposed to 8-MOP/UVA [62].

The inconsistencies reflect the inadequacies of a simply binary Th1/Th2 model and the complexity of biologic effects of ECP. Crucially when interpreting these cytokine "readout" studies of diseases treated with ECP, including GVHD, we need to ascertain whether perceived Th1/Th2 re-balancing reflects a therapeutic mechanism or simply a marker of disease improvement. In ECP treatment of CTCL the re-balancing of the Th1/Th2 relationship may be more reflective of normalisation rather than driving the process [63].

3.3.7 Emergence of Regulatory T cell Populations during ECP Treatment

An elegant animal model reported by Maeda and colleagues in 2005 provided a landmark study in aiding understanding of the tolerogenic mechanisms generated by ECP. This model of contact hypersensitivity demonstrated that the intravenous infusion of syngeneic apoptotic cells by photopheresis induced antigen-specific regulatory T cells (Tregs), whose depletion caused the loss of transfer of tolerance from the primary recipients into naïve animals [64]. The significance of these observations is clear when considering that an imbalance of Tregs and effector T cells is thought to underpin GVHD development [65, 66]. It has been established that the simultaneous injection of purified Tregs and donor effector cells suppresses the early expansion of alloreactive donor T cells, preventing GVHD in a murine model. A number of clinical studies have shown that increased numbers of Tregs in the graft, possessing the regulatory intraplasmic marker, Foxp3, are associated with a reduced risk of GVHD and that the ratio of Treg to effector T cells is significantly reduced in patients with GVHD [65–67].

The induction of Tregs by ECP may provide an explanation why the therapy promotes immune tolerance in a number of conditions without generalized immunosuppression. The observation that regulatory T cells may be generated via tolerogenic dendritic cells following phagocytosis of apoptotic cells was concordant with the earlier observations of the mechanism of action of ECP.

Clinical evidence of regulatory T cell generation in response to ECP was initially provided by a small study of cardiothoracic transplant patients which showed emergence of CD25+ CD69- T cells in all 4 patients treated. This was associated by the authors with a tolerogenic dendritic cell phenotype in DCs co-cultured with ECP-treated PBMC [68]. Subsequently, CD62L+ GITR+ subset of FoxP3+ Tregs were reportedly elevated rapidly in both acute and chronic GVHD patients receiving ECP and the cells were capable of inhibiting alloreactive responses in a contact-dependant manner [69]. Similar expansion of CD4+CD25+ Tregs was found in 3 patients undergoing ECP treatment for post-lung transplant bronchiolitis obliterans syndrome with stabilizing disease [70]. In contrast, patients with worsening symptoms exhibited a falling Treg count. Increases in Treg numbers or Treg associated markers have also been reported following ECP treatment pre-renal transplant, and in recent onset type 1 diabetes [71, 72]. We have reported a deficiency of absolute T regulatory cell numbers in 9 chronic GVHD patients pre-ECP and that at 3 months of treatment Treg levels did normalize; however, although T regulatory cell absolute numbers did increase, no selective increase in T regulatory cell numbers could be demonstrated [57]. The Biagi group built upon their initial observations by demonstrating in a cohort of 9 acute GVHD and 18 chronic GVHD patients that ECP-response is associated with increased levels of regulatory T cells which maintained STAT-5 pathway activity and that higher levels of Tregs in ECP-responding patients correlated with a decreased frequency of circulating Th-17 cells which have been incriminated in chronic inflammation and GVHD [73, 74]. Augmentation in Treg suppression by ECP was also reported by Schmitt and colleagues [75].

These clinical observations were further supported by a recognized animal model of GVHD, illustrating that the transfer of cells treated with ECP reversed established disease by increasing donor regulatory T cells whilst indirectly reducing the number of donor effector lymphocytes that themselves had never been exposed to ECP [76]. Another murine GVHD model suggested that infusion of ECP-treated splenocytes indirectly modulated T cell-mediated alloreactivity via IL-10–producing DCs not in the ECP-treated inocula, resulting in the expansion of Tregs which abrogated the disease [7].

3.3.8 Dysregulation of B Cell Homeostasis and Hallmarks of Improvement in ECP Treatment in GVHD

Whilst acute GVHD is widely accepted to be driven by T cell alloreactivity there is substantial evidence that chronic GVHD encompasses many features of autoimmune disease and immune dysregulation. The role of B cells in the pathogenesis of GVHD is only recently becoming appreciated and investigated. After myeloablative allogeneic hematopoietic cell transplantation (HCT), B cell reconstitution is slow and appears to recapitulate B cell ontogeny [78]. Control of B cell development appears deranged with evidence of breakdown in peripheral B cell tolerance. It has been recognized that dysregulation of the B cell compartment is a hallmark of chronic GVHD and this observation is complemented by the high incidence of autoantibodies found in patients with active chronic GVHD [79]. Greinix and coworkers reported that chronic GVHD is associated with elevated numbers of CD21 negative immature transitional B cells and a defiency of CD27+ memory B cells [80]. Subsequently, a correlation between low numbers of pre-treatment CD21 negative B cells and a good response to ECP therapy was described by the same group [81]. The preponderance of CD21 negative cells remained in evidence in non-responding patient cohorts up to 21 months of treatment. This was the first time that alterations in the behavior of the B cell compartment had been associated with ECP treatment response.

Parallel studies of the Sarantopoulos group in Boston, identified perturbed B cell homeostasis and elevated levels of B cell activating factor (BAFF) in patients with chronic GVHD which appear to correlate with disease activity [82, 83]. BAFF cytokine has defined roles in the survival of naïve B cells and in excess, the promotion of autoantibodies and autoimmune disease [84–86]. Recently we have provided evidence that high levels of serum BAFF (above 4 ng/mL) after 1 month of ECP for chronic GVHD are associated with inferior skin disease response after 3 and 6 months of treatment whilst 1 month ECP low BAFF levels (below 4 ng/mL) are associated with a significant improvement in median skin score and more complete and partial visceral organ responses [87]. The predictive qualities of BAFF measurement were strengthened by BAFF level measurement after 6 months of ECP which suggested that high serum levels were associated with an increased likelihood of both disease flare and the need to re-escalate steroid dose [88]. The ratio between B cell number and BAFF level may also be a key to understanding the dynamics of B cell compartment homeostasis in GVHD (Figure 3.11) [83, 89].

How ECP treatment may influence the BAFF level is not currently understood although work by us and other groups illustrate that ECP modulates APC cytokine production [35, 52, 90, 91], and BAFF cytokine production could logically also be affected. Regardless of mechanism, lower BAFF levels would theoretically serve to promote coherent negative selection of B cells in contrast to the dysregulation and inadequate tolerance present in chronic GVHD [92].

Whilst biomarkers such as BAFF level and B cell phenotype monitoring can provide us with clues to the mechanism of action of ECP, further investigation remains necessary, firstly to understand how the therapy delivers its immunomodulation and secondly to provide us with robust biomarker tools to aid in the prediction of response. In so doing these tools may assist us in providing individualized patient-orientated approaches to improve upon the already impressive treatment benefits of photopheresis. A summary of evidence for the mechanism of action of ECP in graft versus-host disease can be found in table 3.1.

3.3 Mechanism of Action of ECP – Clinical Evidence

Mechanism of Action	Immunological Consequences	Strength and Consistency of Evidence	Evidence Type	References
Apoptosis of treated lymphocytes	Proportion of effector cells inactivated. Antigenic apoptotic cell load available for processing and presentation.	Strong, consistent	CL, IV, AM	17–25, 28
Engulfment of apoptotic lymphocytes by antigen presenting cells	Antigenic load processed in non-inflammatory context. Potential for APC modulation.	Strong, consistent	CL, IV, AM	17, 24
Generation of anti-clonotypic response	Alloreactive and autoreactive effector T cell receptor antigens become target for anti-idiotypic response.	Limited and indirect	CL	12
Modulation of cytokine production in monocytes exposed to ECP-treated cells	Increase in anti-inflammatory cytokines. Decrease in pro-inflammatory cytokines. Attenuation of inflammatory processes.	Strong, consistent	CL, IV, AM	51–54
Apoptosis of treated monocytes	Monocyte function curtailed. Anti-genic apoptotic cell load available for processing & presentation.	Limited, inconsistent	IV	17, 33–36
Survival and direct differentiation of immature dendritic cells from ECP-treated monocytes	Immature, tolerogenic antigen presenting cell population generated.	Limited, inconsistent	IV	37, 47–49
Generation of immature dendritic cell phenotype by exposure to ECP-treated cells	Immature, tolerogenic APC population generated.	Modest, inconsistent	IV, AM	50, 51, 78
Skewing of untreated T cell phenotype	Rebalancing from pro-inflammatory to anti-inflammatory milieu. Population normalization.	Modest, inconsistent	CL, IV	35, 46, 56–62
Regulatory T cell generation	Improved control of auto- and alloreactivity.	Strong, consistent	CL, AM	57, 64–70, 74–78
B cell compartment normalisation	Coherent B cell selection. Attenuation of autoantibody production.	Modest, consistent	CL	82, 88, 89

CL = Clinical data, IV = in-vitro data, AM = animal model, APC = antigen presenting cell.

Table 3.1. Summary of Mechanisms of Action of Extracorporeal Photopheresis in the Treatment of Graft-versus-Host Disease.

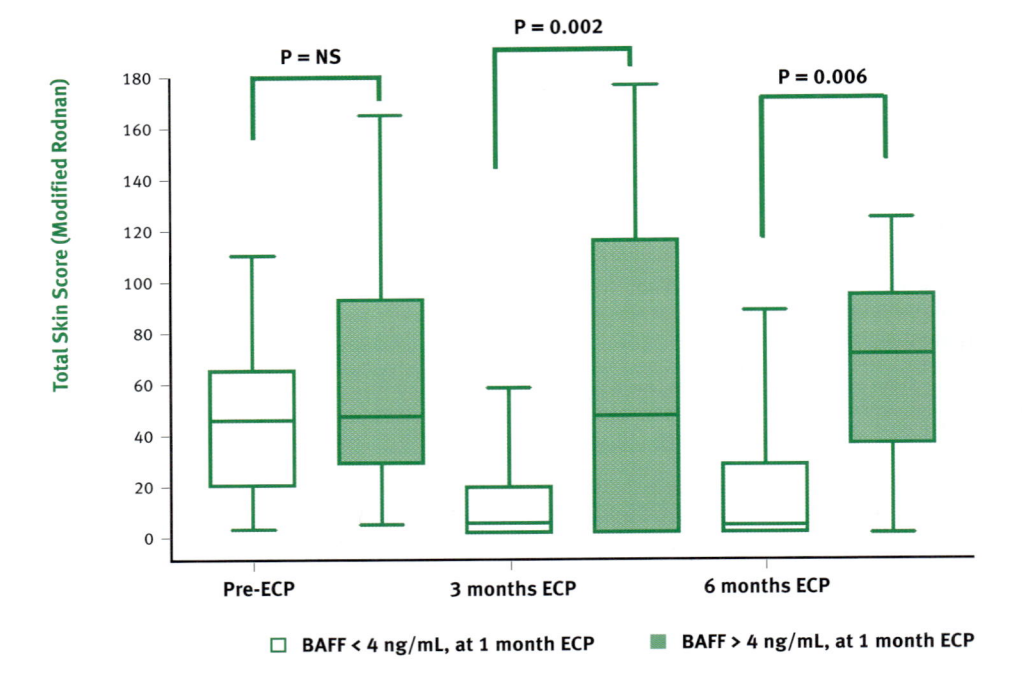

Fig. 3.11. Relationship Between B Cell Activating Factor (BAFF) and ECP Treatment Outcome for Chronic GVHD.
Serum BAFF level in the early stages of ECP treatment predicted response of chronic cutaneous GVHD. Patients grouped into serum BAFF levels either less than 4 ng/mL (white bars, n= 24) or more than 4 ng/mL (green bars, n=11) after 2 paired treatments (1 month) of ECP had similar total skin scores (TSS) (median, 47 vs 48.5) before starting ECP. After 3 months of ECP, patients with early lower BAFF levels demonstrated significant improvement in their skin disease compared with those with higher BAFF 2 months earlier (median TSS, 4.5 vs 46, $P=0.002$). The disparity in disease improvement between the low and high serum BAFF groups at 3 months was still evident after 6 months of ECP (median TSS, 3.5 vs 76, $P=0.006$) [87].

References

[1] Suchin KR, Cassin M, Washko R, et al. Extracorporeal photochemotherapy does not suppress T- or B-cell responses to novel or recall antigens. J Am Acad Dermatol 1999;41:980–6.
[2] Ben Nun A, Werkerle H, Cohen IR. Vaccination against autoimmune encephalomyelitis with T lymphocytes line cells reactive against myelin basic protein. Nature 1981;292:60–1
[3] Holoshitz J, Frenkel A, Ben-Nun A, Cohen IR. Autoimmune encephalomyelitis (EAE) mediated or prevented by T lymphocyte lines directed against diverse antigenic determinants of myelin basic protein. Vaccination is determinant specific. J Immunol 1983;131:2810–3.
[4] Khavari PA, Edelson RL, Lider O, Gasparro FP, Weiner HL, Cohen IR. Specific vaccination against photoinactivated cloned T cells. Clin Res 1988;36:662.
[5] Morison WL, Parrish JA, McAuliffe DJ, Bloch KJ. Sensitivity of mononuclear cells to PUVA: effect on subsequent stimulation with mitogens and on exclusion of typan blue dye. Clin Exp Dermatol 1981;6:273–7.

[6] Edelson R, Berger C, Gasparro F, et al. Treatment of cutaneous T cell lymphoma by extracorporeal photochemotherapy: preliminary results. N Engl J Med 1987;316:297–303.
[7] Perez M, Edelson R, LaRoche L, Berger C. Inhibition of antiskin allograft immunity by infusions with syngeneic photoinactivated effector lymphocytes. J Invest Dermatol 1989;92:669–76. 946–57.
[8] Hanlon DJ, Berger CL, Edelson RL. Photoactivated 8-methoxypsoralen treatment causes a peptide-dependent increase in antigen display by transformed lymphocytes. Int J Cancer 1998;78:70–5.
[9] Bellone M, Iezzi G, Rovere P, et al. Processing of engulfed apoptotic bodies yields T cell epitopes. J Immunol 1997;159:5391–9.
[10] Zang YC, Hong J, Rivera VM, Killian J, Zhang JZ. Preferential recognition of TCR hypervariable regions by human anti-idiotypic T cells induced by T cell vaccination. J Immunol 2000;164:4011–7.
[11] Rook AH, Suchin KR, Kao DMF, et al. Photopheresis: clinical applications and mechanism of action. J Investig Dermatol Symp Proc 1999;4:85–90.
[12] French LE, Lessin SR, Addya K, et al. Identification of clonal T cells in the blood of patients with systemic sclerosis: positive correlation with response to photopheresis. Arch Dermatol 2001;137:1309–13.
[13] French LE, Alcindor T, Shapiro M, et al. Identification of amplified clonal T cell populations in the blood of patients with chronic graft-versus-host disease: positive correlation with response to photopheresis. Bone Marrow Transplant 2002;30:509–15.
[14] Berger CL, Perez M, Laroche L, Edelson RL. Inhibition of autoimmune disease in a murine model of systemic lupus erythematosus induced by exposure to syngeneic photoinactivated lymphocytes. J Invest Dermatol 1990;94:52–7.
[15] Cavaletti G, Perseghin P, Buscemi F, et al. Immunomodulating effects of extracorporeal photochemotherapy in rat experimental allergic encephalomyelitis. Int J Tissue React. 2001;23:21–31.
[16] Girardi M, Herreid P, Tigelaar R. Specific suppression of lupus-like graft versus host disease using extracorporeal photochemical attenuation of effector lymphocytes. J Invest Dermatol 1995;104:177–82.
[17] Yoo EK, Rook AH, Elenitsas R, Gasparro FP, Vowels BR. Apoptosis induction of ultraviolet light A and photochemotherapy in cutaneous T-cell lymphoma: relevance to mechanism of therapeutic action. J Invest Dermatol 1996;107:235–42.
[18] Bladon J, Taylor PC. Extracorporeal photopheresis induces apoptosis in the lymphocytes of cutaneous T-cell lymphoma and graft-versus-host-disease patients. Br J Haematol 1999;107:707–11.
[19] Marks DI, Fox RM. Mechanisms of photochemotherapy induced apoptotic cell death in lymphoid cells. Biochem Cell Biol 1991;69:754–60.
[20] Aringer M, Graninger WB, Smolen JS, et al. Photopheresis treatment enhances CD95 (fas) expression in circulating lymphocytes of patients with systemic sclerosis and induces apoptosis. Br J Rheumatol 1997;36:1276–82.
[21] Bladon J, Taylor PC. The expression of CD10 by apoptotic lymphocytes is preceded by a pronounced externalization of phosphatidylserine. Blood 2000; 96:4009.
[22] Bladon J, Taylor PC. Extracorporeal photopheresis, in cutaneous T-cell lymphoma and graft-versus-host-disease, induces both immediate and progressive apoptotic processes. Br J Dermatol 2002;146:59–68.
[23] Gerber A, Bohne M, Rasch J, Struy H, Ansorge S, Gollnick H. Investigation of annexin V binding to lymphocytes after extracorporeal photoimmunotherapy as an early marker of apoptosis. Dermatology 2000;201:111–7.
[24] Bladon J, Taylor PC. Lymphocytes treated by extracorporeal photopheresis demonstrate a drop in the Bcl-2/Bax ratio: a possible mechanism involved in extracorporeal-photopheresis-induced apoptosis. Dermatology 2002;204:104–7.
[25] Di Renzo M, Rubegni P, Sane P, et al. ECP-treated lymphocytes of chronic graft-versus-host disease patients undergo apoptosis which involves both the Fas/FasL system and the Bcl-2 protein family. Arch Derm Res 2003;295:175–82.

[26] Just U, Dimou E, Knobler R, et al. Leukocyte scintigraphy with 111In-oxine for assessment of cell trafficking after extracorporeal photopheresis. Exp Dermatol 2012; DOI: 10.1111/j.1600-0625.2012.01491.x

[27] Morelli AE, Larregina AT, Shufesky WJ, et al. Internalization of circulating apoptotic cells by splenic marginal zone dendritic cells: dependence on complement receptors and effect on cytokine production. Blood 2003;101:611–20.

[28] Heng AE, Sauvezie B, Genestier L, Demeocq F, Dosgilbert A, Deteix P. PUVA apoptotic response in activated and resting human lymphocytes. Transfus Apher Sci 2003;28:43–50.

[29] Ullrich SE. Photoinactivation of T-cell function with psoralen and UVA irradiation suppresses the induction of experimental murine graft-versus-host disease across major histocompatibility barriers. J Invest Dermatol 1991;96:303–8.

[30] Truitt RL, Johnson BD, Hanke C, Talib S, Hearst JE. Photochemical treatment with S-59 psoralen and ultraviolet A light to control the fate of naive or primed T lymphocytes in vivo after allogeneic bone marrow transplantation. J Immunol 1999;163:5145–56.

[31] Fadok VA, Voelker DR, Campbell PA, Cohen JJ, Bratton DL, Henson PM. Exposure of phosphatidlyserine on the surface of apoptotic lymphocytes triggers specific recognition and removal by macrophages. Journal of Immunol 1992;48:2207–16.

[32] Marshall SR. Technology insight: ECP for the treatment of GvHD– Can we offer selective immune control without generalized immunosuppression? Nat Clin Pract Oncol 2006;3:302.

[33] Tambur AR, Ortegel JW, Morales A, Klingemann H, Gebel HM, Tharp MD. Extracorporeal photopheresis induces lymphocyte but not monocyte apoptosis. Transplant Proc 2000;32:747–8.

[34] Hannani D, Gabert F, Laurin D, et al. Photochemotherapy induces the apoptosis of monocytes without impairing their function. Transplantation 2010;89:492–9.

[35] Holtick U, Marshall SR, Wang XN, et al. Impact of psoralen/UVA treatment on survival, activation, and immunostimulatory capacity of monocyte-derived dendritic cells. Transplantation 2008;85:757–66.

[36] Setterblad N, Garban F, Weigl R, et al. Extracorporeal photopheresis increases sensitivity of monocytes from patients with graft-versus-host disease to HLA-DR-mediated cell death. Transfusion 2008;48:169–77.

[37] Legitimo A, Consolini R, Failli A et al. In vitro treatment of monocytes with 8-methoxypsoralen and ultraviolet A light induces dendritic cells with a tolerogenic phenotype. Clin Exp Immunol 2007;148:564–72.

[38] Schwarz A, Maeda A, Kernebeck K, van Steeg H, Beissert S, Schwarz T. Prevention of UV radiation-induced immunosuppression by IL-12 is dependent on DNA repair. J Exp Med 2005;201:173–9.

[39] Savill J, Dransfield I, Gregory C, Haslett C. A blast from the past: clearance of apoptotic cells regulates immune responses. Nat Rev Immunol 2002;2:965–75.

[40] Voll RE, Herrmann M, Roth EA, Stach C, Kalden JR, Girkontaite I. Immunosuppressive effects of apoptotic cells. Nature 1997;390:350–1.

[41] Albert ML. Death-defying immunity: do apoptotic cells influence antigen processing and presentation? Nat Rev Immunol 2004;4:223–31.

[42] Steinman RM, Hawiger D, Liu K, et al. Dendritic cell function in vivo during the steady state: a role in peripheral tolerance. Ann N Y Acad Sci. 2003;987:15–25. Review.

[43] Mahnke K, Knop J, Enk AH. Induction of tolerogenic DCs: "you are what you eat". Trends Immunol 2003;24:646–51. Review.

[44] Fadok VA, Bratton DL, Konowal A, et al. Macrophages that have ingested apoptotic cells in vitro inhibit proinflammatory cytokine production through autocrine/paracrine mechanisms involving TGF-beta, PGE2, and PAF. J Clin Invest 1998;101:890–8.

[45] Lanzavecchia A, Sallusto F. The instructive role of dendritic cells on T cell responses: lineages, plasticity and kinetics. Curr Opin Immunol 2001;13:291–8. Review.

[46] Alcindor T, Gorgun G, Miller KB, et al. Immunomodulatory effects of extracorporeal photochemotherapy in patients with extensive chronic graft-versus-host disease. Blood 2001;98:1622–5.
[47] Spisek R, Gasova Z, Bartunkova J. Maturation state of dendritic cells during the extracorporeal photopheresis and its relevance for the treatment of chronic graft-versus-host disease. Transfusion 2006;46:55–65.
[48] Korholz D, Kunst D, Hempel L, et al. Decreased interleukin 10 and increased interferon-gamma production in patients with chronic graft-versus-host disease after allogeneic bone marrow transplantation. Bone Marrow Transplant 1997;19:691–5.
[49] Di Renzo M, Rubegni P, Pasqui AL et al. Extracorporeal photopheresis affects IL10 and IL12 monocyte production in chronic graft-versus-host-disease patients. Br J Dermatol 2005;153:59–65.
[50] Legitimo A, Consolini R, Failli A, et al. In vitro treatment of monocytes with 8-methoxypsoralen and ultraviolet A light induces dendritic cells with a tolerogenic phenotype. Clin Exp Immunol 2007;148:564–72.
[51] Craciun LI, Stordeur P, Schandene L, et al. Increased production of interleukin-10 and interleukin-1 receptor antagonist after extracorporeal photochemotherapy in chronic graft-versus-host disease. Transplantation 2002;74:995–1000.
[52] Bladon J, Taylor PC. Lymphocytes treated by extracorporeal photopheresis can down-regulate cytokine production in untreated monocytes. Photodermatol Photoimmunol Photomed 2005;21:293–302.
[53] Bladon J, Taylor PC. The down-regulation of IL1a and IL6, in monocytes exposed to extracorporeal photopheresis (ECP)-treated lymphocytes, is not dependent on lymphocyte phosphatidylserine externalisation. Transpl Int 2006;19:319–24.
[54] Gerner M, Holig K, Wehner R, et al. Extracorporeal photopheresis efficiently impairs the proinflammatory capacity of human 6-sulfo LacNAc dendritic cells. Transplantation 2009;8:1134–8.
[55] Trepel F; Number and distribution of lymphocytes in man. A critical analysis. J Mol Med 1974; 52:511–5.
[56] Seaton ED, Szydlo RM, Kanfer E, Apperley JF, Russell-Jones R. Influence of extracorporeal photopheresis on clinical and laboratory parameters in chronic graft-versus-host disease and analysis of predictors of response. Blood 2003;102:1217–23.
[57] Bladon J, Taylor PC. Extracorporeal photopheresis normalizes some lymphocyte subsets (including T regulatory cells) in chronic graft-versus-host-disease. Ther Apher Dial 2008;12:311–8.
[58] Silva MG, Ferreira Neto L, Guimarães A, Machado A, Parreira A, Abecasis M. Long-term follow-up of lymphocyte populations and cellular cytokine production in patients with chronic graft-versus-host disease treated with extracorporeal photopheresis. Haematologica 2005;90:565–7.
[59] Yamashita K, Horwitz ME, Kwatemaa A, et al Unique abnormalities of CD4+ and CD8+ central memory cells associated with chronic graft-versus-host disease improve after extracorporeal photopheresis. Biol Blood Marrow Transplant 2006;12:22–30.
[60] Darvay A, Salooja N, Russell-Jones R. The effect of extracorporeal photopheresis on intracellular cytokine expression in chronic cutaneous graft-versus-host disease. J Eur Acad Dermatol Venereol 2004;18:279–84.
[61] Gorgun G, Miller KB, Foss FM. Immunologic mechanisms of extracorporeal photochemotherapy in chronic graft-versus host-disease. Blood 2002;100:941–7.
[62] Klosner G, Trautinger F, Knobler R, Neuner P. Treatment of peripheral blood mononuclear cells with 8-methoxypsoralen plus ultraviolet A radiation induces a shift in cytokine expression from a Th1 to a Th2 response. J Invest Dermatol 2001;116:459–62.
[63] Di Renzo M, Rubegni P, De Aloe G, et al. Extracorporeal photochemotherapy restores Th1/Th2 imbalance in patients with early stage cutaneous T cell lymphoma. Immunol 1997;92:99–103.
[64] Maeda A, Schwarz A, Kernebeck K, Gross N, Aragane Y, Peritt D, et al. Intravenous infusion of syngeneic apoptotic cells by photopheresis induces antigen-specific regulatory T cells. J Immunol 2005;174:5968–76.

[65] Rezvani K, Mielke S, Ahmadzadeh M, et al. High donor FOXP3-positive regulatory T-cell (Treg) content is associated with a low risk of GVHD following HLA-matched allogeneic SCT. Blood 2006;108:1291–7.
[66] Edinger M, Hoffmann P, Ermann J, et al. CD4+CD25+ regulatory T cells preserve graft-versus-tumor activity while inhibiting graft-versus-host disease after bone marrow transplantation. Nat Med. 2003;9:1144–50.
[67] Magenau JM, Qin X, Tawara I, et al. Frequency of CD4(+)CD25(hi)FOXP3(+) regulatory T cells has diagnostic and prognostic value as a biomarker for acute graft-versus-host-disease. Biol Blood Marrow Transplant. 2010;7:907–14.
[68] Lamioni A, Parisi F, Isacchi G, et al. The immunological effects of extracorporeal photopheresis unraveled: induction of tolerogenic dendritic cells in vitro and regulatory T cells in vivo. Transplantation. 2005;79:846–50.
[69] Biagi E, Di Biaso I, Leoni V, et al. Extracorporeal photochemotherapy is accompanied by increasing levels of circulating CD4+CD25+GITR+Foxp3+CD62L functional regulatory T-cells in patients with graft-versus-host disease. Transplantation 2007;84:31–9.
[70] Meloni F, Cascina A, Miserere S, Perotti C, Vitulo P, Fietta AM. Peripheral CD4+CD25+ Treg cell counts and the response to extracorporeal photopheresis in lung transplant recipients. Transpl Proc 2007;39:213–7.
[71] Jonson CO, Pihl M, Nyholm C, Cilio CM, Ludvigsson J, Faresjö M. Regulatory T cell-associated activity in photopheresis-induced immune tolerance in recent onset type 1 diabetes children. Clin Exp Immunol 2008;153:174–81.
[72] Lamioni A, Carsetti R, Legato A,et al. Induction of regulatory T cells after prophylactic treatment with photopheresis in renal transplant recipients. Transplantation 2007;83:1393–6.
[73] Di Biaso I, Di Maio L, Bugarin C, et al. Regulatory T cells and extracorporeal photochemotherapy: correlation with clinical response and decreased frequency of proinflammatory T cells. Transplantation 2009;87:1422–5.
[74] Chen X, Vodanovic-Jankovic S, Johnson B, Keller M, Komorowski R, Drobyski WR. Absence of regulatory T-cell control of TH1 and TH17 cells is responsible for the autoimmune-mediated pathology in chronic graft-versus-host-disease. Blood 2007;110:3804–13.
[75] Schmitt S, Johnson TS, Karakhanova S, Näher H, Mahnke K, Enk AH. Extracorporeal photopheresis augments function of CD4+CD25+FoxP3+ regulatory T cells by triggering adenosine production. Transplantation 2009;88:411–6.
[76] Gatza E, Rogers CE, Clouthier SG, et al. Extracorporeal photopheresis reverses experimental graft-versus-host disease through regulatory T cells. Blood 2008;112:1515–21.
[77] Capitini CM, Davis JEP, Larabee SM, Herby S, Nasholm NM, Fry TJ. Extracorporeal photopheresis attenuates murine graft-versus-host disease via bone marrow–derived interleukin-10 and preserves responses to dendritic cell vaccination. Biol Blood Marrow Transplant 2011; 17:790–9.
[78] Storek J, Ferrara S, Ku N, Giorgi JV, Champlin RE, Saxon A. B cell reconstitution after human bone marrow transplantation: recapitulation of ontogeny? Bone Marrow Transplant 1993;12: 387–98.
[79] Shimabukuro-Vornhagen A, Hallek MJ, Storb R, von Bergwelt-Baildon MS. The role of B cells in the pathogenesis of graft-versus-host disease. Blood 2009;114:4919–27.
[80] Greinix HT, Pohlreich D, Kouba M, et al. Elevated numbers of immature/transitional CD21- B lymphocytes and deficiency of memory CD27+ B cells specify patients with active chronic graft versus-host disease. Biol Blood Marrow Transplant 2008;14:208–19.
[81] Kuzmina Z, Greinix HT, Knobler R, et al. Proportions of immature CD19+CD21- B lymphocytes predict the response to extracorporeal photopheresis in patients with chronic graft-versus-host disease. Blood 2009;114:744–6.
[82] Sarantopoulos S, Stevenson KE, Kim HT, et al. High levels of B-cell activating factor in patients with active chronic graft-versus-host disease. Clin Cancer Res 2007;13:6107–14.

[83] Sarantopoulos S, Stevenson KE, Kim HT, et al. Altered B-cell homeostasis and excess BAFF in human chronic graft-versus-host disease. Blood 2009;113:3865–74.
[84] Mariette X, Roux S, Zhang J, et al. The level of BLyS (BAFF) correlates with the titre of autoantibodies in human Sjogren's syndrome. Ann Rheum Dis 2003;62:168–71.
[85] Mackay F, Woodcock SA, Lawton P, et al. Mice transgenic for BAFF develop lymphocytic disorders along with autoimmune manifestations. J Exp Med 1999;190:1697–1710.
[86] Thien M, Phan TG, Gardam S, et al. Excess BAFF rescues self-reactive B cells from peripheral deletion and allows them to enter forbidden follicular and marginal zone niches. Immunity 2004;20:785–98.
[87] Whittle R, Taylor PC. Circulating B-cell activating factor level predicts clinical response of chronic graft-versus-host disease to extracorporeal photopheresis. Blood 2011;118:6446–9.
[88] Whittle R, Taylor PC. Circulating B-cell activating factor level predicts likelihood of chronic GVHD flare and probability of successful steroid taper during extracorporeal photopheresis therapy. Bone Marrow Transplant 2012;47(S1):S63.
[89] Kuzmina Z, Greinix HT, Weigl R, et al. Significant differences in B-cell subpopulations characterize patients with chronic graft-versus-host disease-associated dysgammaglobulinemia. Blood 2011;117:2265–74.
[90] Neuner P, Charvat B, Knobler R, et al. Cytokine release by peripheral blood mononuclear cells is affected by 8-methoxypsoralen plus UV-A. Photochem Photobiol 1994;59:182–8.
[91] Bladon J, Taylor PC. Extracorporeal photopheresis reduces the number of mononuclear cells that produce pro-inflammatory cytokines, when tested ex-vivo. J Clin Apher 2002; 17:177–82.
[92] Socie G. Chronic GVHD: B cells come of age. Blood 2011;117:2086–7.

Section 4: **Extracorporeal Photopheresis in Acute Graft-versus-Host Disease**

Andrea Bacigalupo and Hildegard T. Greinix
4 Extracorporeal Photopheresis in Acute Graft-versus-Host Disease

Acute graft-versus-host disease (GVHD) is a serious complication of allogeneic hematopoietic cell transplantation (HCT) affecting 20% to 80% of patients [1]. It occurs more frequently and is more severe after HCT from an unrelated or HLA-nonidentical stem cell donor or a female donor graft given to a male recipient [2]. Furthermore, conditioning intensity, use of total body irradiation and graft source reportedly have an effect on risk of acute GVHD [3]. The underlying pathophysiology is complex and is thought to consist of several interrelated phases including dysregulated and uncontrolled activation of immune mediators and effector cells [4].

Severe acute GVHD and its treatment have a negative impact on patients' survival and are associated with serious opportunistic infections and severe organ toxicities.

4.1 First-Line Therapy of Acute GVHD

4.1.1 When to Start First-Line Therapy

There is no consensus on whether GVHD grade I should be treated with corticosteroids: in one study looking at transplant-related mortality (TRM) in two centers [5], results were said to be biased by the fact that patients with GVHD grade I were treated in one institution whereas in the other only patients with GVHD grade ≥ II were included. A prospective randomized trial is currently comparing no treatment with corticosteroids at 1 mg/kg/day (unpublished).

4.1.2 What First-Line Therapy to Use

Currently, acute GVHD grade II is treated in all centers with corticosteroids (usually methylprednisolone) at 2 mg/kg/day. This is considered to be the standard first-line systemic therapy for acute GVHD grades II to IV, resulting in complete response (CR) rates of 25% to 54% [6]. There seems to be no advantage of using a higher dose of corticosteroids, as shown in a randomized study comparing 10 mg/kg/day versus 2 mg/kg/day [7]. To date, we have no prospective study comparing corticosteroids at 2 mg/kg/day versus 1 mg/kg/day as first-line therapy. In a retrospective study on patients with mainly acute GVHD grades I to II 1 mg/kg/day achieved similar rates of CR, non-relapse mortality and survival compared to 2 mg/kg/day [8] However, in this retrospective study, more patients receiving 2 mg/kg had GVHD involving the gut, and were therefore "selected" for a higher dose of steroids. Standard therapy remains 2 mg/kg/day, until a lower dose is shown to be equivalent in a prospective randomized trial.

4.1.3 Duration of First-Line Therapy and Response

The initial dose of cortisteroids is intended to be given for 5–10 days, after which time it is usually tapered slowly, when patients respond. Thus, duration of first-line therapy and response are somehow correlated: when a patient responds it is easy to taper corticosteroids; when a patient does not respond or shows progression, corticosteroids are continued and second-line treratment is initiated. Achieving a CR to first-line treatment is of central importance since responses correlate with survival. Patients with no response to initial therapy at day 28 were 2.78 times more likely to experience TRM before 2 years than patients with a response [9].

The Italian cooperative group GITMO has shown in two prospective randomized trials that day +5 can also be an early time point to identify responders. In a first study a significantly higher TRM (49 % versus 27 %, p=0.009) and worse overall survival (35 % versus 53 %, p=0.007) were observed in patients not responding to corticosteroids by day +5 [7]. Response was assessed as the ability of patients to taper steroid dose as per protocol. Thus, tapering of steroids was taken as a surrogate of clinical response, as judged by the attending physician. Although this may seem rather "subjective", a second prospective randomized trial on 211 patients confirmed that patients able to taper steroids on day +5 have a lower TRM of 27 % compared to 49 % for patients unable to undergo steroid taper by day+5 [10]. Thus, long-term outcome of patients with acute GVHD is determined early after start of initial treatment with corticosteroids.

Response to first-line therapy with corticosteroids varies and no consistent predictors of response are currently available. Most data suggest a decreasing likelihood of CR to first-line therapy with increasing grade of acute GVHD and increasing numbers of organs involved. All reports, so far, support inferior survival in those patients who fail to respond to first-line therapy [11].

4.1.4 Combination First-Line Therapy

So far, combining other immunosuppressive agents with corticosteroids has neither improved response rates nor overall survival of patients with acute GVHD and therefore, is not to be considered as standard of care and should be limited to patients participating in well-designed prospective phase II or phase III clinical trials [6]. In one large "pick the winner" study mycophenolate mofetil (MMF) in addition with steroids, showed best outcome, when compared to steroids and etanercept, denileukin diftitox or pentostatin as first-line therapy of acute GVHD [12]. However, in a subsequent prospective study, the winner (MMF+steroids) was compared to steroids alone and the study has been closed prematurely because of lack of any advantage for the MMF+steroid arm (unpublished).

4.2 Predicting GVHD Severity

Knowing in advance whether a patient, presenting with a modest skin rash will develop 2 litres of bloody diarrhea and a bilirubin of 20 mg/dL, would be highly desirable. Unfortunately, extensive studies with single nucleotide polymorphisms (SNPs) of inflammatory cytokines have shown predictive value in some centers but not in others, and we are currently lacking a validated method to predict GVHD and most of all its severity. Validated biomarkers for early detection of high-risk acute GVHD patients with dismal prognosis are highly warranted to allow intensified systemic first-line treatment aiming at improving patients' outcome. Recently, Ferrara and colleagues observed that high regenerating islet-derived 3-alpha (REG3α) concentrations at diagnosis of acute gastrointestinal (GI) GVHD, advanced clinical stage and severe histologic damage independently predicted 1-year nonrelapse mortality (NRM) [13]. The prognostic value of REG3α has to be confirmed in additional patients before being recommended for use in daily clinical routine. Currently, no biomarker panels are available for clinical use that could predict upfront patients who will develop steroid-refractory acute GVHD and thus, have the worst prognosis.

4.3 Second-line Therapy of Corticosteroid-Refractory Acute GVHD

4.3.1 Defining Steroid-Refractory Acute GVHD

There is limited consensus regarding the definition of steroid refractoriness with variations in dose and duration of first-line corticosteroid therapy administered and time allotted to assess treatment response in the HCT community [11]. Pidala and Anasetti [14] proposed the following definition of steroid-refractory acute GVHD: a progression of at least 1 overall grade within 3 days, failure to demonstrate any overall grade improvement over 5 to 7 days, or incomplete response by 14 days of 1 to 2 mg/kg/day of corticosteroid therapy. In the two prospective GITMO studies, steroid refractory GVHD was defined as the inability to taper the dose of steroids by day +5 [7, 10].

4.3.2 Second-line Therapy with Immunosuppressive Agents

To date, no consensus on the optimal choice of agents for secondary therapy of acute GVHD has been reached and treatment choices are based on physician's experience, risk of toxicity and potential exacerbation of pre-existing comorbidity, interactions with other agents as well as ease of use [6].

Recently, Martin and colleagues performed a literature review on 67 prospective and retrospective studies on second-line therapy of acute GVHD published between 1990 and 2011 [6]. The frequency of reported treatments in these reports is shown in Figure 4.1. Investigating immunosuppressive agents targeting T cells (antithymocyte globulin), interleukin-2 receptor (Daclizumab, Basiliximab, Denileukin diftitox), tumour necrosis factor receptor (Etanercept), CD52 (Alemtuzumab), or enacting mTOR inhibition (Sirolimus) in prospective studies CR rates ranged from 8% to 63% as summarized in Table 4.1 [10, 15–30]. Main side-effects reportedly were serious infections, myelosuppression, Epstein-Barr virus lymphoproliferative disease and transplant-associated microangiopathy impacting negatively overall survival rates. Thus, substantial improvements in second-line treatment of acute GVHD are highly warranted to improve patients' long-term prognosis.

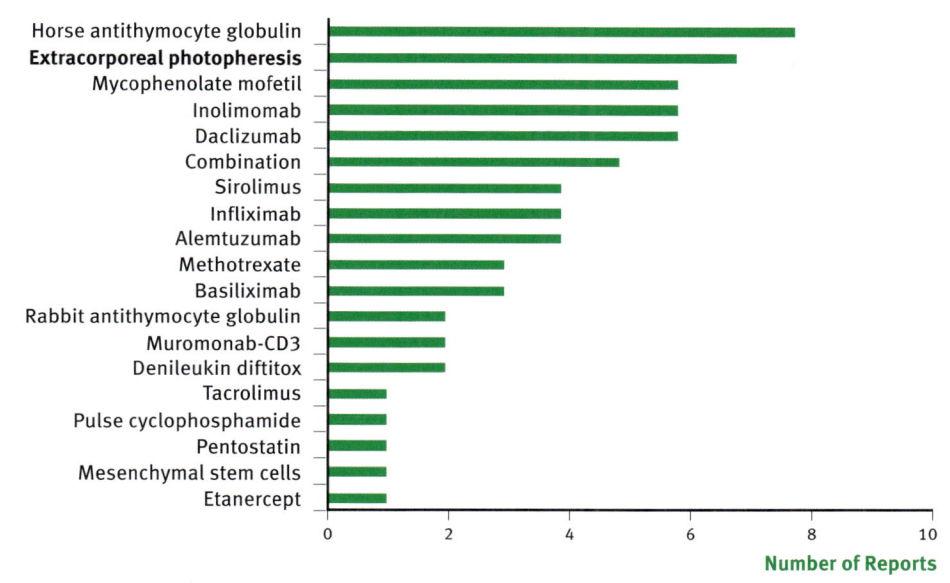

Fig. 4.1. **Treatments Evaluated in Prospective and Retrospective Studies on Secondary Therapy of Acute GVHD and Published Between 1990 and 2011.**
Individual second-line therapies are shown in order of frequency reported. (modified according to Martin et al, Reference 6).

4.3.3 ECP in Corticosteroid-Refractory Acute GVHD

During the last years, more and more HCT centers have administered ECP to patients with corticosteroid-refractory acute GVHD (Figure 4.2). Summarizing 24 publications including 297 patients CR and partial resolution (PR) of cutaneous, hepatic and gastrointestinal manifestations reportedly was achieved in 75% (range, 50% to 100%), 47% (range, 0% to 100%) and 58% (range, 0% to 100%) of patients, respectively. Median overall survival of patients was 60% (range, 37.5% to 85%).

Results of larger prospective studies on the use of ECP in steroid-refractory acute GVHD patients are shown in Table 4.2. After a pilot study the Medical University of Vienna performed a prospective phase II study intensifying the ECP schedule to 2 to 3 treatments per week on a weekly basis until resolution of steroid-refractory acute

Agent	Author	No of Patients	CR No (%)	Survival
ATG	Van Lint 06 [7]	27	9/27 (33)	
	MacMillan 07 [15]	47	15/47 (32)	45% at 18 mo
MMF	Kim 04 [16]	13	2/13 (15)	2-yr 33%
	Furlong 09 [17]	19	6/19 (31)	1-yr 16%
Daclizumab	Anasetti 94 [18]	20	4/20 (20)	med. OS 76 d
	Przepiorka 00 [19]	43	29–47%	120 d OS 29–53%
	Willenbacher 01 [20]	12	1/12 (8)	17% alive at 1 yr
	Bordigoni 06 [21]	62	42/62 (68)	
Sirolimus	Benito 01 [22]	21	5/21 (24)	33% after 1–2 yrs
Alemtuzumab	Gomez-Almaguer 08 [23]	18	6/18 (33)	
	Martinez 09 [24]	10	2/10 (20)	all died after 4–88 d
Basiliximab	Massenkeil 02 [25]	17	9/17 (53)	
	Schmidt-Hieber 05 [26]	23	4/23 (17.5)	
Denileukin diftitox	Ho 04 [27]	32	10/30 (33)	33% alive at 7 mo
	Shaughnessy 05 [28]	22	9/22 (41)	23% at med 496 d
Pentostatin	Bolanos-Meade [29]	23	14/22 (63)	26% at 1 yr
Daclizumab+Etanercept	Wolff 05 [30]	21	8/21 (38)	19% alive med 586 d

Abbreviations: no=number, CR=complete resolution, ATG=antithymocyte globulin, MMF=mycophenolate mofetil, mo=months, yr=year, med=median, OS=overall survival, d=day.

Table 4.1. Results of Second-Line Treatment of Acute GVHD Using Immunosuppressive Agents in Prospective Studies.

GVHD [34, 35, 42]. All patients had received corticosteroids at ≥2 mg/kg body weight (b.w.) for a median of 17 (range, 4 to 49) days prior to initiation of ECP in addition to immunosuppression with cyclosporine A. In the phase II study ECP was initiated significantly earlier than in the pilot study after a median of 15 (range, 4 to 43) compared to a median of 21 (range, 9 to 49) days on corticosteroid medication (p=0.03). Figure 4.3 shows the response to ECP according to grade of steroid-refractory acute GVHD. Intensified ECP in the phase II study resulted in increased CR rates in patients with GI involvement (73% versus 25%) and grade IV acute GVHD (60% versus 12%), respectively. In patients responding to ECP treatment duration was short with best responses achieved after a median of 4 (range, 1 to 13) cycles of ECP equalling a median of 1.3 (range, 0.5 to 6) months of treatment. Corticosteroids could be discontinued after a median of 55 (range, 17 to 284) days.

The cumulative incidence of TRM at 4 years was overall 36% (95% confidence interval, CI 10–31%) and significantly lower for patients achieving a CR to ECP (14%

versus 73%). A shorter interval between day 0 of HCT and start of ECP, a corticosteroid dose below 1 mg/kg b.w. at 4 weeks and below 0.5 mg/kg b.w. at 8 weeks after initiation of ECP were significantly associated with lower TRM whereas a higher grade of GVHD during first-line treatment and at start of ECP, more organs involved and higher corticosteroid dose at initiation of ECP and failure to achieve a CR 3 months after initiation of ECP were significantly associated with higher TRM.

Overall survival at 4 years was significantly better in patients completely responding to ECP compared to those not achieving a CR (59% versus 11%, p<0.0001). A higher grade of acute GVHD during first-line treatment and at initiation of ECP, a higher corticosteroid dose and more organs affected by GVHD at start of ECP, and failure to achieve a CR to ECP at 3 months were significantly associated with worse survival.

Meantime more patients with corticosteroid-refractory acute GVHD received ECP as second-line treatment at the Medical University of Vienna confirming initially achieved high response rates and favourable overall survival of ECP-responders after a median of 6 (range, 0.5 to 15) years of follow-up. Figures 4.4a and 4.4b show results in 96 patients with corticosteroid-refractory acute GVHD given ECP as second-line therapy. Of note, no increase in relapse rates was observed indicating no negative impact of ECP on the graft-versus-leukemia effect. ECP was tolerated excellently with few side-effects consisting mainly of reversible drops of peripheral blood cell counts in the early phase after HCT [41].

Perotti and colleagues recently reported an overall response rate of 68% using ECP in 50 patients with steroid-refractory acute GVHD including 35% CR and confirmed the corticosteroid-sparing effect of ECP [41]. Response rates were similar for

Author	No of Patients	CR Skin No (%)	CR Liver No (%)	CR Gut No (%)	OS %
Salvaneschi 01 [31]	9	6/9 (67)	1/3 (33)	3/5 (60)	67
Dall'Amico 02 [32]	14	10/14 (71)	4/7 (57)	6/10 (60)	57
Messina 03 [33]	33	25/33 (76)	9/15 (60)	15/20 (75)	69 at 5 yrs
Greinix 06 [34, 35]	59	47/57 (82)	14/23 (61)	9/15 (60)	47 at 5 yrs
Garban 06 [36]	12	8/12 (67)	0/2 (0)	2/5 (40)	42
Kanold 07 [37]	12	9/10 (90)	5/9 (55.5)	5/6 (83)	75 at 8.5 mo
Calore 08 [38]	15	12/13 (92)		14/14 (100)	85 at 5 yrs
Perfetti 08 [39]	23	15/23 (65)	3/11 (27)	8/20 (40)	48 at 37 mo
Gonzalez-Vicent 08 [40]	8	8/8 (100)	2/2 (100)	4/7 (57)	37.5
Perotti 10 [41]	50	39/47 (83)*	16/24 (67)*	8/11 (73)*	64 at 1 yr

Abbreviations: No=number, CR=complete resolution, OS=overall survival, yrs=years, mo=months.
* results were provided as complete and partial resolution.

Table 4.2. Results of Second-Line Treatment of Acute GVHD Using Extracorporeal Photopheresis.

90 — 4 Extracorporeal Photopheresis in Acute Graft-versus-Host Disease

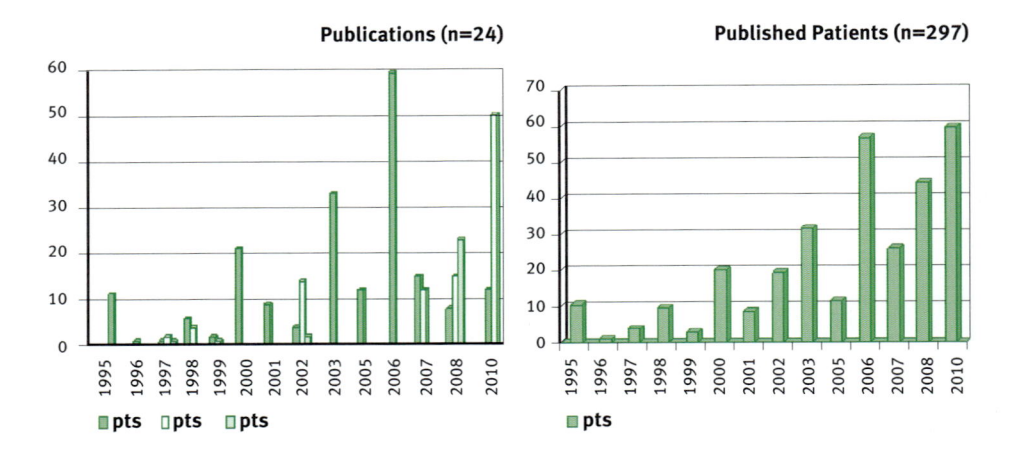

Fig. 4.2. Number of Publications on the Use of Extracorporeal Photopheresis in Patients With Steroid-refractory Acute GVHD According to Years of Publication (left) and Number of Patients Reported (right).

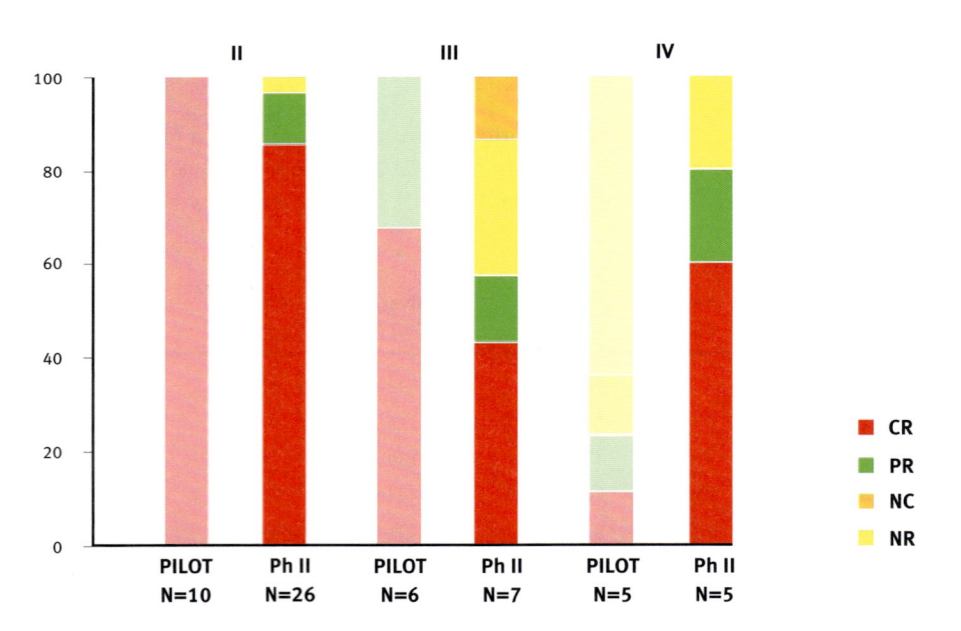

Fig. 4.3. Response of Patients With Steroid-Refractory Acute GVHD to Extracorporeal Photopheresis According to Grade of Graft-versus-Host Disease at Initiation of ECP.
The left columns show the responses in the pilot study (PILOT) and the right columns the responses of patients in the phase II study (Ph II) according to grade at initiation of ECP. CR = complete resolution of GVHD defined as resolution of all organ manifestations; PR = partial resolution of GVHD defined as greater than 50 % response; NC = no change of GVHD defined as stable organ involvement despite tapering of corticosteroids by at least 50 %; NR = no response of GVHD defined as progressive worsening of GVHD and the inability to taper corticosteroids.

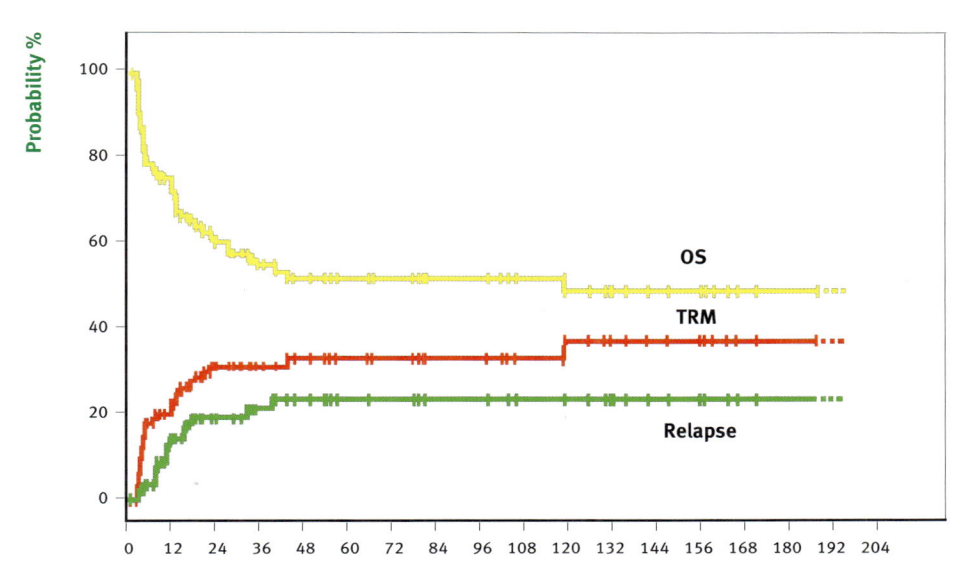

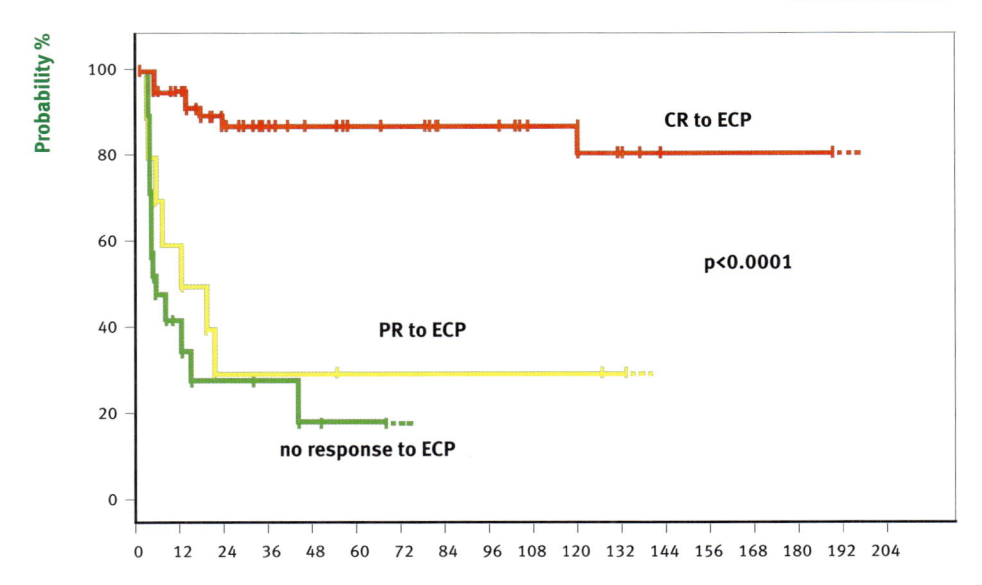

Fig. 4.4. Results of ECP in Corticosteroid-Refractory Acute GVHD.
(a) Kaplan-Meier probability of overall survival of 96 patients with corticosteroid-refractory acute graft-versus-host disease given extracorporeal photopheresis as second-line therapy. OS = overall survival, TRM = transplant-related mortality; (b) Kaplan-Meier probability of overall survival of 96 patients with corticosteroid-refractory acute GVHD according to response to ECP. Overall survival is shown for patients with complete resolution of acute GVHD (CR to ECP), partial resolution of acute GVHD (PR to ECP) and no response to ECP (no response to ECP), respectively.

the different organ systems (skin 83 %, liver 67 %, GI 73%). Furthermore, ECP-responders had a significantly improved survival of 62% compared to 6% in patients not responding to ECP. Ability to decrease the corticosteroid dose 30 days after start of ECP was associated with significantly decreased mortality confirming the importance of steroid-sparing in acute GVHD.

In a retrospective analysis on 23 patients with steroid-refractory acute GVHD given ECP for a median of 7 (range, 1 to 33) months Perfetti and colleagues observed a CR in 12 patients (52%) and reduction of the average grade of GVHD from 2.8 on the first day of ECP to 1.4 on day 90 from ECP [39]. Complete responses of skin, liver and gut manifestations were obtained in 66 %, 27 % and 40 %. Patients treated within 35 days from onset of acute GVHD had higher response rates (83% versus 47%, p=0.1). Of note, the average dose of corticosteroids was significantly reduced from 2.17 mg/kg/day at start of ECP to 0.2 mg/kg/day (p=0.004) on day 90 from ECP. A trend for improved survival at 4 years was observed in patients with acute GVHD grades III to IV treated with ECP as compared to matched controls (38 % versus 16 %, p=0.08).

Several studies of ECP have been conducted in pediatric patients with acute GVHD and have shown similar results to those obtained in adults. Messina and colleagues performed a multicentre, retrospective study on 33 pediatric patients with steroid-refractory acute GVHD observing 54 % CR and 21% partial resolution (PR) [33]. CR rates for skin, GI and liver involvement were 76%, 75%, and 60%, respectively. The 5-year OS rate was significantly better for ECP-responders (69%) than non-responders (12%). As a result of ECP, immunosuppressive therapy could be discontinued in 8 patients (42%) and reduced in seven (36%), respectively. The median Karnofsky performance score improved significantly from 60 % before ECP to 100 % (range, 80–100 %) after completing ECP therapy.

Supporting data come from subsequent smaller studies using the twice-weekly ECP treatment regimen [31, 37, 38, 40]. Calore and colleagues performed a comparison of ECP and steroid therapy in pediatric patients revealing CR rates by day 100 of 73 % and 56 %, respectively [38]. CR to ECP therapy was observed in 92% of patients with skin manifestations, 71% with GI and 100 % with liver disease. TRM at day 100 of treatment was 6% for steroid therapy, but no patients had died in the ECP cohort, and 2-year OS rates were numerically, but not significantly, higher for ECP (85%) than for steroid therapy (57 %) [38].

Several authors have pointed out that use of ECP in children presents specific challenges, such as patients' low body weight, vascular access, extracorporeal volume, metabolic and hematological problems, and psychological tolerance [33, 37, 43]. Nevertheless, Messina and colleagues were able to treat patients with a body weight as low as 10 kg without significant side-effects [33]. In contrast to many groups that have used an "offline", two-stage technique for mononuclear cell collection and irradiation [37, 40, 41], Schneiderman and colleagues reported the use of a sterile, closed-loop procedure, in which patients received fluid boluses of normal saline or 5% albumin to boost blood volume before, and if needed during, ECP procedures

[43]. The process was well tolerated by patients, and therefore, could extend the use of continuous-flow ECP to these patients with low body weight.

In 2007, Kanold and colleagues published clinical practice guidelines recommending ECP in pediatric patients with acute GVHD not responding to corticosteroids, defined as absence of clinical improvement after 1 week of steroid therapy (up to 2–5 mg/kg/day) [37]. In addition, ECP was considered to be a reasonable choice as first-line therapy for pediatric patients with grade IV acute GVHD in association with conventional immunosuppressive therapy. Furthermore, recommendations were provided on vascular access and ECP technique in children, and the recommended schedule was to start with ECP at three times a week until maximal response is achieved.

Recently, Martin and colleagues published recommendations of the American Society of Blood and Marrow Transplantation (ASBMT) for treatment of acute GVHD based on a comprehensive and critical review of published reports [6]. Data on 6-month survival and CR and PR of acute GVHD in 67 reports summarizing results of second-line treatment did not support the choice of any specific agent for second-line therapy. Amongst the 5 studies with outliers in 6-month survival, Messina and colleagues' clinical trial on ECP was cited with an outlier high survival [33]. Since only children were treated, with a median age of 9.6 years, Martin and colleagues concluded that these outliers could reflect age differences between patient cohorts since the benchmark study using horse ATG included a patient cohort with a median age of 27 years (6). The ASBMT described ECP's limited toxicity, including blood loss from the extracorporeal circuit, hypocalcemia due to anticoagulant, mild cytopenia and catheter-associated bacteremia but no increased risk for infections beyond standard therapy, and specifically mentioned no concerns for increased viral reactivations during ECP treatment. A typical ECP schedule of 3 times per week during the first week followed by 2 per week on a weekly basis was described. According to the ASBMT recommendations, choice of second-line regimen should be guided by considerations of potential toxicity, interactions with other agents, familiarity of physician with the agent, prior experience of physician with the agent, convenience and costs.

4.4 Conclusions on the Use of ECP in Acute GVHD

In patients with corticosteroid-refractory acute GVHD decisions to initiate ECP should be made soon e. g. after 3 days with progressive manifestations of GVHD, after 1 week with persistent grade III GVHD and after 2 weeks with persistent grade II GVHD as recently recommended by Martin and colleagues [6]. Timely initiation of ECP reportedly was associated with improvement of response rates especially in patients with steroid-refractory acute GVHD of the gut and grade IV manifestations [34, 35, 39].

In patients responding to ECP corticosteroid medication can be tapered rapidly without flare-ups of acute GVHD activity. Thus, a corticosteroid-sparing effect of ECP has frequently been reported in patients with acute GVHD [31, 33, 34, 36, 39, 42].

Response to ECP corresponded favourably with improved survival rates [33, 34, 38, 39, 41, 42]. ECP has an excellent safety profile, does not cause generalized immunosuppression [44] and does not negatively impact on the graft-versus-leukemia effect since no increase in relapse rates has been reported after use of ECP in steroid-refractory acute GVHD patients [34, 42]. Therefore, use of ECP as second-line therapy of acute GVHD can be recommended as recently published by the American Society of Blood and Marrow Transplantation [6].

In view of the poor prognosis of patients with steroid-refractory acute GVHD and the excellent safety profile of ECP, it is tempting to assume that ECP in first-line therapy will be able to improve patients' outcome. However, data on prospective clinical trials are currently lacking and thus, studies investigating ECP in first-line therapy are highly warranted.

References

[1] Greinix HT. Graft-versus-host disease. Uni-Med Science 2008.
[2] Flowers MED, Inamoto Y, Carpenter PA, et al. Comparative analysis of risk factors for acute graft-versus-host disease and for chronic graft-versus-host disease according to National Institute of Health consensus criteria. Blood 2011;117:3214–9.
[3] Jagasia M, Arora M, Flowers MED et al. Risk factors for acute GVHD and survival after hematopoietic cell transplantation. Blood 2012;119:296–307.
[4] Ferrara JL, Levine JE, Reddy P, Holler E. Graft-versus-host disease. Lancet 2009;373:1550–61.
[5] Remberger M, Storer B, Ringdén O, Anasetti C. Association between pretransplant thymoglobulin and reduced non-relapse mortality rate after marrow transplantation from unrelated donors. Bone Marrow Transplant 2002;29:391–7.
[6] Martin PJ, Rizzo JD, Wingard JR, et al. First and second-line systemic treatment of acute graft-versus-host disease: Recommendations of the American Society of Blood and Marrow Transplantation. Biol Blood Marrow Transplant 2012; doi:10.1016/j.bbmt.2012.04.005
[7] Van Lint MT, Uderzo C, Locasciulli A, et al. Early treatment of graft-versus-host disease with high- or low-dose 6-methylprednisolone: a multicenter randomized trial from the Italian Group for Bone Marrow Transplantation. Blood 1998;92:2288–93.
[8] Mielcarek M, Storer BE, Boeckh M, et al. Initial therapy of acute graft-versus-host disease with low-dose prednisone does not compromise patient outcomes. Blood 2009;113:2888–94.
[9] MacMillan M, DeFor TE, Weisdorf DJ. The best endpoint for acute GVHD treatment trials. Blood 2010;115:5412–7.
[10] Van Lint MT, Milone G, Leotta S, et al. Treatment of acute graft-versus-host disease with prednisolone: significant survival advantage for day +5 responders and no advantage for nonresponders receiving anti-thymocyte globulin. Blood 2006;107:4177–81.
[11] Deeg HJ. How I treat refractory acute GVHD. Blood 2007;109:4119–26.
[12] Alousi AM, Weisdorf DJ, Logan BR, et al. Etanercept, mycophenolate, denileukin, or pentostatin plus corticosteroids for acute graft-versus-host disease: a randomized phase 2 trial from the Blood and Marrow Transplant Clinical Trials Network. Blood 2009;114:511–7.
[13] Ferrara JLM, Harris AC, Greenson JK, et al. Regenerating islet-derived 3-alpha is a biomarker of gastrointestinal graft-versus-host disease. Blood 2011;118:6702–8.
[14] Pidala J, Anasetti C. Glucocorticoid-refractory acute graft-versus-host disease. Biol Blood Marrow Transplant 2010;16:1504–18.

[15] MacMillan mL, Couriel D, Weisdorf DJ, et al. A phase 2/3 multicenter randomized clinical trial of ABX-CBL versus ATG as secondary therapy for steroid-resistant acute graft-versus-host disease. Blood 2007;109:2657–62.
[16] Kim JG, Sohn SK, Kim DH, et al. Different efficacy of mycophenolate mofetil as salvage treatment for acute and chronic GVHD after allogeneic stem cell transplant. Eur J Haematol 2004;73:56–61.
[17] Furlong T, Martin P, Flowers MED, et al. Therapy with mycophenolate mofetil for refractory acute and chronic graft-versus-host disease. Bone Marrow Transplant 2009;44:739–48.
[18] Anasetti C, Hansen JA, Waldmann TA, et al. Treatment of acute graft-versus-host disease with humanized anti-Tac: an antibody that binds to the interleukin-2 receptor. Blood 1994;84:1320–7.
[19] Przepiorka D, Kernan NA, Ippoliti C, et al. Daclizumab, a humanized anti-interleukin-2 receptor alpha chain antibody, for treatment of acute graft-versus-host disease. Blood 2000;95:83–9.
[20] Willenbacher W, Basara N, Blau IW, Fauser AA, Kiehl MG. Treatment of steroid refractory acute and chronic graft-versus-host disease with daclizumab. Br J Haematol 2001;112:820–3.
[21] Bordigoni P, Dimicoli S, Clement L, et al. Daclizumab, an efficient treatment for steroid-refractory acute graft-versus-host disease. Br J Haematol 2006;135:382–5.
[22] Benito AI, Furlong T, Martin PJ, et al. Sirolimus (rapamycin) for the treatment of steroid-refractory acute graft-versus-host disease. Transplantation 2001;72:1924–9.
[23] Gomez-Almaguer D, Ruiz-Arguelles GJ, Carmen Tarin-Arzaga L, et al. Alemtuzumab for the treatment of steroid-refractory acute graft-versus-host disease. Biol Blood Marrow Transplant 2008;14:10–5.
[24] Martinez C, Solano C, Ferra C, Sampol A, Valcarcel D, Perez-Simon JA. Alemtuzumab as treatment of steroid-refractory acute graft-versus-host disease: results of a phase II study. Biol Blood Marrow Transplant 2009;15:639–42.
[25] Massenkeil G, Rackwitz S, Genvresse I, Rosen O, Dorken B, Arnold R. Basiliximab is well tolerated and effective in the treatment of steroid-refractory acute graft-versus-host disease after allogeneic stem cell transplantation. Bone Marrow Transplant 2002;30:899–903.
[26] Schmidt-Hieber M, Fietz T, Knauf W, et al. Efficacy of the interleukin-2 receptor antagonist basiliximab in steroid-refractory acute graft-versus-host disease. Br J Haematol 2005;130:568–74.
[27] Ho VT, Zahrieh D, Hochberg E, et al. Safety and efficacy of denileukin diftitox in patients with steroid-refractory acute graft-versus-host disease after allogeneic hematopoietic stem cell transplantation. Blood 2004;104:1224–6.
[28] Shaughnessy PJ, Bachier C, Grimley M, et al. Denileukin diftitox for the treatment of steroid-resistant acute graft-versus-host disease. Biol Blood Marrow Transplant 2005;11:188–93.
[29] Bolanos-Meade J, Jacobsohn DA, Margolis J, et al. Pentostatin in steroid-refractory acute graft-versus-host disease. J Clin Oncol 2005;23:2661–8.
[30] Wolff D, Roessler V, Steiner B, et al. Treatment of steroid-resistant acute graft-versus-host disease with daclizumab and etanercept. Bone Marrow Transplant 2005;35:1003–10.
[31] Salvaneschi L, Perotti C, Zecca M, et al. Extracorporeal photochemotherapy for treatment of acute and chronic GVHD in childhood. Transfusion 2001;41:1299–1305.
[32] Dall'Amico R, Messina C. Extracorporeal photochemotherapy for the treatment of graft-versus-host disease. Ther Apher 2002;6:296–304.
[33] Messina C, Locatelli F, Lanino E, et al. Extracorporeal photochemotherapy for paediatric patients with graft-versus-host disease after haematopoietic stem cell transplantation. Br J Haematol 2003;22:118–27.
[34] Greinix HT, Knobler RM, Worel N, et al. The effect of intensified extracorporeal photochemotherapy on long-term survival in patients with severe acute graft-versus-host disease. Haematologica 2006;91:405–8.
[35] Greinix HT, Worel N, Knobler R. Role of extracorporeal photopheresis (ECP) in treatment of steroid-refractory acute graft-versus-host disease. Biol Blood Marrow Transplant 2010;16:1747–8.

[36] Garban F, Drillat P, Makowski C, et al. Extracorporeal photochemotherapy for the treatment of graft-versus-host disease: hematologic consequences of short-term, intensive courses. Haematologica 2005;90:1096–1101.

[37] Kanold J, Merlin E, Halle P, et al. Photopheresis in pediatric graft-versus-host disease after allogeneic marrow transplantation: clinical practice guidelines based on field experience and review of the literature. Transfusion 2007;47:2276–89.

[38] Calore E, Calo A, Tridello G, et al. Extracorporeal photochemotherapy may improve outcome in children with acute GVHD. Bone Marrow Transplant 2008;42:421–5.

[39] Perfetti P, Carlier P, Strada P, et al. Extracorporeal photopheresis for the treatment of steroid refractory acute GVHD. Bone Marrow Transplant 2008;42:609–17.

[40] Gonzalez-Vicent M, Ramirez M, Perez A, Lassaletta A, Sevilla J, Angel Diaz M. Extracorporeal photochemotherapy for steroid-refractory graft-versus-host disease in low-weight pediatric patients. Immunomodulatory effects and clinical outcome. Haematologica 2008;93:1278–80.

[41] Perotti C, Del Fante C, Tinelli C, et al. Extracorporeal photochemotherapy in graft-versus-host disease: a longitudinal study on factors influencing the response and survival in pediatric patients. Transfusion 2010;50:1359–69.

[42] Greinix HT, Volc-Platzer B, Kalhs P, et al. Extracorporeal photochemotherapy in the treatment of severe steroid-refractory acute graft-versus-host disease: a pilot study. Blood 2000;96:2426–31.

[43] Schneiderman J, Jacobsohn DA, Collins J, Thormann K, Kletzel M. The use of fluid boluses to safely perform extracorporeal photopheresis (ECP) in low-weight children: a novel procedure. J Clin Apher 2010;25:63-9.

[44] Suchin KR, Cassin M, Washko R, et al. Extracorporeal photochemotherapy does not suppress T- or B-cell responses to novel or recall antigens. J Am Acad Dermatol 1999;41:980–6.

Section 5: Extracorporeal Photopheresis in Chronic Graft-versus-Host Disease

5 Extracorporeal Photopheresis in Chronic Graft-versus-Host Disease

Yoshihiro Inamoto and Mary E.D. Flowers

5.1 Results of ECP in Cutaneous Manifestations of Chronic GVHD

5.1.1 Cutaneous Manifestations of Chronic GVHD

Skin is the most commonly involved organ by chronic GVHD, with more than 60% of the patients having cutaneous manifestations (Figure 5.1) [1, 2]. According to the 2005 National Institutes of Health Consensus Criteria [3], diagnostic manifestations for chronic GVHD include poikiloderma, lichen planus-like eruption and sclerotic features. Depigmentation represents a distinctive feature of chronic GVHD (not present in acute GVHD) but it is insufficient for the initial diagnosis of chronic GVHD without histological documentation or other diagnostic manifestations. Other cutaneous features of chronic GVHD include sweat gland impairment, ichthyosis, keratosis pilaris, hypopigmentation and hyperpigmentation. Erythema, maculopapular rash and pruritus are common manifestations encountered in both acute and chronic GVHD [3].

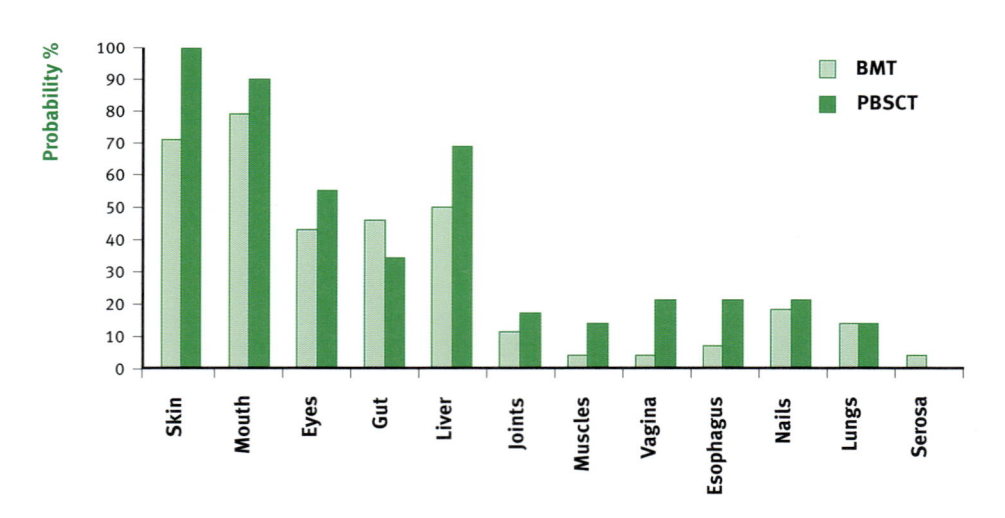

Fig. 5.1. Sites Affected by Chronic GVHD.
Columns show the proportions of patients with organs affected by chronic GVHD at any time. Adapted from Flowers, MED et al. in Blood 2002;100:415–9, Reference 1. BMT is bone marrow transplantation, PBSCT is peripheral blood stem cell transplantation.

5.1.2 Results of Phase II Studies with Non-ECP Therapies for Cutaneous Chronic GVHD

A variety of second-line agents including thalidomide, clofazimine, mycofenolate mofetil, hydroxychloroquine, sirolimus, methotrexate, rituximab, imatinib and pentostatin have been used to treat patients with cutaneous chronic GVHD refractory or resistant to initial corticosteroid treatment [4–16]. Response rates of cutaneous chronic GVHD after non-ECP therapies have ranged from 25% to 100%, with response rates for sclerotic chronic GVHD features ranging from 0% to 73% (Table 5.1). Such results, however, need to be taken with caution considering that eligibility criteria, time of assessment, measures used to grade skin severity and response criteria were not standardized, precluding valid comparison of response rates among reported studies [17].

Agent	Author	Year	Number of patients	Skin response %	Sclerosis response %
Thalidomide	Parker et al. [4]	1995	80	25	
	Browne et al. [5]	2000	37	38	
Clofazimine	Lee et al. [6]	1997	22	56	50
Mycofenolate mofetil	Busca et al. [7]	2000	15	33	14
	Busca et al. [8]	2003	21	53	
Hydroxychloroquine	Gilman et al. [9]	2000	40	38	0
Sirolimus	Couriel et al. [10]	2005	35	68	73
	Johnston et al. [11]	2005	19	67	50
Methotrexate	Huang et al. [12]	2005	21	100	
Rituximab	Cutler et al. [13]	2006	21	60	Yes*
	Kim et al. [14]	2010	37	77	
Imatinib	Olivieri et al. [15]	2009	19	89	Yes*
Pentostatin	Jacobsohn et al. [16]	2009	51	54	59

*Response was reported for sclerotic manifestations.
Table 5.1. Complete and Partial Response Rates of Cutaneous Chronic GVHD in Prospective Phase II Studies of Immunosuppressive Agents.

5.1.3 Results of Phase II Studies with ECP Treatment for Cutaneous Chronic GVHD

Results of phase II studies of ECP treatment for steroid-refractory or steroid-dependent chronic GVHD reported in the past 15 years are summarized in Table 5.2 [18–26]. The number of patients in these studies ranged from 11 to 48. Skin was reported to be involved in 80% to 100% of the patients enrolled into these studies. Physician-assessed rates of skin responses ranged from 40% to 100%, with the time of assessment prespecified only in 3 studies [19, 22, 25] and responses still somewhat subjective albeit not much different than those reported for non-ECP studies in similar setting. The change of skin score across time was evaluated in 4 studies [19, 21, 22, 25], but instruments used to grade severity of cutaneous GVHD were not uniform. For these reasons, comparison of response rates are difficult among the reports.

Author	Year	Number of patients	Skin response %	Sclerosis response %
Greinix et al. [18]	1998	15	100	100
Child et al. [19]	1999	11	60 at week 14 89 at week 30	
Salvaneschi et al. [20]	2001	14	83	
Messina et al. [21]	2003	44	73	
Seaton et al. [22]	2003	28	38 at week 12 48 at week 24	
Foss et al. [23]	2005	25	60	
*Couriel et al. [24]	2006	71	59	67
Flowers et al. [25]	2008	48	40 at week 12	Yes†
Perotti et al. [26]	2010	23	96	

†The response rate was not reported.
*Retrospective study.

Table 5.2. Complete and Partial Response Rates in Cutaneous Chronic GVHD in Prospective Phase II Studies of Extracorporeal Photopheresis.

5.1.4 Results of Two Phase II Randomized, Single-Blind, Multicenter Studies of ECP for Treatment of Cutaneous Chronic GVHD

To date, only one prospective randomized study has been published using ECP therapy for patients with steroid-refractory, dependent or intolerant chronic GVHD [25]. This report was a phase II randomized, single-blind, multicenter clinical trial of ECP combined with conventional therapy versus conventional therapy alone for treatment of steroid-refractory/dependent chronic GVHD with cutaneous involvement. This is the first study to use the Vienna Total Skin Score (TSS), a 50-point scale developed to grade skin involvement in chronic GVHD [27]. The TSS grades 10 separate regions of the body according to 4 skin features raging from normal (score 0) to hidebound skin/unmovable sclerosis (score 4) (Figure 5.2). The TSS was obtained at baseline and subsequently at pre-specified time points during the study by a blinded observer who was unaware of the treatment arm the patient was randomized to. Crossover to the ECP treatment arm was allowed if response was not observed by 3 months after study enrollment or, earlier, if progression of chronic GVHD as defined by pre-specified study criteria occurred.

Grades:

0 = Normal
1 = Hypopigmentation, hyperpigmentation, erythematous rash or alopecia
2 = Lichenoid plaque, thickening, able to move
3 = Thickened, limited motion, able to pinch
4 = Hidebound, unable to move, unable to pinch

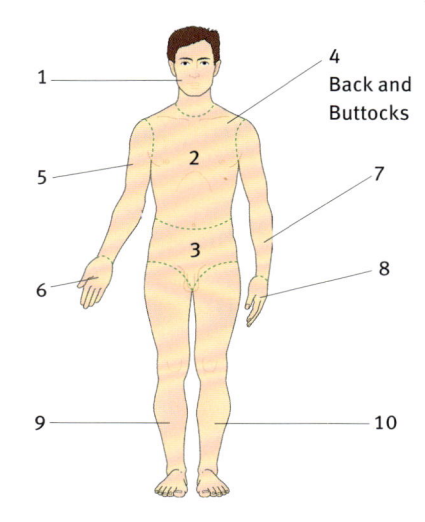

Fig. 5.2. Total Skin Score (TSS) according to Vienna GVHD Grading System [27].
Numbers indicated the 10 body surface areas.

5.1.4.1 Eligibility

Patients with histologically confirmed chronic GVHD with cutaneous manifestations that were steroid-refractory, steroid-dependent or steroid-intolerant were eligible. Steroid refractoriness was defined as lack of response or disease progression after administration of at least 1 mg/kg of methylprednisolone equivalent. Steroid dependence was defined as requiring more than 10 mg methylprednisolone equivalent to control skin manifestations. Steroid intolerance was defined as avascular necrosis, severe myopathy, uncontrolled diabetes, or systemic viral or fungal infections.

5.1.4.2 Treatment

Patients were randomized in a 1:1 ratio to receive conventional treatment alone (control arm), or to receive 12 weeks of ECP treatment in addition to conventional treatment (ECP arm). Patients in the control arm were treated with corticosteroid and calcineurin inhibitor with or without mycofenolate mofetil (conventional treatment). Discontinuation of these agents was not permitted during the course of the study except for safety reasons. Patients in the ECP arm received conventional treatment plus

ECP 3 times during week 1, and twice weekly on consecutive days during weeks 2 through 12. Responding patients in the ECP arm could continue ECP treatment twice monthly until week 24.

5.1.4.3 Crossover
Patients in the control arm were permitted to crossover to the ECP arm (1) before week 12 if they had progressive skin disease defined as greater than 25% worsening in the TSS from baseline, or (2) after week 12 if they had an inadequate skin response defined as less than 15% improvement in the TSS from baseline or a less than 25% reduction in corticosteroid dose from baseline.

5.1.4.4 Primary Endpoint
The percentage of change in the TSS after 12 weeks of treatment compared with the baseline by the blinded assessor was the primary endpoint of this prospective phase II study.

5.1.4.5 Results
A total of 100 patients were randomized into the study from 23 transplant centers in North and South America, Europe and Australia. Characteristics of patients and chronic GVHD between the arms were well-balanced. The improvement in the TSS from baseline until week 12 appeared greater in the ECP arm (−14.5%) than the control arm (−8.5%), but did not differ significantly between the arms ($P = 0.48$). Analyses of secondary endpoints showed that by week 12, more patients in the ECP arm had both a 50% or greater reduction in daily steroid dose and a 25% or greater improvement in the TSS than those in the control arm (8.3% vs 0%, $P=0.04$). At week 12, 40% of the patients in the ECP arm had a skin response as assessed by the unblinded investigator, compared with 10% of the patients in the control arm ($P=0.002$). Improvement rates in extra-cutaneous manifestations at week 12 were 53% for the mouth, 21% for the liver, 11% for the lung, 30% for the eyes, 22% for the joints and 50% for the gastrointestinal tract. At week 12, the median improvement in Targeted Symptoms Assessment quality of life self-evaluation from baseline was 19% in the ECP arm and 2.5% in the control arm ($P=0.01$). During the entire 24 weeks of ECP treatment, improvement in the TSS continued by time (Figure 5.3a). Skin sclerosis also responded to ECP treatment.

5.1.4.6 Results of Crossover Study
Twenty-nine patients in the control arm who had worsening before week 12 or an inadequate response of cutaneous GVHD after week 12 were enrolled in the crossover study [28]. Progressive improvement in skin manifestations of chronic GVHD was observed after a 24-week course of ECP treatment (Figure 5.3b).

5.1 Results of ECP in Cutaneous Manifestations of Chronic GVHD — 103

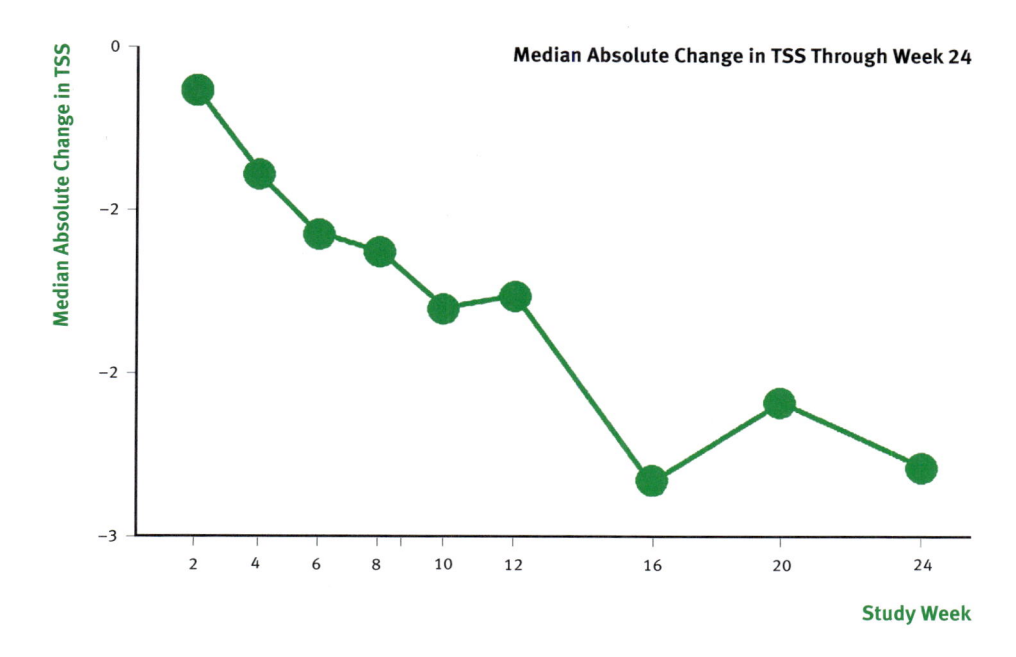

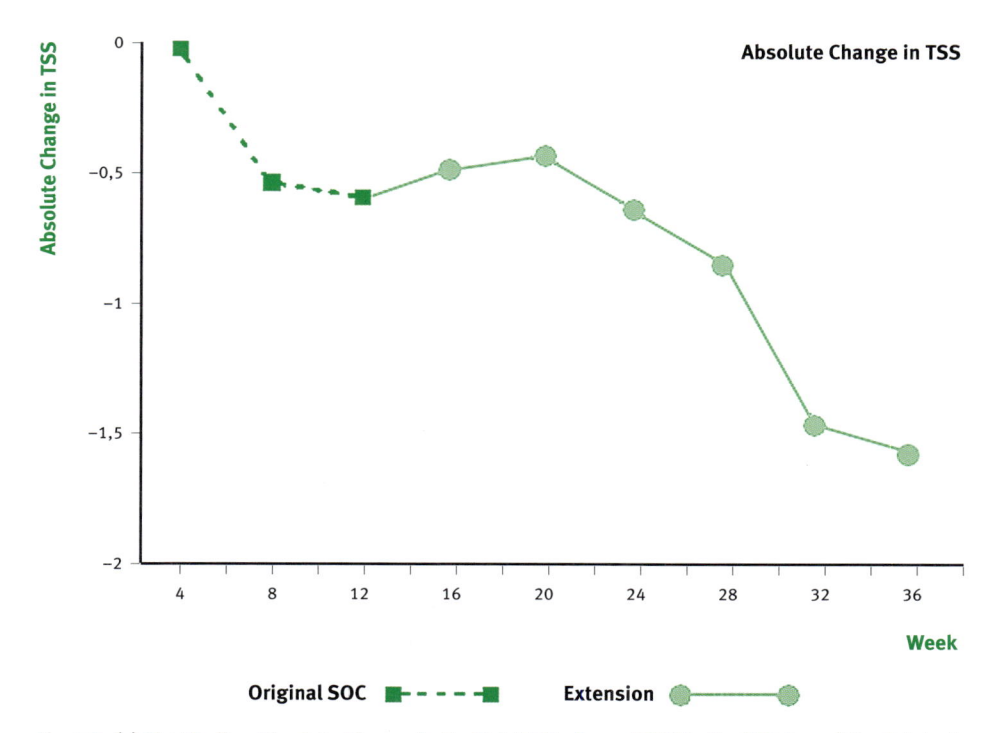

Fig. 5.3. (a) The Median Absolute Change in the Total Skin Score (TSS) in the ECP Arm of the Original Study and (b) in the Crossover Study.

5.1.4.7 Interpretation and Conclusions

While no statistically significant improvement in the TSS was observed at 12 weeks after ECP in combination with conventional treatment, as compared with conventional treatment alone, continued improvement in TSS was observed by 24 weeks, indicating that 12 weeks may be too early to evaluate efficacy of ECP treatment in cutaneous chronic GVHD. The results of the ECP crossover study confirmed that response in cutaneous chronic GVHD required longer duration of ECP treatment. Other secondary end points of the ECP randomized study showed that this therapy had a steroid-sparing effect and was associated with an improvement in quality of life. Consistent with previous studies, ECP for treatment of chronic GVHD was well tolerated and was not associated with an increased risk of infection [18–21]. ECP represents an alternative treatment for steroid-refractory, dependent or intolerant cutaneous chronic GVHD.

5.1.5 Summary

Many evidences of ECP treatment for cutaneous chronic GVHD have been published, but the comparison of the efficacy of ECP treatment with other agents is difficult due to the wide variety in eligibility criteria, treatment schedule, time of assessment and response measures [17]. Nevertheless, the current evidences show that some patients with chronic GVHD will benefit from treatment with ECP. For steroid-refractory cutaneous chronic GVHD, at least 24 weeks of treatment with ECP is necessary to achieve adequate response [25, 28]. Advantages of ECP include no increased risk of infection compared to other therapies and an excellent safety profile. Limitation of ECP includes the need for specialized service and the time required to deliver the treatment and its cost compared to other treatments. Further studies are warranted to characterize the optimal indication, regimen and duration of ECP for treatment of cutaneous chronic GVHD.

References

[1] Flowers ME, Parker PM, Johnston LJ, et al. Comparison of chronic graft-versus-host disease after transplantation of peripheral blood stem cells versus bone marrow in allogeneic recipients: long-term follow-up of a randomized trial. Blood 2002;100:415–9.
[2] Arai S, Jagasia M, Storer B, et al. Global and organ-specific chronic graft-versus-host disease severity according to the 2005 NIH Consensus Criteria. Blood 2011;118:4242–9.
[3] Filipovich AH, Weisdorf D, Pavletic S, et al. National Institutes of Health consensus development project on criteria for clinical trials in chronic graft-versus-host disease: I. Diagnosis and staging working group report. Biol Blood Marrow Transplant 2005;11:945–56.
[4] Parker PM, Chao N, Nademanee A, et al. Thalidomide as salvage therapy for chronic graft-versus-host disease. Blood 1995;86:3604–9.
[5] Browne PV, Weisdorf DJ, DeFor T, et al. Response to thalidomide therapy in refractory chronic graft-versus-host disease. Bone Marrow Transplant 2000;26:865–9.

[6] Lee SJ, Wegner SA, McGarigle CJ, Bierer BE, Antin JH. Treatment of chronic graft-versus-host disease with clofazimine. Blood 1997;89:2298–302.
[7] Busca A, Saroglia EM, Lanino E, et al. Mycophenolate mofetil (MMF) as therapy for refractory chronic GVHD (cGVHD) in children receiving bone marrow transplantation. Bone Marrow Transplant 2000;25:1067–71.
[8] Busca A, Locatelli F, Marmont F, Audisio E, Falda M. Response to mycophenolate mofetil therapy in refractory chronic graft-versus-host disease. Haematologica 2003;88:837–9.
[9] Gilman AL, Chan KW, Mogul A, et al. Hydroxychloroquine for the treatment of chronic graft-versus-host disease. Biol Blood Marrow Transplant 2000;6:327–34.
[10] Couriel DR, Saliba R, Escalon MP, et al. Sirolimus in combination with tacrolimus and corticosteroids for the treatment of resistant chronic graft-versus-host disease. Br J Haematol 2005;130:409–17.
[11] Johnston LJ, Brown J, Shizuru JA, et al. Rapamycin (sirolimus) for treatment of chronic graft-versus-host disease. Biol Blood Marrow Transplant 2005;11:47–55.
[12] Huang XJ, Jiang Q, Chen H, et al. Low-dose methotrexate for the treatment of graft-versus-host disease after allogeneic hematopoietic stem cell transplantation. Bone Marrow Transplant 2005;36:343–8.
[13] Cutler C, Miklos D, Kim HT, et al. Rituximab for steroid-refractory chronic graft-versus-host disease. Blood 2006;108:756–62.
[14] Kim SJ, Lee JW, Jung CW, et al. Weekly rituximab followed by monthly rituximab treatment for steroid-refractory chronic graft-versus-host disease: results from a prospective, multicenter, phase II study. Haematologica 2010;95:1935–42.
[15] Olivieri A, Locatelli F, Zecca M, et al. Imatinib for refractory chronic graft-versus-host disease with fibrotic features. Blood 2009;114:709–18.
[16] Jacobsohn DA, Gilman AL, Rademaker A, et al. Evaluation of pentostatin in corticosteroid-refractory chronic graft-versus-host disease in children: a Pediatric Blood and Marrow Transplant Consortium study. Blood 2009;114:4354–60.
[17] Martin PJ, Inamoto Y, Carpenter PA, Lee SJ, Flowers ME. Treatment of chronic graft-versus-host disease: Past, present and future. Korean J Hematol 2011;46:153–63.
[18] Greinix HT, Volc-Platzer B, Rabitsch W, et al. Successful use of extracorporeal photochemotherapy in the treatment of severe acute and chronic graft-versus-host disease. Blood 1998;92:3098–104.
[19] Child FJ, Ratnavel R, Watkins P, et al. Extracorporeal photopheresis (ECP) in the treatment of chronic graft-versus-host disease (GVHD). Bone Marrow Transplant 1999;23:881–7.
[20] Salvaneschi L, Perotti C, Zecca M, et al. Extracorporeal photochemotherapy for treatment of acute and chronic GVHD in childhood. Transfusion 2001;41:1299–305.
[21] Messina C, Locatelli F, Lanino E, et al. Extracorporeal photochemotherapy for paediatric patients with graft-versus-host disease after haematopoietic stem cell transplantation. Br J Haematol 2003;122:118–27.
[22] Seaton ED, Szydlo RM, Kanfer E, Apperley JF, Russell-Jones R. Influence of extracorporeal photopheresis on clinical and laboratory parameters in chronic graft-versus-host disease and analysis of predictors of response. Blood 2003;102:1217–23.
[23] Foss FM, DiVenuti GM, Chin K, et al. Prospective study of extracorporeal photopheresis in steroid-refractory or steroid-resistant extensive chronic graft-versus-host disease: analysis of response and survival incorporating prognostic factors. Bone Marrow Transplant 2005;35:1187–93.
[24] Couriel DR, Hosing C, Saliba R, et al. Extracorporeal photochemotherapy for the treatment of steroid-resistant chronic GVHD. Blood 2006;107:3074–80.
[25] Flowers ME, Apperley JF, van Besien K, et al. A multicenter prospective phase 2 randomized study of extracorporeal photopheresis for treatment of chronic graft-versus-host disease. Blood 2008;112:2667–74.

[26] Perotti C, Del Fante C, Tinelli C, et al. Extracorporeal photochemotherapy in graft-versus-host disease: a longitudinal study on factors influencing the response and survival in pediatric patients. Transfusion 2010;50:1359–69.
[27] Greinix HT, Pohlreich D, Maalouf J, et al. A single-center pilot validation study of a new chronic GVHD skin scoring system. Biol Blood Marrow Transplant 2007;13:715–23.
[28] Greinix HT, van Besien K, Elmaagacli AH, et al. Progressive improvement in cutaneous and extracutaneous chronic graft-versus-host disease after 24-week course of extracorporeal photopheresis – Results of a crossover randomized study. Biol Blood Marrow Transplant 2011;17:1775–82.

Madan Jagasia, Kavita Raj and Emma Das-Gupta

5.2 Results of ECP in Extracutaneous Manifestations of Chronic GVHD

5.2.1 Introduction

Graft-versus-host disease (GVHD) remains an important complication of allogeneic stem cell transplantation (HCT) and impacts not only survival but contributes to late effects of HCT and affects quality of life [1–3]. The organ specificity of acute and chronic GVHD has some overlap but the phenotypes are different [4]. Extracutaneous involvement is seen in both acute and chronic GVHD. In the former, liver and the gastrointestinal tract are most commonly affected. In chronic GVHD, the manifestations of extra-cutaneous involvement are protean and include eyes, mouth, esophagus, liver, lung and rarely other organ involvement [5]. Figure 5.4 outlines the incidence of various organs affected in chronic GVHD, as defined by the NIH consensus criteria [4] using a prospectively assembled cohort of patients who required systemic treatment for chronic GVHD [6]. Although skin is a major target site for chronic GVHD, extra-cutaneous manifestations contribute to the symptom burden and affect survival and quality of life [2].

Treatment of both acute and chronic GVHD has been dependent on systemic steroids. Recent data suggests that almost 50% of patients with acute GVHD will not respond to initial systemic steroid therapy when response is assessed at day 28 [7]. Similarly, in chronic GVHD, steroid therapy remains the gold standard, without prospective randomized evidence that addition of any other agent modulates the natural history of chronic GVHD [5, 8]. Extracorporeal photopheresis (ECP) therapy is a well established modality to treat chronic GVHD and its role in the management of acute GVHD continues to evolve [9–12].

In this chapter, we describe the role of ECP in extracutaneous manifestations of chronic GVHD. The NIH definition of overlap chronic GVHD includes a component of acute GVHD that co-exists with chronic GVHD and the relevant data is encompassed in this chapter. As ECP is used in combination with systemic immunosuppression and other supportive measures, the relevant aspects of non-ECP therapy are included to provide a comprehensive approach to management of the patient who is initiated on ECP therapy. Organs that are affected rarely with chronic GVHD are beyond the scope of the chapter.

5.2.2 Liver and Gastrointestinal (GI) GVHD

GI and liver GVHD are common complications of HCT. Until recently, hepatic and GI GVHD was classified as either acute or chronic, based on whether the GVHD was di-

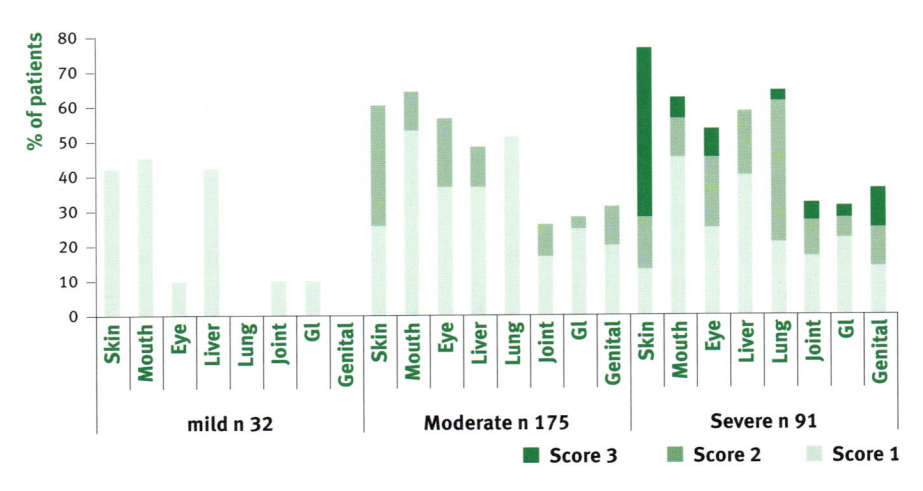

Fig. 5.4. Incidence of Organs Affected in Chronic GVHD Stratified by NIH Severity (mild, moderate and severe).
Within each category, colors represent individual organ system severity based on a score of 0–3. (Reference 6, © the American Society of Hematology).

agnosed before or after 100 days from HCT. The NIH consensus conference recognized the clinical reality that patients continue to present with features of acute GVHD beyond day 100 [4]. It therefore introduced the term "persistent, recurrent, or late-onset acute GVHD" for hepatic or GI involvement occurring beyond day 100, in the absence of other diagnostic or distinctive manifestations of chronic GVHD [4].

Hepatic GVHD typically presents as cholestasis, with increased bilirubin or alkaline phosphatase but may also present as acute hepatitis [4]. Diagnosis may require a liver biopsy due to the wide differential diagnosis that includes hepatic sinusoidal obstructive disease (SOS), infection and drug-induced toxicity. This is particularly important in the absence of other features of GVHD. The severity of acute hepatic GVHD can be assessed by the Glucksberg grading system or the IBMTR severity index [13, 14]. Chronic GVHD of the liver can manifest in various ways: Portal fibrosis and bile duct drop out are associated with progressive cholestatic jaundice [15]. Asymptomatic elevation of serum transaminases, gamma-glutamyl-transferase (GGT) and alkaline phosphatase as isolated laboratory abnormalities in the absence of jaundice are often seen in patients with chronic GVHD elsewhere in the body [16]. An acute hepatitis picture can also occur, commonly after donor lymphocyte infusions (DLI) or at the time of tapering of immunosuppressive medication [16].

The main sign of acute GVHD of the gut is diarrhea, the volume of which is proportional to the severity of GVHD. In the most severe cases abdominal pain and ileus are also present. Upper GI symptoms can also occur and include anorexia, nausea and emesis. Occasionally patients present with these symptoms alone without diarrhea and this situation was recognized as grade 1 GVHD by the 1994 Keystone consensus criteria [17]. Gastrointestinal involvement is uncommon in chronic GVHD, and apart from esophageal involvement, gut GVHD occurring beyond day 100 behaves as persistent or protracted acute GVHD [16]. This form of GVHD is often associated with other more typical features of chronic GVHD. Esophageal chronic GVHD may present as insidious weight loss, dysphagia and pain [18]. Radiologically, web formation and esophageal narrowing may be seen. Upper gut GVHD can also cause nausea, vomiting and satiety. Mid-gut and colonic GVHD can be protracted and is variable in its presentation. Symptoms often wax and wane. Diarrhea, abdominal pain and malabsorption are all features [16]. The NIH chronic GVHD activity assessment grades the features of gut GVHD from 0 to 3 and classifies symptoms as upper GI (early satiety, anorexia, nausea and vomiting), esophageal (dysphagia, odynophagia) and lower GI (diarrhea).

5.2.2.1 Role of ECP Therapy

ECP is an established effective second line treatment for chronic GVHD of the gut and liver [9, 12, 19, 22, 23] and is now a recommended treatment by the Haemato-oncology Task Force of the British Committee for Standards in Haematology (BCSH) and the British Society for Blood and Marrow Transplantation (BSBMT) and the German-Austrian-Swiss Consensus Group on Clinical Practice in Chronic GVHD [24, 25] Flowers and colleagues published the first randomized controlled prospective phase II trial of ECP for the treatment of patients with chronic GVHD [26]. In this study, assessment at week 12 of treatment demonstrated a response in 3/14 (11%) patients with liver GVHD and 1/2 (50%) patients with gut involvement. By week 24, an additional 4 patients (29%) with liver GVHD had responded. In a following open-label cross-over ECP study in 29 eligible participants randomized initially to the standard of care non-ECP arm, 3 of 6 patients (50%) with liver and 1 of 2 (50%) with GI involvement demonstrated response defined as CR or partial resolution (PR) to ECP by week 12 [23]. Overall, the response to ECP reported for chronic visceral GVHD is variable between studies. Greinix and colleagues reported a complete resolution (CR) rate of 68% to 70% for chronic liver GVHD [9, 27]. Couriel and colleagues reported responses in 71% of patients with liver involvement [12]. Chronic GVHD involving the gut tends to be less responsive to ECP [9, 21]. Response of chronic GVHD to ECP has been associated with increased survival and a reduction in the use of corticosteroids [28]. Flowers and colleagues also demonstrated an improvement in quality of life [26]. Treatment schedules vary, but the most commonly used consists of ECP treatment on 2 consecutive days every two weeks, tapering according to response based on 3-monthly assessments. This schedule has been endorsed in the UK consensus statement [29].

In conclusion, ECP is an efficacious treatment for both acute and chronic GVHD affecting the liver and gut. It is well tolerated with few side effects and is less immunosuppressive than alternative treatments making it a safe and ideal steroid sparing therapy.

5.2.2.2 Role of Non-ECP Therapy

Liver and GI GVHD are often seen in the context of overlap chronic GVHD. The therapeutic approach is similar to acute GVHD affecting liver and GI tract. As the time to response with ECP can be several weeks, judicious integration of non-ECP therapy is paramount. There is almost no literature based evidence to guide the style of combination of non-ECP therapy with ECP, and data is often extrapolated from the non-ECP literature. Corticosteroids remain the standard first-line treatment of liver and GI GVHD. Response rates are generally higher for gut (40–50%) than liver (15–35%) involvement [30]. Steroids, both systemic or in combination with topical (budenoside or beclomethasone dipropionate) have been used for GI GVHD [30–33]. MacMillan and colleagues found that the occurrence of lower GI involvement (with or without other organ manifestations) predicted a lower response rate to treatment with corticosteroids [7].

There is no clear consensus on the optimal second-line therapy for acute GVHD of the liver or gut. Second-line options have recently been reviewed by a joint working group of the BCSH/BSBMT [33] as well as the American Society of Blood and Marrow Transplantation [34].

The management of chronic liver and GI GVHD has recently been reviewed by both the BCSH/BSBMT and the German-Austrian-Swiss Consensus Group on Clinical Practice in Chronic GVHD [24, 25, 35, 36]. Since the 1980s the standard first-line treatment of chronic GVHD of the gut or liver has been corticosteroids. The standard dose used is 1 mg/kg/day of prednisolone or an equivalent dose of methylprednisolone [24, 34, 36]. The Seattle group suggested maintaining the starting dose for 2 weeks or until there is objective evidence of improvement and then tapering slowly using an alternate day dosing regimen over a period of months [37]. The routine use of calcineurin inhibitors (CNIs) for the treatment of newly diagnosed chronic GVHD is not recommended, although they may be of use as steroid sparing agents [24, 36].

Drugs commonly used for second-line therapy of chronic GVHD include CNIs, mycophenolate mofetil (MMF) and mTOR inhibitors [24, 25]. MMF is less suited to the treatment of GI GVHD as the drug itself has GI toxicity. One phase II study has shown that hydroxychloroquine is beneficial in the treatment of liver GVHD but has little efficacy in the treatment of gastrointestinal GVHD [38]. Ursodeoxycholic acid, a hydrophilic dihydroxy bile acid has also been shown in small studies and case reports to have efficacy in the treatment of chronic liver GVHD when given in addition to immunosuppressive agents [39].

Supportive care is an important aspect of the successful management of acute and chronic GVHD of the liver and GI tract. Infection is a major cause of death in patients receiving immunosuppressive therapy for GVHD and systemic infection prophylaxis should be used. Patients with acute GI GVHD may benefit from short term "gut rest" [40]. Nutritional support is an important component of the treatment of acute and chronic gut GVHD. Enteral nutrition is preferable, but in the case of acute GVHD with large volumes of diarrhea, parenteral nutritional support should be provided [40, 41]. Anti-diarrheal agents including loperamide, codeine and octreotide may be helpful in addition to systemic immunosuppression [41].

5.2.3 Ocular and Oral GVHD

5.2.3.1 Ocular GVHD
Ocular GVHD is a distinctive criterion for chronic GVHD per the NIH consensus criteria. Distinctive features of ocular GVHD include new onset of dry, gritty or painful eyes, cicatricial conjunctivitis, keratoconjunctivitis sicca (KCS) and confluent areas of punctuate keratopathy. The global severity criteria consider the functional impact of the ocular symptoms and offer a guide to treatment. In the presence of distinctive features of chronic GVHD in at least one other organ, a Schirmer's test that is ≤5 mm or new onset KCS by slit lamp examination with a Schirmer score of 6–10 mm are confirmatory of ocular GVHD [4]. The Schirmer's test, performed on day 100 after HCT has only a positive predictive value of 41% and a negative predictive value of 82% and therefore, comprehensive ocular screening is recommended [42, 43]. In about 80% of patients with conjunctival involvement, pseudomembranes develop and in a third progress to corneal epithelial sloughing. Histopathologically keratinisation of the conjunctiva and cornea, hemorrhage and epithelial thinning of the conjunctiva may occur [44]. Chronic GVHD may affect the periorbital skin and/or eyelids with hyperpigmentation, loss of eyelashes, ectropion, poikiloderma, poliosis, madarosis, inflammation of the eyelids (blepharitis) and/or vitiligo [43]. The nasolacrimal duct and canalicular ducts may be obstructed.

Ocular GVHD occurs in approximately 40% of allograft recipients. Under half of these cases develop by day 100 whereas the rest may manifest later. In 80% of patients ocular GVHD is preceded by GVHD at other sites particularly cutaneous GVHD. Recognized independent risk factors for developing ocular GVHD include prior cutaneous GVHD and male recipient from a female donor [42].

5.2.3.2 Oral GVHD
After the skin, the oral cavity is the most common site affected by chronic GVHD [6, 45]. Diagnostic clinical features for oral chronic GVHD include lichen-like lesions and sclerotic GVHD [4]. Xerostomia, mucoceles, mucosal atrophy, pseudomembranes, and ulcers are distinctive clinical features of chronic GVHD. Secondary infections such as herpes simplex, yeast, or malignancy need to be excluded. Dryness of the oral mucosa may also result in ulcerations, and secondary infections. Chronic GVHD and secondary infection may occur simultaneously and treatment of the latter may be necessary while oral chronic GVHD persists and immunosuppressive therapy is ongoing. Symptoms such as gingivitis, mucositis, erythema and pain may occur in both

acute and chronic GVHD [4]. Oral GVHD may affect the mucosa or the salivary glands or both. Untreated it is likely to be associated with a reduced nutritional intake, and predisposes to oral malignancy. Xerostomia also predisposes to poorer dental hygiene and dental caries. It is a reflection of salivary gland inflammation and destruction. If destruction of glands has occurred then reversal of xerostomia is unlikely. Often xerostomia and xerophthalmia occur together in patients. In a study of sicca symptoms and signs in 101 patients with chronic GVHD, 77% reported xerostomia and concurrent dry eyes occurred in all but one patient [46].

5.2.3.3 Role of ECP Therapy in Ocular and Oral GVHD

Various schedules of ECP have been used for treatment of patients with chronic GVHD ranging from 2–4 sessions per week either weekly or fortnightly. In several studies ECP was used late in the course of chronic GVHD which may have tempered responses. Additionally, patients were treated simultaneously with steroids/cyclosporine or other immunosuppressive agents making it difficult to attribute success to any one treatment.

In a study of steroid-refractory chronic GVHD, patients were treated with 2–4 treatments of ECP weekly until a partial response when the numbers of sessions were tapered [12]. Of 71 patients treated, 59 (79%) had cutaneous, 21 (30%) liver, 11 (15%) lung seen as bronchiolitis obliterans, 9 (13%) oral, 6 (8%) ocular and 3 (4%) GI manifestations of chronic GVHD. Mucocutaneous and liver GVHD responded best with 15 patients (71%) with liver, 7 (77%) with oral mucosa, 4 (67%) with ophthalmic and 33 (59%) with cutaneous involvement by chronic GVHD responding. The median time to response was 116 days for ocular (range, 17–280 days) and 42 (range, 11–231) days for oral GVHD, respectively [12].

A prospective phase II study in 95 patients with steroid-intolerant, steroid-dependent or steroid-refractory chronic GVHD randomized patients to receive standard treatment (prednisone plus CNI, n=47) or standard treatment plus ECP [26]. At 12 weeks improvement in the total skin score was evident in modest numbers of patients treated with ECP compared to the control arm (8.3% versus 0). Responses in ocular GVHD were improved by ECP (30% ECP versus 7% control arm, p=0.04) and there was a trend to improved responses in oral GVHD (53% ECP versus 27% control arm, p=0.06) as well [26].

An open-labeled cross-over extension of the study allowed 29 patients on the standard arm to crossover to the ECP arm if there was progression of chronic GVHD, less than 15% improvement in cutaneous GVHD or less than 25% reduction in steroid dose within 12 weeks [23]. A third (31%) of these patients responded to ECP by week 24 and 33% were able to reduce steroids by ≥50%. Seventy percent of patients with oral GVHD responded to ECP with CR or PR by week 24. This suggests that prolonged treatment with ECP is necessary for maximal response and even delayed introduction of ECP is of additional benefit to standard therapy [23].

In view of the safety of ECP it has been recommended as second-line therapy of chronic GVHD, and it would probably be beneficial to introduce ECP earlier into the algorithm for treatment of chronic GVHD before irreversible changes occur [25].

5.2.3.4 Role of Non-ECP Therapy in Ocular GVHD

Treatment of ocular GVHD is directed at limiting immune damage, symptomatic alleviation of dry eyes and prevention of secondary complications. Ideally, an ophthalmologist with knowledge and experience of HCT and ocular GVHD should be part of the multidisciplinary team caring for these patients. Systemic immunosuppressive therapy is indicated based on a global severity score of moderate/severe. Topical immunosuppression to decrease ocular surface inflammation or in cases of severe ocular GVHD may be necessary. Topical steroid therapy is best coordinated by an experienced ophthalmologist to minimize its side effects including rise of intraocular pressure, cataract formation and infectious keratitis [43, 47]. Topical cyclosporine and autologous serum eye drops have been used to achieve symptomatic improvement, increase tear formation and reduce areas of corneal dryness [36, 43, 47]. To lubricate the eyes, preservative free artificial tears may be used.

Slow dissolving 5 mg pellets of hydroxypropyl methylcellulose inserted into the lower eye lid may also be beneficial. Topical transilast may alter the increased fibroblast activity in ocular GVHD [48]. Other causes of dry eyes such as medications with anticholinergic side effects have to be considered and then, may need to be altered. The use of eye protection such as moisture chamber glasses that decrease evaporation or scleral lenses, for patients with severe corneal epithelial defects, that are gas permeable but retain fluid may enable healing.

In severe cases tarsorrhaphy may be needed to decrease the exposed surface area. In patients with severe ocular sicca (< 5 mm tear film on Schirmer's) blocking the drainage of tears by occlusion of the lacrimal puncta either with plugs or permanently with thermal cauterization may be used.

5.2.3.5 Role of Non-ECP Therapy in Oral GVHD

For non severe oral chronic GVHD local therapies may be useful [36, 47]. Localized, discrete mucosal lesions may be treated with the application of high potency steroid gel (such as clobetasol, betamethasone or fluocinonide). Asymptomatic mucosal ulcers may also need treating with these agents to enable restoration of mucosal barrier integrity. Alternatively, topical tacrolimus ointment or rinse may be useful and preferred over topical steroids for dry lesions on the lips as steroids cause permanent atrophy if applied to the vermillion of the lips.

In lesions that persist for 3–4 weeks despite topical therapy, intralesional steroid injections (triamcinolone) weekly are a useful alternative. Local treatment with dexamethasone mouth wash for oral sensitivity or 0.1 % tacrolimus in water as an oral rinse may be helpful. The use of toothpaste such as biotene may be helpful. Artificial saliva may ameliorate symptoms but use of pilocarpine may increase salivary secretion.

For more generalised disease, mouth washes with steroids such as dexamethasone, prednisone or triamcinolone 4 times a day may be used. Alternatively, cyclosporine or tacrolimus mouth wash may also be used. Because of the risk of developing oral candida, patients need to be on appropriate anti-fungal prophylaxis. The use of azathioprine is associated with an increased risk of developing secondary malignancies: hence, its use for oral GVHD is best limited to under a year of treatment. Topical lidocaine may be used to ameliorate painful lesions that hinder nutrition and communication.

Patients with persistent mucosal oral GVHD or who develop new lesions after three years from transplant are at an increased risk of developing a secondary squamous cell cancer. These most often occur from leukoplakia lesions. Thus, these lesions need to be biopsied at intervals to recognize cancer early. Treatment of leukoplakia with oral clobetasol may result in resolution or softening of these lesions. However, if they persist or get worse a biopsy is indicated.

In severe cases systemic therapy with prednisolone and cyclosporine may be necessary. As oral GVHD often accompanies systemic chronic GVHD, treatment may be commenced based on the overall severity of chronic GVHD.

5.2.4 Chronic GVHD of the Lungs

Lung injury is a frequent complication after HCT and non-infectious pulmonary death accounts for significant proportion of post-transplantation morbidity and mortality [49–51]. Bronchiolitis obliterans syndrome (BOS) is one of the more common non-infectious pulmonary complications and is now considered as a diagnostic criterion of chronic GVHD [4, 51]. Incidence of BOS is variable in the literature [51–54]. Recent data suggests that 10 %–20 % of all long term survivors with chronic GVHD may develop BOS [55]. BOS tends to be underdiagnosed as detection is delayed by low sensitivity of spirometry. BOS is currently defined using a combination of spirometric, imaging and histologic criteria [4]. Infections may mimic BOS or be superimposed on BOS and need to be ruled out. Obliterative bronchiolitis is a histologic diagnosis with changes affecting the small airways in a patchy distribution.

Patients typically present with otherwise unexplained decline in pulmonary function tests (PFT) with or without symptoms of cough and worsening dyspnea. Chest radiographs may be normal or may show attenuated pulmonary vessels, bronchial cuffing, subsegmental atelectasis and irregular linear opacities [51, 56]. Lung volume can be normal or mildly increased. Computed tomography (CT) scan shows bronchial dilation, bronchial wall thickening and mosaic attenuation that are most marked in the lower lobes. Air trapping is frequently depicted on expiratory CT scans. Presence of air trapping is of limited sensitivity for early diagnosis of obliterative bronchiolitis.

Progress in BOS therapy has been limited due to the lack of accurate and early identification of the disease process. Implementation of screening PFT on day 100 and then monitoring on a quarterly basis during the first year after HCT has been suggested [56, 57]. If serial PFTs show a clinically significant decline, further diagnostic work up using high resolution CT scan and judicious use of invasive procedures can be undertaken.

5.2.4.1 Role of ECP Therapy

ECP has been used for BOS after lung transplant [58–64]. Morrell and colleagues studied a cohort of 60 patients and showed that the slope of forced expiratory volume in 1 sec (FEV_1) decline decreased to –28.9 mL/month during the 6 months period after initiation of ECP, compared to –116 mL/month prior to ECP [59]. The mean difference in rate of decline was 87.1 mL/month (95% CI, 57.3 to 116.9, P<0.0001). No clinical risk factors could predict ECP responsiveness.

The Regensburg Consensus Conference on Clinical Practice in Chronic GVHD [56] endorsed the use of ECP as first-line therapy for BOS after HCT based on 3 studies [21, 65, 66]. Two of these studies were not specific to BOS. Couriel and colleagues reported on the outcome of 63 patients with chronic GVHD [66]. Eleven patients had BOS and 54% responded to ECP including 1 CR and 5 PR. Child and colleagues reported on outcome of five patients treated with chronic GVHD of the lungs [21]. Two patients (40%) showed an improvement of diffusion capacity without change in their restrictive defect whereas 2 other patients had no change in PFTs. One patient was not evaluable as PFT was not repeated after ECP therapy. Lucid and colleagues reported on the use of ECP in a series of 9 patients with a median follow-up of 23 months who had BOS refractory to conventional treatment [65]. The median number of prior treatments was 5 and the median time to onset of BOS was 17 months after HCT. Response was defined as symptomatic improvement, decreased dependency on supplemental oxygen (if patient was requiring oxygen therapy for BOS) and improvement in PFTs. Figure 5.5 details the stabilization of PFTs. Six of the 9 patients (67%) had stabilization of lung function, but annualized change in FEV_1 from the onset of ECP to end of follow-up was not compared to annualized change in FEV_1 from the end of previous therapy to the onset of ECP.

Dall'Amico and colleagues treated 11 patients with BOS with ECP achieving responses in 54% including 4 CR and 2 PR [22]. Treating 14 pediatric BOS patients with ECP, Messina and colleagues observed responses in 43% with 4 CR and 2 PR, respectively [67]. In the prospectively randomized phase II study in steroid-refractory/dependent/intolerant chronic GVHD, 2 of 9 BOS patients in the ECP study arm (22%) responded to ECP [26]. In the following open-label crossover ECP, study 3 of 4 BOS patients (75%) achieved a CR or PR by week 12 [23].

In conclusion, about half of the 100 patients with lung involvement reportedly responded to ECP including 14 CR, 20 PR and 17 improvements. Thus, ECP is a promising therapeutic modality for these patients with otherwise dismal prognosis. However, well-designed prospective studies on the use of ECP therapy for BOS are highly warranted including identification of early onset of BOS prior to development of irreversible lung damage and definition of biomarkers of response. Furthermore, the integration of non-ECP therapy with ECP could optimize individual patient's outcome.

5.2.4.2 Role of Non-ECP Therapy

The Regensburg conference report addressed and summarized the literature on therapy of chronic GVHD of the lungs [56]. It is clear that the quality of data supporting prevalent practices is generally poor. Recently, Sengsayadeth and colleagues summarized non-ECP therapy in a review [68]. Management of BOS patients should include comprehensive vaccination (influenza, pneumococcal), antibiotic prophylaxis, and management of hypogammaglobulinemia to decrease risk of sinopulmonary infections. Pulmonary rehabilitation therapy should be encouraged.

5.2.5 Summary

Unfortunately, very few randomized controlled studies have been undertaken assessing treatment options for patients with chronic GVHD during the last several years. Heterogeneity of chronic GVHD, lack of a prospectively validated classification system, lack of uniform response criteria or surrogate endpoints for use in clinical trials, lack of uniform immunosuppressive therapeutic approaches have been important hurdles. With the advent of the NIH consensus criteria and emerging prospective validation, a renewed synchronized and well orchestrated international collaborative effort was started to support clinical trials in chronic GVHD. ECP has demonstrated promising results in extracutaneous manifestations of chronic GVHD with a favorable safety profile. However, to better define the role of ECP in chronic GVHD additional prospective controlled studies with optimal tissue sampling should be performed to identify biomarkers and phenotypic subsets of chronic GVHD patients that best respond to ECP therapy.

References

[1] Jagasia M, Arora M, Flowers ME et al. Risk factors for acute GVHD and survival after hematopoietic cell transplantation. Blood 2012;119:296–307.
[2] Pidala J, Kurland B, Chai X et al. Patient-reported quality of life is associated with severity of chronic graft-versus-host disease as measured by NIH criteria: report on baseline data from the Chronic GVHD Consortium. Blood 2011;117:4651–7.
[3] Lee SJ, Klein JP, Barrett AJ et al. Severity of chronic graft-versus-host disease: association with treatment-related mortality and relapse. Blood 2002;100:406–14.

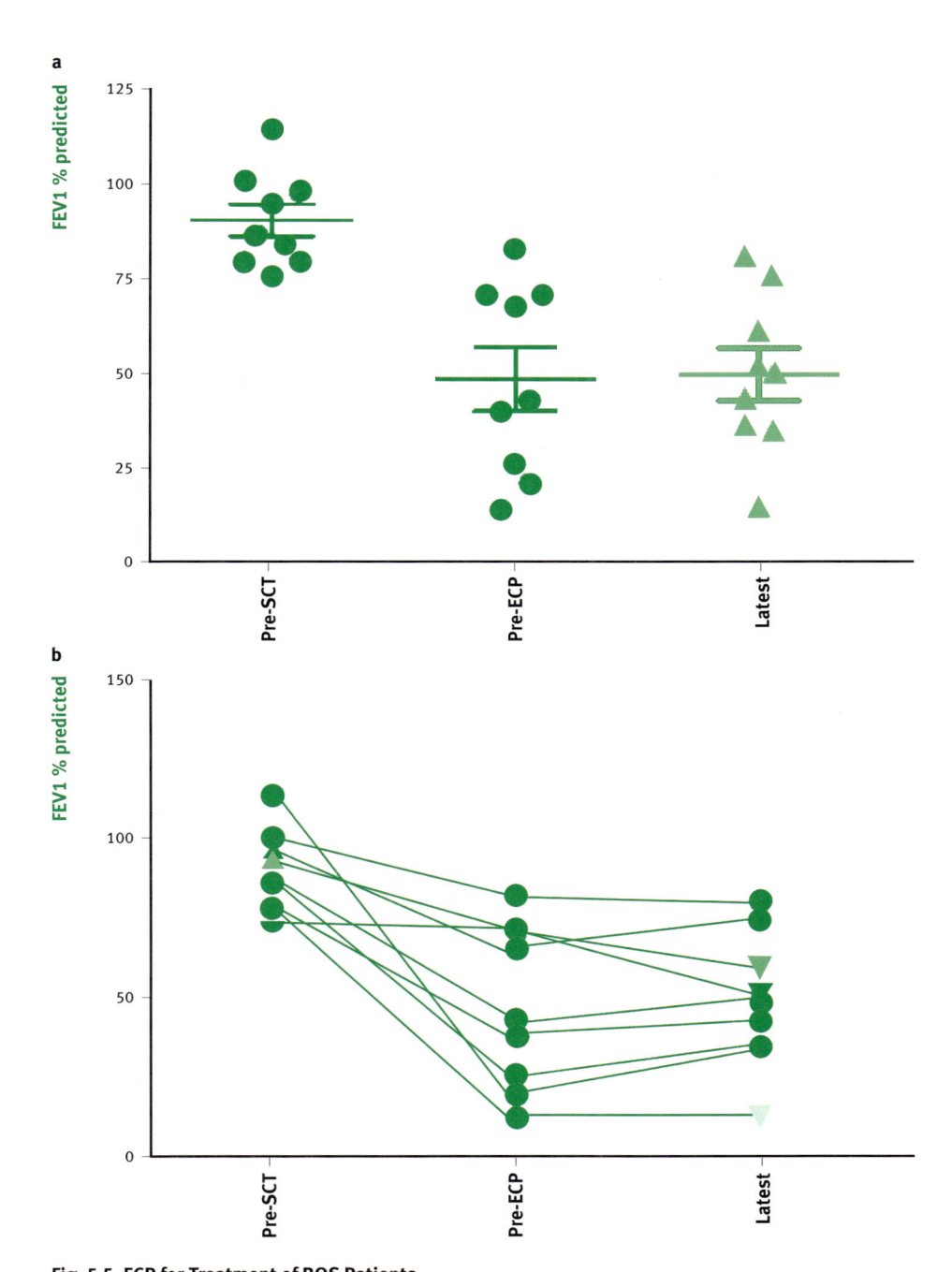

Fig. 5.5. ECP for Treatment of BOS Patients.
(a) Serial pulmonary function tests (forced expiratory volume in 1s, FEV$_1$): pretransplantation (pre-SCT), pre-ECP and at latest follow up. **(b)** Response to ECP, median time 25 days post ECP (range, 20–958 days). (Reference 65, © Bone Marrow Transplantation).

[4] Filipovich AH, Weisdorf D, Pavletic S et al. National Institutes of Health consensus development project on criteria for clinical trials in chronic graft-versus-host disease: I. Diagnosis and staging working group report. Biol Blood Marrow Transplant 2005;11:945–56.
[5] Lee SJ, Vogelsang G, Flowers ME. Chronic graft-versus-host disease. Biol Blood Marrow Transplant 2003;9:215–33.
[6] Arai S, Jagasia M, Storer B et al. Global and organ-specific chronic graft-versus-host disease severity according to the 2005 NIH Consensus Criteria. Blood 2011;118:4242–9.
[7] MacMillan ML, Weisdorf DJ, Wagner JE et al. Response of 443 patients to steroids as primary therapy for acute graft-versus-host disease: comparison of grading systems. Biol Blood Marrow Transplant 2002;8:387–94.
[8] Martin PJ, Inamoto Y, Carpenter PA, Lee SJ, Flowers ME. Treatment of chronic graft-versus-host disease: Past, present and future. Korean J Hematol 2011;46:153–63.
[9] Greinix HT, Volc-Platzer B, Rabitsch W et al. Successful use of extracorporeal photochemotherapy in the treatment of severe acute and chronic graft-versus-host disease. Blood 1998;92:3098–104.
[10] Greinix HT, Volc-Platzer B, Kalhs P et al. Extracorporeal photochemotherapy in the treatment of severe steroid-refractory acute graft-versus-host disease: a pilot study. Blood 2000;96:2426–31.
[11] Jagasia MH, Savani BN, Stricklin G et al. Classic and overlap chronic graft-versus-host disease (cGVHD) is associated with superior outcome after extracorporeal photopheresis (ECP). Biol Blood Marrow Transplant 2009;15:1288–95.
[12] Couriel DR, Hosing C, Saliba R et al. Extracorporeal photochemotherapy for the treatment of steroid-resistant chronic GVHD. Blood 2006;107:3074–80.
[13] Glucksberg H, Storb R, Fefer A et al. Clinical manifestations of graft-versus-host disease in human recipients of marrow from HLA-matched sibling donors. Transplantation 1974;18:295–304.
[14] Rowlings PA, Przepiorka D, Klein JP et al. IBMTR Severity Index for grading acute graft-versus-host disease: retrospective comparison with Glucksberg grade. Br J Haematol 1997;97:855–64.
[15] Shulman HM, Sharma P, Amos D, Fenster LF, McDonald GB. A coded histologic study of hepatic graft-versus-host disease after human bone marrow transplantation. Hepatology 1988;8:463–70.
[16] Kida A, McDonald GB. Gastrointestinal, hepatobiliary, pancreatic, and iron-related diseases in long-term survivors of allogeneic hematopoietic cell transplantation. Semin Hematol 2012;49:43–58.
[17] Przepiorka D, Weisdorf D, Martin P et al. 1994 Consensus Conference on Acute GVHD Grading. Bone Marrow Transplant 1995;15:825–8.
[18] McDonald GB, Sullivan KM, Schuffler MD, Shulman HM, Thomas ED. Esophageal abnormalities in chronic graft-versus-host disease in humans. Gastroenterology 1981;80:914–21.
[19] Apisarnthanarax N, Donato M, Korbling M et al. Extracorporeal photopheresis therapy in the management of steroid-refractory or steroid-dependent cutaneous chronic graft-versus-host disease after allogeneic stem cell transplantation: feasibility and results. Bone Marrow Transplant 2003;31:459–65.
[20] Bisaccia E, Palangio M, Gonzalez J et al. Treatment of extensive chronic graft-versus-host disease with extracorporeal photochemotherapy. J Clin Apher 2006;21:181–7.
[21] Child FJ, Ratnavel R, Watkins P et al. Extracorporeal photopheresis (ECP) in the treatment of chronic graft-versus-host disease (GVHD). Bone Marrow Transplant 1999;23:881–7.
[22] Dall'Amico R, Messina C. Extracorporeal photochemotherapy for the treatment of graft-versus-host disease. Ther Apher 2002;6:296–304.
[23] Greinix HT, van Besien K, Elmaagacli AH et al. Progressive improvement in cutaneous and extracutaneous chronic graft-versus-host disease after a 24-week course of extracorporeal photopheresis-results of a crossover randomized study. Biol Blood Marrow Transplant 2011;17:1775–82.
[24] Dignan FL, Amrolia P, Clark A et al. Diagnosis and management of chronic graft-versus-host disease. Br J Haematol 2012;158:46–61.

[25] Wolff D, Schleuning M, von Harsdorf S et al. Consensus Conference on Clinical Practice in Chronic GVHD: Second-line treatment of chronic graft-versus-host disease. Biol Blood Marrow Transplant 2011;17:1–17.
[26] Flowers ME, Apperley JF, van Besien K et al. A multicenter prospective phase 2 randomized study of extracorporeal photopheresis for treatment of chronic graft-versus-host disease. Blood 2008;112:2667–74.
[27] Greinix HT, Socie G, Bacigalupo A et al. Assessing the potential role of photopheresis in hematopoietic stem cell transplant. Bone Marrow Transplant 2006;38:265–73.
[28] Foss FM, Gorgun G, Miller KB. Extracorporeal photopheresis in chronic graft-versus-host disease. Bone Marrow Transplant 2002;29:719–25.
[29] Scarisbrick JJ, Taylor P, Holtick U et al. U.K. consensus statement on the use of extracorporeal photopheresis for treatment of cutaneous T-cell lymphoma and chronic graft-versus-host disease. Br J Dermatol 2008;158:659–78.
[30] Martin PJ, Schoch G, Fisher L et al. A retrospective analysis of therapy for acute graft-versus-host disease: initial treatment. Blood 1990;76:1464–72.
[31] Van Lint M, Uderzo C, Locasciulli A et al. Early treatment of acute graft-versus-host disease with high- or low-dose 6-methylprednisolone: a multicenter randomized trial from the Italian Group for Bone Marrow Transplantation. Blood 1998; 92:2288–93.
[32] Hockenbery DM, Cruickshank S, Rodell TC et al. A randomized, placebo-controlled trial of oral beclomethasone dipropionate as a prednisone-sparing therapy for gastrointestinal graft-versus-host disease. Blood 2007;109:4557–63.
[33] Dignan FL, Clark A, Amrolia P et al. Diagnosis and management of acute graft-versus-host disease. Br J Haematol 2012;158:30–45.
[34] Martin PJ, Rizzo JD, Wingard JR, et al. First and second-line systemic treatment of acute graft-versus-host disease: Recommendations of the American Society of Blood and Marrow Transplant. Biol Blood Marrow Transplant 2012. doi: 10.1016/j.bbmt.2012.04.005.
[35] Greinix HT, Loddenkemper C, Pavletic SZ et al. Diagnosis and staging of chronic graft-versus-host disease in the clinical practice. Biol Blood Marrow Transplant 2011;17:167–75.
[36] Wolff D, Gerbitz A, Ayuk F et al. Consensus conference on clinical practice in chronic graft-versus-host disease (GVHD): first-line and topical treatment of chronic GVHD. Biol Blood Marrow Transplant 2010;16:1611–28.
[37] Lee SJ, Flowers ME. Recognizing and managing chronic graft-versus-host disease. Hematology Am Soc Hematol Educ Program 2008;134–141.
[38] Gilman AL, Chan KW, Mogul A et al. Hydroxychloroquine for the treatment of chronic graft-versus-host disease. Biol Blood Marrow Transplant 2000;6:327–34.
[39] Fried RH, Murakami CS, Fisher LD, Willson RA, Sullivan KM, McDonald GB. Ursodeoxycholic acid treatment of refractory chronic graft-versus-host disease of the liver. Ann Intern Med 1992;116:624–9.
[40] Deeg HJ. How I treat refractory acute GVHD. Blood 2007;109:4119–26.
[41] Dignan FL, Scarisbrick JJ, Cornish J et al. Organ-specific management and supportive care in chronic graft-versus-host disease. Br J Haematol 2012;158:62–78.
[42] Jacobs R, Tran U, Chen H et al. Prevalence and risk factors associated with development of ocular GVHD defined by NIH consensus criteria. Bone Marrow Transplant 2012 Epub ahead of print.
[43] Dietrich-Ntoukas T, cursiefen C, Westekemper H, et al. Diagnosis and treatment of ocular chronic graft-versus-host disease: report from the German-Austrian- Swiss Consensus Conference on Clinical Practice in chronic GVHD. Cornea 2012;31:299–310.
[44] Jabs DA, Hirst LW, Green WR, Tutschka PJ, Santos GW, Beschorner WE. The eye in bone marrow transplantation. II. Histopathology. Arch Ophthalmol 1983;101:585–90.
[45] Kuzmina Z, Eder S, Böhm A, et al. Significantly worse survival of patients with NIH-defined chronic graft-versus-host disease and thrombocytopenia or progressive onset type: results of a prospective study. Leukemia 2012;26:746–56.

[46] Imanguli MM, Atkinson JC, Mitchell SA et al. Salivary gland involvement in chronic graft-versus-host disease: prevalence, clinical significance, and recommendations for evaluation. Biol Blood Marrow Transplant 2010;16:1362–9.

[47] Couriel D, Carpenter PA, Cutler C et al. Ancillary therapy and supportive care of chronic graft-versus-host disease: National Institutes of Health consensus development project on criteria for clinical trials in chronic graft-versus-host disease: V. Ancillary Therapy and Supportive Care Working Group Report. Biol Blood Marrow Transplant 2006;12:375–96.

[48] Ogawa Y, Dogru M, Uchino M et al. Topical tranilast for treatment of the early stage of mild dry eye associated with chronic GVHD. Bone Marrow Transplant 2010;45:565–9.

[49] Savani BN, Griffith ML, Jagasia S, Lee SJ. How I treat late effects in adults after allogeneic stem cell transplantation. Blood 2011;117:3002–9.

[50] Savani BN, Montero A, Wu C et al. Prediction and prevention of transplant-related mortality from pulmonary causes after total body irradiation and allogeneic stem cell transplantation. Biol Blood Marrow Transplant 2005;11:223–30.

[51] Williams KM, Chien JW, Gladwin MT, Pavletic SZ. Bronchiolitis obliterans after allogeneic hematopoietic stem cell transplantation. JAMA 2009;302:306–14.

[52] Dudek AZ, Mahaseth H, DeFor TE, Weisdorf DJ. Bronchiolitis obliterans in chronic graft-versus-host disease: analysis of risk factors and treatment outcomes. Biol Blood Marrow Transplant 2003;9:657–66.

[53] Au BK, Au MA, Chien JW. Bronchiolitis obliterans syndrome epidemiology after allogeneic hematopoietic cell transplantation. Biol Blood Marrow Transplant 2011;17:1072–8.

[54] Chien JW, Duncan S, Williams KM, Pavletic SZ. Bronchiolitis obliterans syndrome after allogeneic hematopoietic stem cell transplantation-an increasingly recognized manifestation of chronic graft-versus-host disease. Biol Blood Marrow Transplant 2010;16(1 Suppl):S106–14.

[55] Bacigalupo A, Chien J, Barisione G, Pavletic S. Late pulmonary complications after allogeneic hematopoietic stem cell transplantation: diagnosis, monitoring, prevention, and treatment. Semin Hematol 2012;49:15–24.

[56] Hildebrandt GC, Fazekas T, Lawitschka A et al. Diagnosis and treatment of pulmonary chronic GVHD: report from the consensus conference on clinical practice in chronic GVHD. Bone Marrow Transplant 2011;46:1283–95.

[57] Chien JW, Martin PJ, Flowers ME, Nichols WG, Clark JG. Implications of early airflow decline after myeloablative allogeneic stem cell transplantation. Bone Marrow Transplant 2004;33:759–64.

[58] Marques MB, Schwartz J. Update on extracorporeal photopheresis in heart and lung transplantation. J Clin Apher 2011;26:146–51.

[59] Morrell MR, Despotis GJ, Lublin DM, Patterson GA, Trulock EP, Hachem RR. The efficacy of photopheresis for bronchiolitis obliterans syndrome after lung transplantation. J Heart Lung Transplant 2010;29:424–31.

[60] Benden C, Speich R, Hofbauer GF et al. Extracorporeal photopheresis after lung transplantation: a 10-year single-center experience. Transplantation 2008;86:1625–7.

[61] Astor TL, Weill D. Extracorporeal photopheresis in lung transplantation. J Cutan Med Surg 2003;7(4 Suppl):20–4.

[62] Villanueva J, Bhorade SM, Robinson JA, Husain AN, Garrity ER, Jr. Extracorporeal photopheresis for the treatment of lung allograft rejection. Ann Transplant 2000;5:44–7.

[63] O'Hagan AR, Stillwell PC, Arroliga A, Koo A. Photopheresis in the treatment of refractory bronchiolitis obliterans complicating lung transplantation. Chest 1999;115:1459–62.

[64] Slovis BS, Loyd JE, King LE, Jr. Photopheresis for chronic rejection of lung allografts. N Engl J Med 1995;332:962.

[65] Lucid CE, Savani BN, Engelhardt BG et al. Extracorporeal photopheresis in patients with refractory bronchiolitis obliterans developing after allo-SCT. Bone Marrow Transplant 2011;46:426–9.

[66] Couriel D, Hosing C, Saliba R et al. Extracorporeal photopheresis for acute and chronic graft-versus-host disease: does it work? Biol Blood Marrow Transplant 2006;12(1 Suppl 2):37–40.
[67] Messina C, Locatelli F, Lanino E, et al. Extracorporeal photochemotherapy for paediatric patients with graft-versus-host disease after haematopoietic stem cell transplantation. Br J Haematol 2003;122:118–27.
[68] Sengsayadeth SM, Srivastava S, Jagasia M, Savani BN. Time to explore preventive and novel therapies for bronchiolitis obliterans syndrome after allogeneic hematopoietic stem cell transplantation. Biol Blood Marrow Transplant 2012 March 24. PMID: 22449611 (Epub ahead of print).

Kari Zureki and Daniel R. Couriel
5.3 ECP in Chronic GVHD: Steroid-Sparing Effect

5.3.1 Introduction

Chronic graft-versus-host disease (GVHD) is the leading long-term complication of allogeneic hematopoietic cell transplantation (HCT), and it affects approximately 50% or more patients and the majority of those with acute GVHD [1–3]. The treatment of chronic GVHD continues to be one of the major challenges in the management of cancer survivors after allogeneic HCT. The disease has very polymorphic clinical manifestations, and its course is highly unpredictable. Furthermore, the lack of biomarkers or consistent early manifestations often result in late diagnosis with fibrotic changes that are largely irreversible. In this setting, corticosteroids are usually required for prolonged periods of time and most secondary therapies are marginally effective. Immune dysfunction due to chronic GVHD and the immunosuppressive agents used for its treatment predispose to infections, the main cause of death of chronic GVHD patients [4]. Long-term toxicity from corticosteroids blends with chronic GVHD manifestations with an impact on non-relapse mortality (NRM), morbidity and quality of life [4–7]. Unfortunately, corticosteroids are, unavoidably, a key component of therapy, and additional agents in the initial treatment of chronic GVHD have not significantly impacted efficacy of therapy or patient's survival [8, 9]. On the other hand, the median duration of steroid therapy is about 2–3 years [10], and patients that do not have an adequate initial response to corticosteroids require secondary therapy. In this situation, both efficacy and steroid-sparing ability are just as important. In this section we will focus on the steroid-sparing capacity of secondary treatments of chronic GVHD, with particular focus on extracorporeal photopheresis (ECP).

5.3.2 Corticosteroids and Other Immunosuppressive Agents in Chronic GVHD

Corticosteroids remain the standard initial therapy for chronic GVHD, and are still considered the single most effective strategy. There are only six randomized studies that evaluated the initial therapy of chronic GVHD [9, 11–15], and all of them included corticosteroids with or without other agents. Koc and colleagues demonstrated benefit in the addition of calcineurin inhibitors to the initial management of chronic GVHD with prednisone [13]. This benefit was manifested as a decrease in the incidence of avascular necrosis in the calcineurin inhibitor arm, although there was no impact on transplant-related mortality (TRM). The combination of corticosteroids and calcineurin inhibitors became standard of care for patients with chronic GVHD that are not enrolled in a clinical trial, based on both the efficacy of steroids and the steroid-sparing potential of the calcineurin inhibitor [13].

Overall, the response rate to initial therapy with corticosteroids is about 50% [16], including complete and partial responses of organ manifestations afflicted by chronic GVHD. Thus, there is a high proportion of patients that will be exposed to the long-term effects of corticosteroids, and where severe complications like myopathy and avascular necrosis of the bone are relatively frequent [7, 17]. Thus, the management of steroid-related complications can become more challenging than that of chronic GVHD itself.

5.3.2.1 Therapy of Chronic GVHD Beyond Corticosteroids

There is currently no standard second-line therapy for steroid-refractory GVHD patients. A variety of new drugs and other immunomodulatory treatments have shown activity as salvage therapy of chronic GVHD, mostly in small pilot and phase II studies. Martin and colleagues performed a comprehensive review of published phase II studies on secondary therapy for chronic GVHD, showing numerous deficiencies [8]. Fewer than 10% of reports documented an effort to minimize patient selection bias, used a consistent treatment regimen, or tested a formal statistical hypothesis that was based on a contemporaneous or historical benchmark. Furthermore, the steroid-sparing effect of these agents has not been reported systematically, and the lack of standardized measures complicates comparisons.

Over the last decade, particularly following the National Institutes of Health (NIH) Consensus Conference [18], there has been increasing awareness of the importance of the steroid-sparing effect as a relevant and objective endpoint in the evaluation of secondary therapies. Other factors that influence the choice of secondary treatment are toxicity profile, organ involvement, patient and health care provider preference, accessibility and costs.

Some commonly used secondary treatments with reported steroid-sparing potential include ECP, rituximab, mycophenolate mofetil (MMF), pentostatin and sirolimus. ECP is one of the most widely studied and utilized treatments for chronic GVHD and will be reviewed in the following sections. Rituximab is particularly effective in mucocutaneous chronic GVHD, and three studies showed median corticosteroid dose-reductions of more than 70% [19–21]. The steroid-sparing effect was more frequent in patients without visceral involvement [19–21].

Furlong and colleagues prospectively evaluated MMF in 23 patients with chronic GVHD that had failed corticosteroids and showed that 26% of these patients had disease resolution and were able to discontinue their immunosuppressive medication after 3 years. However, the majority of patients received other immunosuppressive agents in addition to MMF [22].

Pentostatin has activity in the treatment of chronic GVHD, mainly in mucocutaneous and musculoskeletal forms [23]. A significant reduction in the median dose of corticosteroids has also been observed in responders to pentostatin [24].

Sirolimus is also effective in the treatment of chronic GVHD, particularly in patients with cutaneous, sclerotic manifestations [25, 26]. One study demonstrated that

3 of 16 evaluable patients treated with sirolimus had a sustained response while tapering all immunosuppressive medications [26].

Overall, the relatively small number of patients in these studies, the limitations in the study design, and the varying criteria for reporting reductions in steroid dosages and other immunosuppressive therapies, prevents definitive conclusions or comparisons of the steroid-sparing potential of each individual therapy.

5.3.3 Overview of ECP in Chronic GVHD and its Steroid-Sparing Effect

Extracorporeal photopheresis has been widely studied as a treatment for chronic GVHD. It is currently approved by the Food and Drug Administration (FDA) for the treatment of cutaneous T-cell lymphoma (CTCL). Although the mechanism of action of ECP in the treatment of chronic GVHD is not yet fully understood, its effectiveness has been demonstrated in different studies.

In an early study by Greinix and colleagues [27], high response rates were observed in patients with cutaneous, oral and liver manifestations of chronic GVHD. Eight of the 15 patients with chronic GVHD had been treated with corticosteroids prior to ECP, and after a median treatment course of 80 days, all of them were able to completely be weaned off steroids.

In a study by Couriel and colleagues [28], a total of 246 patients with steroid refractory chronic GVHD were evaluated retrospectively. Overall, 63 of these patients received ECP treatment after up to 3 lines of immunosuppression, and 83% of them were on corticosteroids. Overall, 61% (n=43) of the patients responded to ECP, and 14 achieved a complete response. Patients with skin, liver, oral or ocular symptoms had the best responses, particularly the ones with sclerodermatous features. After 6 months, 28 of the 44 patients still alive had a sustained response. Of these, 12 patients were able to successfully taper off corticosteroids, with a cumulative incidence of steroid discontinuation at 1 year of 22%, respectively.

A phase 2 randomized study conducted by Flowers and colleagues [29], targeted patients with cutaneous chronic GVHD after failing corticosteroids, and compared ECP for 12–24 weeks along with standard treatment (n=48) versus standard treatment alone (n=47). Response to treatment after 12 weeks was higher in the ECP arm (14.5% of improvement in Vienna Total Skin Score (TSS) from baseline) compared to the control (8.5% improvement), although the difference was not statistically significant. At 12 weeks, 8.3% of patients in the ECP group had a 50% reduction in the steroid dose and a 25% decrease in the Vienna TSS, compared to 0% in the control group. Furthermore, significantly more patients in the ECP study arm achieved more than 50% reduction in the corticosteroid dose and a final steroid dose below 10 mg/day (10 versus 3, p=0.04) by week 12. Thus, this is the first randomized study to report a significant difference in the steroid-sparing capacity of a study agent versus standard therapy of chronic GVHD.

Greinix and colleagues recently reported a follow-up to this study [30], focusing on 29 patients that experienced either lack of response or progressive chronic GVHD in the control arm, and were crossed over to the ECP arm at week 12. After a 24-week course of ECP at a similar schedule as the one used in patients on the initial ECP study arm, the median decrease in TSS score was 25.8%, and 33% of patients (n=8) had 50% or greater reduction in their corticosteroid dose.

Seaton and colleagues [31] studied 28 patients, 27 of whom had previously received therapy with 2 or more immunosuppressive agents. Patients with cutaneous, liver and oral manifestations of chronic GVHD had objective improvement, and amount of systemic immunosuppression including corticosteroids was either stable or decreased in 86% of the patients treated.

In a study by Dignan and colleagues [32], 69 out of 82 patients evaluated received ECP treatment for 6 months. Of these, 65 patients experienced a greater than 50% improvement in symptoms. Improvement in skin involvement was evident with 11% of patients reaching a complete and 81% a partial response. Those patients with oral involvement demonstrated a lower response rate with 1 out of 32 achieving a complete response and 88% a partial one, respectively. Steroid dose could be reduced in 80% of these patients, with 27.5% completely discontinued steroid therapy.

Other clinical investigators reported promising results on the steroid-sparing potential of ECP both in adult as well as pediatric patients with steroid-refractory chronic GVHD [33–35].

5.3.4 Conclusions

Clinical studies addressing second-line therapy for chronic GVHD have several limitations. Most of them are pilot or phase II studies with a relatively small number of patients and frequent deficiencies in their study design. The lack of objective, valid and reliable tools to measure the disease further complicates the interpretation of these results including comparisons between different immunosuppressive strategies. In this setting, significant dose reductions or discontinuation of corticosteroids became a more objective, surrogate marker of treatment success or failure. Transplant physicians have increasingly recognized this reality and reporting on steroid-sparing potential of secondary therapy for acute or chronic GVHD is becoming an essential, unavoidable component of efficacy, just as important as rates of complete response or progression. Treatments that are commonly used in chronic GVHD patients who fail corticosteroids seem to have some degree of steroid-sparing potential. In the case of ECP, this effect has been more consistently demonstrated in a relatively larger number of studies and patients, and, more importantly, in a randomized study against a control arm investigating conventional immunosuppressive therapy. Our analysis of the literature underscores the importance of standardizing and validating measures for the reduction or discontinuation of corticosteroids over time.

References

[1] Socie G, Ritz J, Martin PJ. Current challenges in chronic graft-versus-host disease. Biol Blood Marrow Transplant 2010; 16(Suppl 1):S146–51.
[2] Couriel D, Caldera H, Champlin R, Komanduri K. Acute graft-versus-host disease: pathophysiology, clinical manifestations, and management. Cancer 2004;101:1936–46.
[3] Thepot S, Zhou J, Perrot A, et al. The graft-versus-leukemia effect is mainly restricted to NIH-defined chronic graft-versus-host disease after reduced intensity conditioning before allogeneic stem cell transplantation. Leukemia 2010;24:1852–8.
[4] Vogelsang GB. How I treat chronic graft-versus-host disease. Blood 2001;97:1196–201.
[5] Lee SJ, Flowers ME. Recognizing and managing chronic graft-versus-host disease. Hematology Am Soc Hematol Educ Program 2008;134–41.
[6] Wang, M, Delasalle K, Feng L et al. CR represents an early index of potential long survival in multiple myeloma. Bone Marrow Transplant, 2010;45:498–504.
[7] Couriel DR. Ancillary and supportive care in chronic graft-versus-host disease. Best Pract Res Clin Haematol 2008;21:291–307.
[8] Martin PJ, Inamoto Y, Carpenter PA, Lee SJ, Flowers MED. Treatment of chronic graft-versus-host disease: Past, present and future. Korean J Hematol 2011;46:153–63.
[9] Martin PJ, Storer BE, Rowley SD et al. Evaluation of mycophenolate mofetil for initial treatment of chronic graft-versus-host disease. Blood 2009;113:5074–82.
[10] Stewart BL, Storer B, Storek J et al. Duration of immunosuppressive treatment for chronic graft-versus-host disease. Blood 2004;104:3501–6.
[11] Sullivan KM, Witherspoon RP, Storb R et al. Prednisone and azathioprine compared with prednisone and placebo for treatment of chronic graft-v-host disease: prognostic influence of prolonged thrombocytopenia after allogeneic marrow transplantation. Blood 1988;72:546–54.
[12] Koc S, Leisenring W, Flowers ME et al. Thalidomide for treatment of patients with chronic graft-versus-host disease. Blood 2000;96:3995–6.
[13] Koc S, Leisenring W, Flowers ME et al. Therapy for chronic graft-versus-host disease: a randomized trial comparing cyclosporine plus prednisone versus prednisone alone. Blood 2002;100:48–51.
[14] Arora M, Wagner JE, Davies SM et al. Randomized clinical trial of thalidomide, cyclosporine, and prednisone versus cyclosporine and prednisone as initial therapy for chronic graft-versus-host disease. Biol Blood Marrow Transplant 2001;7:265–73.
[15] Gilman AL, Schultz KR, Goldman FD et al. Randomized trial of hydroxychloroquine for newly diagnosed chronic graft-versus-host disease in children: a Children's Oncology Group study. Biol Blood Marrow Transplant 2012;18:84–91.
[16] Arora M. Therapy of chronic graft-versus-host disease. Best Pract Res Clin Haematol 2008;21: 271–9.
[17] Lee HJ, Oran B, Saliba RM et al. Steroid myopathy in patients with acute graft-versus-host disease treated with high-dose steroid therapy. Bone Marrow Transplant 2006;38: 299–303.
[18] Pavletic SZ, Martin P, Lee SJ et al. Measuring therapeutic response in chronic graft-versus-host disease: National Institutes of Health Consensus Development Project on Criteria for Clinical Trials in Chronic Graft-versus-Host Disease: IV. Response Criteria Working Group report. Biol Blood Marrow Transplant 2006;12:252–66.
[19] Zaja F, Bacigalupo A, Patriarca F et al. Treatment of refractory chronic GVHD with rituximab: a GITMO study. Bone Marrow Transplant 2007;40:273–7.
[20] Cutler C, Miklos D, Kim HT et al. Rituximab for steroid-refractory chronic graft-versus-host disease. Blood 2006;108:756–62.
[21] Mohty M, Marchetti N, El-Cheikh J, Faucher C, Fürst S, Blaise D. Rituximab as salvage therapy for refractory chronic GVHD. Bone Marrow Transplant 2008;41:909–11.

[22] Furlong T, Martin P, Flowers ME et al. Therapy with mycophenolate mofetil for refractory acute and chronic GVHD. Bone Marrow Transplant 2009;44:739–48.
[23] Jacobsohn DA, Chen AR, Zahurak M et al. Phase II study of pentostatin in patients with corticosteroid-refractory chronic graft-versus-host disease. J Clin Oncol 2007;25:4255–61.
[24] Jacobsohn DA, Gilman AL, Rademaker A et al. Evaluation of pentostatin in corticosteroid-refractory chronic graft-versus-host disease in children: a Pediatric Blood and Marrow Transplant Consortium study. Blood 2009;114:4354–60.
[25] Couriel DR, Saliba R, Escalon MP et al. Sirolimus in combination with tacrolimus and corticosteroids for the treatment of resistant chronic graft-versus-host disease. Br J Haematol 2005;130:409–17.
[26] Johnston LJ, Brown J, Shizuru JA et al. Rapamycin (sirolimus) for treatment of chronic graft-versus-host disease. Biol Blood Marrow Transplant 2005;11:47–55.
[27] Greinix HT, Volc-Platzer B, Rabitsch W et al. Successful use of extracorporeal photochemotherapy in the treatment of severe acute and chronic graft-versus-host disease. Blood 1998;92:3098–104.
[28] Couriel DR, Hosing C, Saliba R et al. Extracorporeal photochemotherapy for the treatment of steroid-resistant chronic GVHD. Blood 2006;107:3074–80.
[29] Flowers ME, Apperley JF, van Besien K et al. A multicenter prospective phase 2 randomized study of extracorporeal photopheresis for treatment of chronic graft-versus-host disease. Blood 2008; 112:2667–74.
[30] Greinix HT, van Besien K, Elmaagacli AH et al. Progressive improvement in cutaneous and extracutaneous chronic graft-versus-host disease after a 24-week course of extracorporeal photopheresis--results of a crossover randomized study. Biol Blood Marrow Transplant 2011;17: 1775–82.
[31] Seaton ED, Szydlo RM, Kanfer E, Apperley JF, Russell-Jones R. Influence of extracorporeal photopheresis on clinical and laboratory parameters in chronic graft-versus-host disease and analysis of predictors of response. Blood 2003;102:1217–23.
[32] Dignan FL, Greenblatt D, Cox M et al. Efficacy of bimonthly extracorporeal photopheresis in refractory chronic mucocutaneous GVHD. Bone Marrow Transplant 19 September 2011. doi:10.1038/bmt.2011.186
[33] Salvaneschi L, Perotti C, Zecca M et al. Extracorporeal photochemotherapy for treatment of acute and chronic GVHD in childhood. Transfusion 2001;41:1299–305.
[34] Foss FM, DiVenuti GM, Chin K et al. Prospective study of extracorporeal photopheresis in steroid-refractory or steroid-resistant extensive chronic graft-versus-host disease: analysis of response and survival incorporating prognostic factors. Bone Marrow Transplant 2005;35: 1187–93.
[35] Jagasia MH, Savani BN, Stricklin G et al. Classic and overlap chronic graft-versus-host disease (GVHD) is associated with superior outcome after extracorporeal photopheresis (ECP). Biol Blood Marrow Transplant 2009;15:1288–95.

Hildegard T. Greinix
5.4 Prediction of Response to ECP

The currently recommended first-line treatment of chronic graft-versus-host disease (cGVHD) based on randomized phase III studies consists of corticosteroids initially at 1 mg/kg/day administered with a calcineurin inhibitor [1, 2]. No uniformly acceptable schedule for tapering the dose of corticosteroids exists to date but most clinical investigators try to use the minimum dose of prednisone sufficient to control cGVHD manifestations to avoid serious side-effects associated with long-term use of corticosteroids. The median duration of immunosuppressive treatment for cGVHD reportedly is approximately 2 years in patients given marrow grafts and approximately 3.5 years in those given peripheral blood stem cell transplants [3]. About half of the patients respond to first-line therapy and prognosis of steroid-refractory cGVHD remains poor [4, 5].

Numerous clinical studies have been performed to evaluate secondary treatment of steroid-refractory cGVHD. However, no single agent or strategy has reportedly been more beneficial compared to others and thus, various treatment modalities have been in clinical use for therapy of steroid-refractory cGVHD patients during the last years [6]. Treatment choices are mainly based on physician experience, ease of use, risk of toxicity, need for monitoring and potential exacerbation of pre-existing co-morbidities. Clinical management of cGVHD patients is generally approached through empirical trial and error since valid biomarkers to identify the drug or treatment strategy effective in an individual patient are lacking.

5.4.1 Identification of Biomarkers in Chronic Graft-versus-Host Disease

Biomarkers have been defined as any characteristic that is objectively measured and evaluated as an indicator of a normal biologic or pathogenic process, a pharmacologic response to a treatment modality, or a surrogate endpoint to substitute for a clinical trial outcome. In cGVHD, biomarkers could be useful to predict the risk of developing cGVHD, objectively diagnose organ manifestations, measure disease activity, distinguish irreversible organ damage from continued disease activity, predict the prognosis of cGVHD and to predict response to therapy. Several candidate biomarkers have been reported in cGVHD including human leukocyte antigen (HLA) class I and class II and minor histocompatibility antigen (mHag) disparities between donors and recipients, cytokine gene polymorphisms, regulatory immune cell populations such as regulatory T cells and dendritic cells and cell populations affecting inflammatory responses [7]. However, none of these have been established as validated biomarkers for cGVHD.

5.4.1.1 B Lymphocyte Subpopulations and BAFF in Chronic GVHD

The pathophysiology of cGVHD is still poorly understood. The importance of autoreactivity is suggested by clinical manifestations of cGVHD that frequently mimic those of autoimmune diseases and by the detection of auto-antibodies derived from B cells after T helper type (TH2) mediated stimulation and cytokine release [8, 9]. Another probable mechanism for cGVHD is dysfunctional T cell selection in the thymus inducing autoimmune diseases [10]. Since cGVHD only occurs in patients after allogeneic hematopoietic cell transplantation (HCT) and can be prevented by T cell depletion from the donor graft, donor T cell responses directed at allogeneic antigens in the patient are of critical important for the development of cGVHD.

Recent studies have provided evidence that B cells also contribute to the clinical manifestations of cGVHD. Gender-mismatched allogeneic HCT was associated with the presence of alloantibody to Y chromosome-associated mHags in male recipients and the presence of this alloantibody correlated with the clinical development of cGVHD [11, 12] Functional asplenia observed in patients with cGVHD also affects homeostasis of memory B lymphocytes circulating in the peripheral blood (PB) [13, 14]. Greinix and colleagues observed a significant increase of $CD19^+CD21^-$ immature transitional B lymphocyte numbers and deficiency of $CD19^+CD27^+$ memory B cells in patients with active cGVHD compared to ones with resolved or never experiencing cGVHD [15]. These abnormalities of B cell function seen as distortion of B cell homeostasis leading to uncontrolled overactivation of B cells recently emigrated from the bone marrow (BM) due to an excess of B cell activating factor (BAFF) characterizes active cGVHD [15–17]. Lack of BAFF consumption by BAFF-R-expressing circulating B cell subpopulations due to lymphopenia after allogeneic HCT is supposed to lead to an imbalance between the amount of bio-available BAFF and BAFF-R-positive B cells. Therefore, large amounts of BAFF act on single B lymphocytes newly emigrated from the BM leading to the expansion of clones which under physiologic BAFF/B cell ratios would have been deleted or ignored [16].

Assessments of different B cell subpopulations and BAFF/B cell ratios in cGVHD patients allowed distinction of different impairments of humoral immunity seen as either immunodeficiency with hypogammaglobulinemia or autoimmunity indicating different pathogenetic mechanisms of cGVHD [17].

Several investigators reported a significant elevation of the tumor necrosis factor family member BAFF in patients with cGVHD [17–19]. However, measurement of BAFF is complicated by several factors including elevated levels in the setting of B lymphopenia and low BAFF levels in patients after administration of high-dose corticosteroids [19, 20].

5.4.2 Biomarkers for Prediction of Response to ECP

In view of the logistical challenges associated with intensified ECP schedules and the rising demands for efficient use of limited resources in costly areas such as allogeneic HCT, biomarkers predicting response to ECP are highly warranted. Furthermore, some patients with cGVHD including sclerodermatous cutaneous manifestations are in need of ECP treatment for prolonged periods of time to achieve clinical response and thus, patients' improvement [21].

5.4.2.1 CD19⁺CD21⁻ Immature Transitional B Lymphocytes

Our group at the Medical University of Vienna investigated CD19⁺CD21⁻ immature transitional B lymphocytes in peripheral blood (PB) of patients with cGVHD before start of ECP and up to 21 months thereafter [22]. Complete (CR) and partial (PR) responses to ECP were observed in 25 of 34 patients (74%) after 12 months. Patients not responding to 6 months of ECP treatment had a significantly (p=0.02) higher percentage of CD19⁺CD21⁻ immature transitional B lymphocytes (mean 22%) in PB prior to start of ECP compared with patients achieving a CR (mean 8%) and PR (mean 16%) as shown in Figure 5.6. Furthermore, the CD21⁻/CD27⁺ B cell ratio was significantly higher (p=0.03) in patients not responding to ECP (mean 17.4) compared with CR patients (mean 1.6), respectively.

During ECP treatment cGVHD patients achieving a CR to ECP had significantly lower percentages of CD19⁺CD21⁻ immature transitional B lymphocytes in PB 6 (mean 5% versus 25%, p<0.001), 12 (mean 6% versus 24%, p<0.001) and 21 (mean 6% versus 26%, p<0.001) months after start of ECP compared with ECP nonresponders as shown in Figure 5.7. In addition, the CD21⁻/CD27⁺ B cell ratio was significantly lower at 6 (mean 2.2 versus 9.6, p=0.001), 12 (mean 2.7 versus 6, p=0.006) and 21 (mean 2 versus 17, p=0.001) months in ECP responders compared with patients not responding to ECP. Thus, relative amounts of CD19⁺CD21⁻ immature transitional B cells represent the first reported cellular biomarkers predicting response to ECP. They can also serve as a novel biomarker for measuring activity of cGVHD objectively and should be investigated in further prospective clinical trials.

5.4.2.2 B Cell Activating Factor

The tumour necrosis factor family member BAFF is a crucial survival factor for peripheral B cells and is a key regulator of normal B cell homeostasis [23]. High BAFF levels have been reported in patients with a variety of autoimmune disorders [24, 25]. In scenarios with high BAFF levels autoreactive B cells are rescued from deletion by attenuating apoptosis during B cell recirculation after germinal center reactions [26]. Elevated BAFF levels reportedly correlated with activity of cGVHD [16, 19].

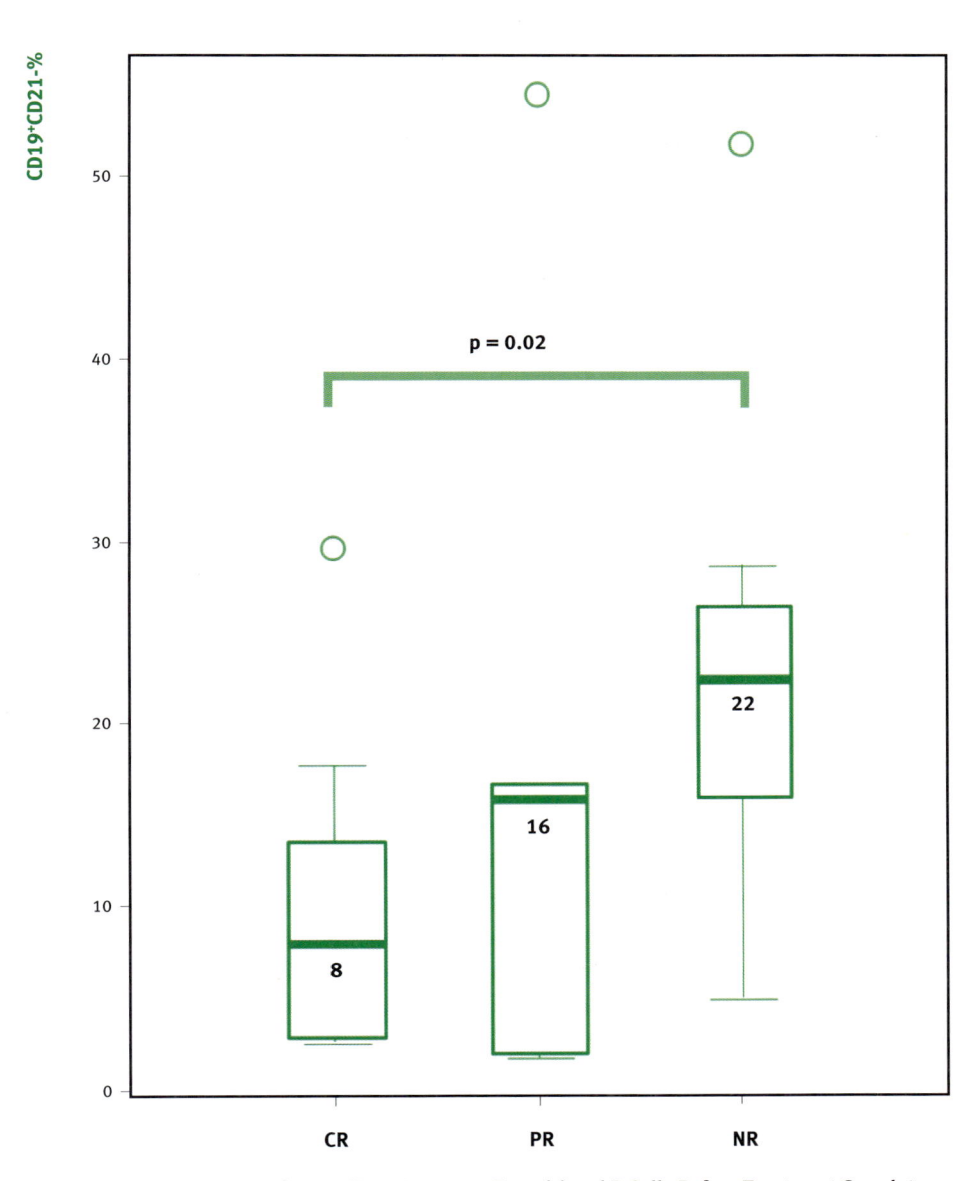

Fig. 5.6. Low Percentages of CD19⁺CD21⁻ Immature Transitional B Cells Before Treatment Correlate Significantly with Complete Resolution of Chronic Graft-versus-Host disease to ECP.
Three groups were analyzed consisting of complete responders (CR, n=6), partial responders (PR, n=6) and nonresponders (NR, n=7) 6 months after initiation of ECP. CD19⁺CD21⁻ immature transitional B cells analyzed before start of ECP are shown in box plot format. Numbers indicate mean percentages (bold horizontal lines), green circles indicate outliers (Reference 22, © American Society of Hematology).

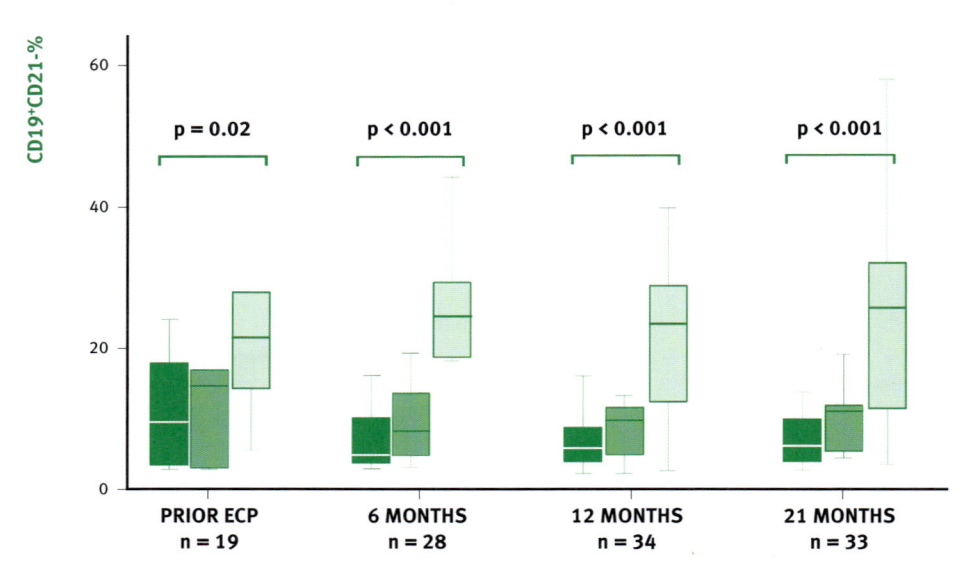

Fig. 5.7. Complete Responders to ECP Have Significantly Lower Percentages of CD19⁺CD21⁻ Immature Transitional B Cells 6, 12 and 21 Months After Initiation of ECP Therapy Compared With Nonresponders.
Patients are divided into complete responders (dark green bars), partial responders (medium green bars) and nonresponders (light green bars) to ECP. Results are shown in box plot format with the bold horizontal line indicating the mean percentages (Reference 22, © American Society Hematology).

Whittle and Taylor measured serum BAFF levels in 46 patients with cGVHD prior to and during ECP and reported that BAFF level at 1 month of ECP predicted cutaneous response at 3 and 6 months [27]. Serum BAFF level below 4 ng/mL at 1 month of ECP was associated with significant improvement of skin involvement seen as reduction of total skin score (TSS) from a median of 47 prior to ECP to 4.5 after 3 months of ECP treatment. In patients with BAFF levels above 4 ng/mL at 1 month no reduction in TSS (median 48.5 prior to ECP versus 46 after 3 months) was observed.

Lower BAFF level at 1 month of ECP was also associated with continuing improvement after 6 months of ECP treatment and complete resolution of cutaneous manifestations in 11 of 20 (55%) patients. In contrast, higher BAFF level at 1 month of ECP was associated with a worsening of TSS and CR of skin involvement in only 1 of 10 (10%) patients, respectively.

Patients with BAFF levels below 4 ng/mL at 1 month of ECP were more likely to achieve at least a 50% reduction of corticosteroid dose between 1 and 6 months of ECP compared to patients with high BAFF levels (70% versus 46%).

In a retrospective analysis of 28 adult patients with cGVHD undergoing ECP treatment all 15 patients with serum BAFF levels above 4 ng/mL following 6 months of ECP therapy experienced GVHD flare between 3 and 18 months of ECP leading to rise of corticosteroid dose in 13 of 15 (87%) patients [28]. However, in the patient cohort with

BAFF level below 4 ng/mL significantly fewer (6 of 13, 46%) presented cGVHD flare between 6 and 18 months (p=0.001) of ECP treatment.

5.4.3 Conclusions

Relative amounts of CD19$^+$CD21$^-$ immature transitional B cells and serum BAFF levels can serve as novel biomarkers for prediction of response to ECP. Whether these findings are ECP-specific is currently unknown since no other treatment cohorts were analyzed and the mechanisms of action of ECP are still subject to further research. Whereas CD19$^+$CD21$^-$ immature transitional B cells significantly correlated with activity of cGVHD and thus, can be used for objective monitoring of disease at various time points during ECP treatment, serum BAFF level is known to be influenced by corticosteroid dose and therefore, could be limited in its clinical usefulness for monitoring disease activity in the treatment course. Well-designed prospective studies with larger patient numbers are warranted to better allow evaluation of the predictive value of these very promising novel biomarkers.

References

[1] Wolff D, Gerbitz A, Ayuk F, et al. Consensus conference on clinical practice in chronic graft-versus-host disease (GVHD): First-line and topical treatment of chronic GVHD. Biol Blood Marrow Transplant 2010;16:1611–28.
[2] Martin PJ, Inamoto Y, Carpenter PA, Lee SJ, Flowers MED. Treatment of chronic graft-versus-host disease: Past, present and future. Korean J Hematol 2011;46:153–63.
[3] Flowers ME, Parker PM, Johnston LJ, et al. Comparison of chronic graft-versus-host disease after transplantation of peripheral blood stem cells versus bone marrow in allogeneic recipients: long-term follow-up of a randomized trial. Blood 2002;100:415–9.
[4] Akpek G, Zahurak mL, Piantadosi S, et al. Development of a prognostic model for grading chronic graft-versus-host disease. Blood 2001;97:1219–26.
[5] Vogelsang GB. How I treat chronic graft-versus-host disease. Blood 2001;97:1196–201.
[6] Wolff D, Schleuning M, von Harsdorf S, et al. Consensus conference on clinical practice in chronic GVHD: Second-line treatment of chronic graft-versus-host disease. Biol Blood Marrow Transplant 2011;17:1–17.
[7] Schultz KR, Miklos DB, Fowler D, et al. Toward biomarkers for chronic graft-versus-host disease: National Institutes of Health Consensus Development Project on criteria for clinical trials in chronic graft-versus-host disease: III. Biomarker Working Group Report. Biol Blood Marrow Transplant 2006;12:126–37.
[8] Tivol E, Komorowski R, Drobyski WR. Emergent autoimmunity in graft-versus-host disease. Blood 2005;105:4885–91.
[9] Hakim FT, Mackall CL. The immune system: effecter and target of graft-versus-host disease. In: Deeg HJ, Burakoff SJ, eds. Graft-vs.Host Disease. New York: Marcel Dekker, Incl; 1997.p. 257–89.
[10] Teshima T, Reddy P, Liu C, et al. Impaired thymic negative selection causes autoimmune graft-versus-host disease. Blood 2003;102:429–35.
[11] Zorn E, Miklos DB, Floyd BH, et al. Minor histocompatibility antigen DBY elicits a coordinated B and T cell response after allogeneic stem cell transplantation. J Exp Med 2004;199:1133–42.

[12] Miklos DB, Kim HT, Miller KH, et al. Antibody responses to H-Y minor histocompatibility antigens correlate with chronic graft-versus-host disease and disease remission. Blood 2005;105: 2793–8.
[13] Kalhs P, Panzer S, Kletter K, et al. Functional asplenia after bone marrow transplantation. A late complication related to extensive chronic graft-versus-host disease. Ann Intern Med 1988;109:461–4.
[14] Kruetzmann S, Rosado MM, Weber H, et al. Human immunoglobulin M memory B cells controlling streptococcus pneumoniae infections are generated in the spleen. J Exp Med 2003;197:939–45.
[15] Greinix HT, Pohlreich D, Kouba M, et al. Elevated numbers of immature/transitional CD21⁻ B lymphocytes and deficiency of memory CD27⁺ B cells identify patients with active chronic graft-versus-host disease. Biol Blood Marrow Transplant 2008;14:208–19.
[16] Sarantopoulos S, Stevenson KE, Kim HT, et al. Altered B-cell homeostasis and excess BAFF in human chronic graft-versus-host disease. Blood 2009:113:3865–74.
[17] Kuzmina Z, Greinix HT, Weigl R, et al. Significant differences in B-cell subpopulations characterize patients with chronic graft-versus-host disease-associated dysgammaglobulinemia. Blood 2011;117:2265–74.
[18] Fujii H, Cuvelier G, She K, et al. Biomarkers in newly diagnosed pediatric extensive chronic graft-versus-host disease: a report from the Children's Oncology Group. Blood 2008;111: 3276–85.
[19] Sarantopoulos S, Stevenson KE, Kim HT, et al. High levels of B-cell activating factor in patients with active chronic graft-versus-host disease. Clin Cancer Res 2007;13:6107–14.
[20] Cambridge G, Isenberg DA, Edwards JC, et al. B cell depletion therapy in systemic lupus erythematosus: relationships among serum B lymphocyte stimulator levels, autoantibody profile and clinical response. Ann Rheum Dis 2008;67:1011–6.
[21] Greinix HT, Volc-Platzer B, Rabitsch W, et al. Successful use of extracorporeal photochemotherapy in the treatment of severe acute and chronic graft-versus-host disease. Blood 1998;92:3098–104.
[22] Kuzmina Z, Greinix HT, Knobler R, et al. Proportions of immature CD19⁺CD21⁻ B lymphocytes predict the response to extracorporeal photopheresis in patients with chronic graft-versus-host disease. Blood 2009;114:744–6.
[23] Tangye SG, Bryant VL, Cuss AK, Good KL. BAFF, APRIL and human B cell disorders. Semin Immunol 2006;18:305–17.
[24] Mariette X, Roux S, Zhang J, et al. The level of BLyS (BAFF) correlates with the titre of autoantibodies in human Sjogren's syndrome. Ann Rheum Dis 2003;62:168–71.
[25] Matsushita T, Hasegawa M, Yanaba K, Kodera M, Takehara K, Sato S. Elevated serum BAFF levels in patients with systemic sclerosis: enhanced BAFF signalling in systemic sclerosis B lymphocytes. Arthritis Rheum 2006;54:192–201.
[26] Goodnow CC, Cyter JG, Hartley SB, et al. Self-tolerance checkpoints in B lymphocyte development. Adv Immunol 1995;59:279–368.
[27] Whittle R, Taylor PC. Circulating B-cell activating factor level predicts clinical response of chronic graft-versus-host disease to extracorporeal photopheresis. Blood 2011;118:6446–9.
[28] Whittle R, Denney H, Alfred A, Taylor PC. Circulating B-cell activating factor level predicts likelihood of chronic GVHD flare and probability of successful steroid taper during extracorporeal photopheresis therapy. Bone Marrow Transplant 2012; 47 (Suppl 1):O320.

Section 6: ECP for the Prevention of Graft-versus-Host Disease

Carrie Kitko and John E. Levine
6 ECP for the Prevention of Graft-versus-Host Disease

6.1 Introduction

Allogeneic hematopoietic cell transplantation (HCT) is one of the most powerful forms of cellular therapy, but graft-versus-host disease (GVHD) remains the main cause of non-relapse mortality following HCT. Current GVHD prevention strategies focus on eliminating or attenuating donor T cell alloreactivity with such techniques as in-vitro or in-vivo T cell depletion or pharmacologic targeting of T cell function [1, 2]. Commonly used GVHD prophylaxis strategies result in rates of GVHD of 40–60% depending on donor source and preparative regimen used, resulting in significant morbidity and mortality for transplant recipients. Novel prevention strategies that target other pathways involved in the development of GVHD are needed. One such approach is extracorporeal photopheresis (ECP), which has been shown to impact on two key components of the GVHD pathway, dendritic cells (DCs) and regulatory T cells (Tregs).

6.2 Standard GVHD Prevention Strategies

In order to highlight the potential role that ECP may add to GVHD prevention, it is important to review which components of the GVHD pathway have been targeted and the success of these strategies.

6.2.1 Methotrexate

GVHD prophylactic treatments have largely focused on the use of alkylators and antimetabolities following HCT. The first widely adopted treatment was methotrexate (MTX), a folate antagonist, which was shown to be effective at reducing GVHD severity and prolonging survival, first in canine models [3] and later in clinical trials [4]. The mechanism of action is thought to be the elimination of recently infused, rapidly proliferating donor lymphocytes that have been activated by recognition of minor or major histocompatibility antigens (MHC) on recipient tissue. After attempting several dosing schedules, the standard treatment regimen used for more than a decade included treatment on days 1, 3, 6 and 11 post-HCT followed by once weekly dosing. Unfortunately, the rates of severe, life-threatening, grades III-IV acute GVHD, were still as high as 25% in the sibling donor setting [5] leading to the introduction of additional agents to MTX for improved GVHD prevention and MTX alone is no longer used.

6.2.2 Cyclophosphamide

However, the approach of targeting activated, proliferating lymphocytes has recently been revisited. Cyclophosphamide (CY) is another chemotherapeutic agent that causes apoptosis of alloreactive T cells and has the advantage of not causing toxicity to the hematopoietic stem cells [6–8]. Following a myeloablative conditioning regimen, 78 related and 39 unrelated HLA-matched HCT recipients received CY 50 mg/kg on days 3 and 4 post-HCT as their sole GVHD prophylaxis. This regimen resulted in successful engraftment in 114 patients (98%) and a day 100 cumulative incidence of grades II-IV GVHD of 43%, with a 10% rate of grades III-IV GVHD. Of note, though these rates of acute GVHD are similar to those reported with other commonly used regimens for prevention, a low 10% cumulative incidence of chronic GVHD was observed [9]. In a subset analysis of 50 patients from the clinical trial, the investigators found higher levels of Foxp3 mRNA levels, a surrogate marker for Treg numbers, in those patients that did not develop GVHD. This was further supported by a smaller subgroup that demonstrated more rapid recovery, as early as day 30, of $CD4^+$ $CD25^+$ $Foxp3^+$ cells in those patients that did not develop GVHD compared to extremely low levels of these cells, even at day 60 in those developing GVHD [10].

6.2.3 Calcineurin Inhibitors

In an effort to improve the efficacy of single agent MTX, combination therapy with calcineurin inhibitors (CNI), which block interleukin-2 (IL-2) mediated T cell expansion and cytotoxicity, was introduced. Initial clinical trials using cyclosporine (CSA), the first clinically available CNI, as monotherapy for GVHD prevention were not successful [11]. However, the combination of an initial brief course of MTX and a prolonged course of CSA proved to be beneficial at both reducing the rates of acute GVHD and improving overall survival in patients with aplastic anemia as well as acute and chronic myelogenous leukemia [12–15]. When this combination was used in the unrelated donor setting, there was still an unacceptably high rate of grades II-IV and grades III-IV acute GVHD of 77% and 35% respectively [16], leading to the introduction of a new CNI, tacrolimus (Tacro), as an alternative. Phase III randomized studies comparing CSA/MTX to Tacro/MTX for prevention of GVHD following allogeneic HCT were performed. In the sibling donor setting, Tacro/MTX had lower rates of acute GVHD grades II-IV (32% vs 44%, p=0.01), though this did not translate into improved disease free survival. Post hoc analyses concluded that the improved GVHD control was offset by increased relapses in the Tacro arm. However, a higher proportion of patients with advanced malignancies (41% vs 29%, p=0.02) was randomized to the tacro arm, suggesting that the increased relapse rate may have been due to imbalances in randomization rather than tacro inhibiting a graft-versus-leukemia effect [17]. A phase III randomized study that evaluated CSA/MTX versus Tacro/MTX following unrelated donor HCT found Tacro/MTX to be superior in terms of occurrence of grades II-IV GVHD (56% vs 74%, p=0.002) which resulted in fewer of the Tacro/MTX patients requiring treatment with glucocorticoids [18].

6.2.4 Mycophenolate Mofetil

Substitutions for MTX have been sought due to the undesirable side effect of delayed engraftment and increased oral mucositis and other gastrointestinal (GI) toxicity. In fact, in the two initial phase III trials comparing CNI combined with MTX, only about 66% of patients were able to receive all four planned doses of MTX due to excessive GI toxicity [17, 18]. In addition, alternative transplant approaches, such as cord blood transplant or non-myeloablative (NMA), raise concern for delayed engraftment or graft failure both of which may be exacerbated by the use of MTX for GVHD prevention. One approach often used in the NMA setting involves replacement of MTX with mycophenolate mofetil (MMF) which is a prodrug, that following hydrolysis to its active form, mycophenolic acid (MPA), leads to reversible inhibition of purine synthesis in T and B lymphocytes, buildup of toxic metabolites, and cell death. Several studies have demonstrated the use of MMF with a CNI following NMA HCT enhances engraftment and reduces rates of grades II–IV GVHD (16–47%) [19–21], but these results have not been as convincingly replicated following myeloablative conditioning [22, 23].

6.2.5 Sirolimus

Another approach has been to substitute MTX with sirolimus, also known as rapamycin, which inhibits the mammalian target of rapamycin (m-TOR), blocking IL-2 signaling and causing effector T cells to become unresponsive and eventually apoptotic [24]. Sirolimus (siro) has several other potentially favorable effects including inhibition of dendritic cell (DC) maturation thereby decreasing antigen presentation to donor T cells and relative sparing of the function of regulatory T cells [25]. Cutler et al reported the outcome of 53 related and 30 unrelated donor myeloablative total body irradiation (TBI)/CY HCT recipients that received tacro/siro without MTX. Outcome for both related and unrelated donors was excellent, with only 5% transplant-related mortality (TRM) by day 100, and cumulative incidence of grades II-IV and grades III-IV acute GVHD of 21% and 5% respectively [26]. Similar results with tacro/siro for GVHD prevention have been reported with other conditioning regimens such as fludarabine/melphalan, etoposide/TBI and busulfan/CY. However, patients that received busulfan based conditioning regimens were more likely to experience severe toxicity such as veno-occlusive disease (VOD) and transplant-associated microangiopathy (TMA) [27]. This concern for increased toxicity of tacro/siro following busulfan-based conditioning was also borne out during a multi-institution phase III study randomizing patients to tacro/siro or tacro/MTX. Higher than expected rates of VOD occurred in recipients of busulfan based conditioning and the combination with tacro/siro was no longer permitted [28].

6.3 GVHD Prevention with ECP: Potential Mechanism of Action

The mechanisms by which ECP is effective for treatment of GVHD are discussed extensively in Section 3 of this book. Briefly, work by Ferrara et al and others have helped establish the framework of our understanding of GVHD pathophysiology [29–31]. The GVHD pathway is initiated by the conditioning regimen which leads to tissue damage, and resultant increases in inflammatory cytokines. This increased inflammatory milieu primes the second phase during which presentation of MHC antigens by host DCs to donor T cells occurs, leading to donor T cell activation and further increases in inflammatory cytokines. In the final phase, the effector immune cells cause direct cytotoxicity of host tissue, which is amplified further by inflammatory mediators such as LPS, tumor necrosis factor (TNF)-α and interleukin (IL)-1 (Figure 6.1a). There are four essential components necessary for this process to proceed, which include 1) Triggers such as MHC mismatch and strength of conditioning, 2) Sensors, largely comprised of antigen presenting cells (APCs) such as DCs, 3) Mediators including donor T cell subsets such as naive CD4+ and CD8+ T cells as well as Tregs, and 4) Effectors of GVHD typically comprising cytotoxic T cells and inflammatory cytokines.

Most GVHD prevention strategies have targeted the effectors of the GVHD process, typically with T cell directed therapies. There is emerging evidence, however, that it is possible to target the sensors and mediators of GVHD to also prevent or lessen the severity of GVHD. Experimental GVHD data from mouse models, as well as results from patients treated with ECP, lend support to the hypothesis that ECP can prevent GVHD by effecting both the DC (sensor) and Treg (mediator) populations.

6.3.1 Targeting Dendritic Cells

Shlomchik et al used a mouse model of allogeneic HCT where strains were MHC-identical, but had multiple minor histocompatibility antigen (miHAs) differences to show that transplantation into a host with recipient DCs unable to present class I restricted peptides resulted in significant reduction in GVHD [32]. Furthermore, after the initiation of GVHD, donor derived APCs continue to contribute to the ongoing severity of disease [33, 34]. Various prevention strategies in mouse models have been employed to impair DC function and/or alter phenotype in order to abrogate GVHD. One such strategy has been the use of histone deacetylase inhibitors (HDACi) to block antigen presentation by DCs. Initial mouse models using HDACi focused on initiation of therapy once GVHD had already been established, with treatment given from days +3 to +7. Mice receiving HDACi demonstrated lower levels of inflammatory cytokines, decreased severity of GVHD and increased overall survival [35]. It was also noted that treatment with HDACi did not diminish the ability of donor T cells to respond to host antigens when exposed to host antigen in vitro. In a subsequent study, the authors treated host-type DCs ex vivo with HDACi followed by infusion of the treated DCs into

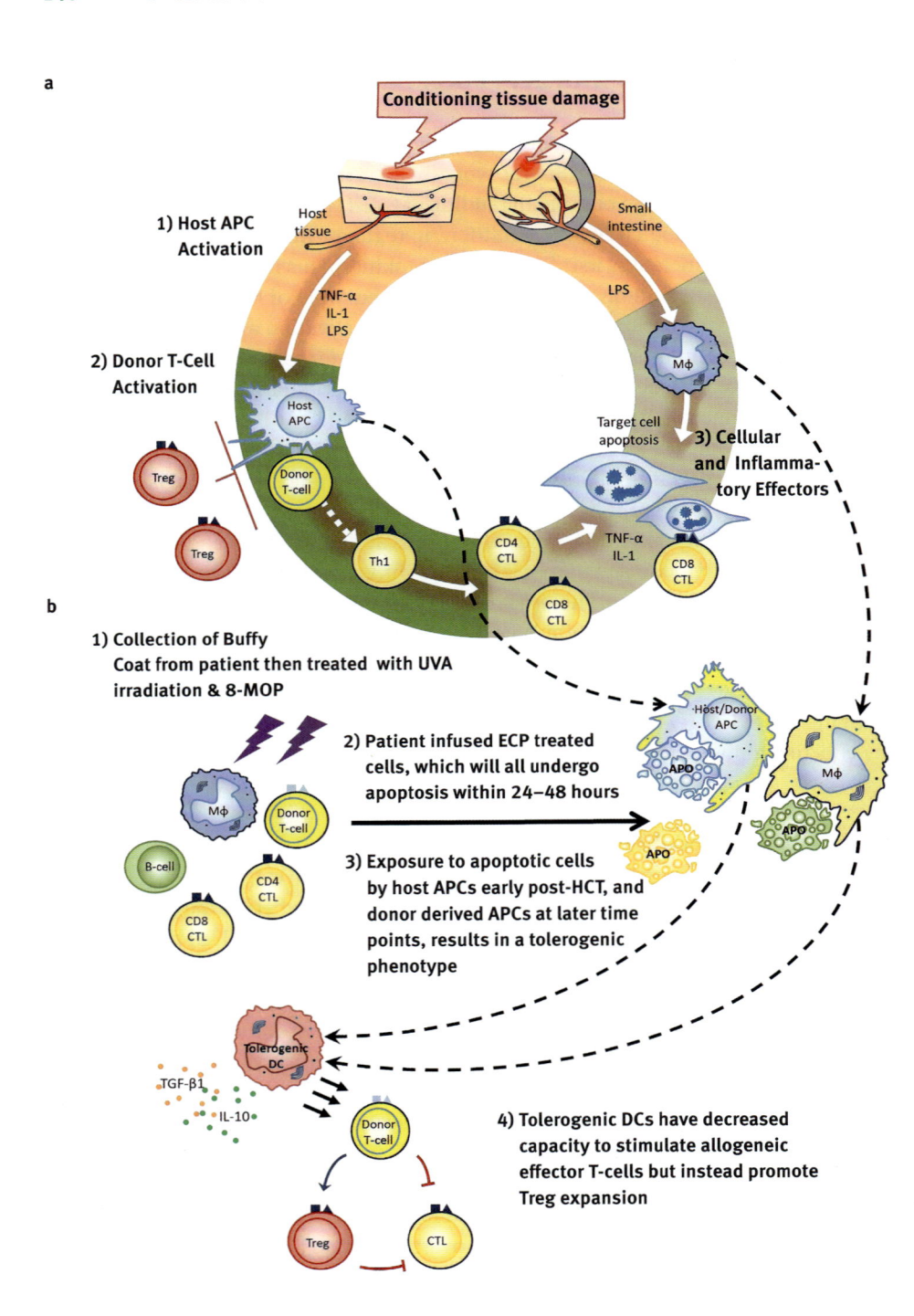

140 — 6 ECP for the Prevention of Graft-versus-Host Disease

Fig. 6.1.

MHC mismatched transplanted mice on days −1, 0 and +2, resulting in reduced inflammatory cytokines, reduced severity of GVHD and increased survival [36]. These results support the hypothesis that modulation of DC function in the early transplant period may successfully reduce rates and severity of GVHD. ECP may result in a similar effect.

Following ECP treatment, 8-methoxypsoralen (8-MOP) and ultraviolet A (UVA) exposed lymphocytes, NK cells and monocytes undergo apoptosis within 24 to 48 hours and when these apoptotic cells are ingested by DCs, the DCs acquire a tolerogeneic phenotype [37]. Several papers have supported the premise that ingestion of apoptotic cells by DCs leads to the development of a tolerant DC phenotype through the promotion of anti-inflammatory cytokine secretion such as transforming growth factor (TGF)-β1, prostaglandin E2 and platelet-activating factor (PAF) [38–42].

6.3.2 Targeting Regulatory T Cells

An important mediator of immunologic tolerance are Tregs, which are also classified as mediators of the GVHD reaction. Several early murine models demonstrated that infusion of donor derived Tregs following both minor and major MHC mismatched HCT resulted in improved GVHD morbidity and survival [43–45]. One pharmacologic approach to increasing Tregs includes post-HCT combination therapy with IL-2 and rapamycin. Shin et al demonstrated, that following an MHC mismatched transplant, combination therapy with IL-2 and rapamycin, starting at the time of HCT, resulted in superior overall survival and decreased GVHD morbidity, compared to either treat-

Fig. 6.1. (a) Pathophysiology of GVHD.
This involves three phases, including 1) damage induced by the HCT preparative regimen which leads to increased inflammatory cytokine secretion which is sensed by host antigen presenting cells (APCs), leading to their activation. 2) Activated host APCs then interact with donor T cells, mediators of GVHD, leading to their activation, proliferation and differentiation. Treatments that promote increases in regulatory T cells (Treg) can suppress this reaction. And finally, if the process is left unchecked, increased activated alloreactive cells cause tissue damage and the release of more inflammatory cytokines that are also harmful to host tissues.
(b) ECP for GVHD Prevention.
1) Patients undergo a leukapheresis during ECP treatment, and these white blood cells are exposed to 8-methoxypsoralen (8-MOP) and ultraviolet A radiation. 2) Treated cells are reinfused to the patient, and all will undergo apoptosis within 24 to 48 hours of treatment. 3) APCs are able to engulf these apoptotic cells. Early post-HCT these APCs will be of host-origin, but at later time points, donor derived APCs will also participate in this process. After apoptotic cell uptake, DCs and macrophages promote tolerance through the secretion of anti-inflammatory cytokines such as TGF-β and IL-10. 4) These tolerogeneic DCs are unable to stimulate the differentiation of donor T cells into cytotoxic lymphocytes, but will promote increased number and function of Tregs. Thus ECP for prophylaxis can potentially modulate the traditional GVHD pathway by changing the DC phenotype to promote tolerance rather than alloreactivity through the generation of increased numbers of Treg.
(Figures courtsey of Lawrence Chang, MD, MPH)

ment in isolation. The improved outcomes were felt to be secondary to a statistically significant increase in absolute number of donor Treg (p<0.05) and reduction in pro-GVHD cytokines such as interferon-gamma (IFN-γ; p<0.001) and TNF-α (p<0.05) [46].

In addition to murine data, there is abundant clinical data to support that Tregs are a key mediator of GVHD following allogeneic HCT. Decreased Treg frequency has been observed in allogeneic HCT recipients at the time of GVHD onset compared to levels at similar time points post-HCT in autologous HCT recipients and allogeneic HCT recipients who never develop GVHD [47]. In addition, patients with the lowest levels of Tregs at onset of GVHD were less likely to respond to treatment, resulting in greater nonrelapse mortality (NRM) [47].

Given the high risk of GVHD and other post-transplant complications such as non-engraftment and immune reconstitution following cord blood and haplo-identical transplant, clinical studies of the potential benefit of post-HCT infusion of ex-vivo expanded Tregs have been performed and demonstrated safety, and potentially some benefit toward reducing rates of GVHD [48, 49]. Rates of acute GVHD following double cord transplantation can be as high as 60%. To attempt to reduce this and improve subsequent overall survival, Brunstein et al performed the first human clinical trial using unrelated donor cord blood expanded Tregs for infusion into patients following double cord blood transplantation. In this trial, 23 patients received a reduced intensity preparative regimen followed by the infusion of two 4–6/6 HLA matched umbilical cord units. The GVHD prophylaxis consisted of MMF and CSA, except for the final six patients who received siro/MMF to further promote long-term survival of Treg. Tregs were isolated from a third 4–6/6 HLA matched cord blood unit by positive selection of CD25+ cells, and then expanded for 18 days in prolonged culture with appropriate growth factors and cytokines such as IL-2, and co-stimulation with anti-CD3/anti-CD28 monoclonal antibody-coated Dynabeads, such that they would be available for infusion on d+1 post-HCT. The median expansion achieved was 211-fold, and all Treg products demonstrated suppressive function in vitro. The targeted cell dose for Treg infusion was 30×10^5/kg, which was achieved in 18 of the 23 patients. The study group was compared to a historical control of 108 adult double cord blood HCT recipients transplanted with the same preparative regimen who received MMF/CSA for GVHD prophylaxis. The authors found that patients receiving Treg infusions had lower rates of GVHD (43% vs 61%, p=0.05). Importantly, Treg infusions did not appear to have a negative impact on rates of infection, relapse or early mortality [48]. This preliminary work demonstrated that expanded Treg infusion following standard double cord transplantation is feasible, although additional studies are needed to better assess efficacy. The challenge to the application of these strategies is obtaining the large number of Tregs needed. ECP may allow an in vivo treatment approach in the peritransplant period, as well as after engraftment, that may allow for enhancement of Treg populations in post-HCT recipients.

As demonstrated by Gatza and Ferrara in a murine model, administration of ECP treated cells after GVHD resulted in improved clinical GVHD score, less GVHD pathology in the liver, gut and skin and most importantly, improved survival by approximately 50%. Treated animals had elevated levels of Tregs in the thymus and spleen, and the beneficial effects of receiving ECP-treated cells was lost if the animals also received anti-CD25 antibody in order to deplete Treg [50]. Several clinical studies have also demonstrated increased levels of Tregs following ECP treatment of acute and chronic GVHD as well as treatment for solid organ rejection. Two small case series that included 10 and 8 patients, respectively demonstrated a significant increase in Tregs from baseline following ECP treatment [51, 52]. In the larger of the two studies, Biagi et al found that after 6 treatments, Tregs increased from 8.9% to 29.1% of total CD4+ cells ($p<0.05$), and this increase was sustained even after 12 procedures [51]. Of note, this patient population included patients with both acute and chronic GVHD, and all patients responded to ECP therapy. In another small case series of lung transplant recipients, Meloni et al found that 6 patients experienced a decline in Treg that seemed to parallel their decline in lung function prior to the initiation of therapy. After ECP was initiated, there was a stabilization or increase in Treg numbers for 3 of 6 patients that paralleled their stabilization in lung function [53].

A recent murine model for GVHD prophylaxis investigated infusion of ECP-treated cells on the same day as donor lymphocyte infusion (DLI). ECP-treated splenocytes were infused in a separate injection just prior to DLI given on days 14 and 28 following a T cell depleted HCT. There was also a comparison "therapeutic" group that received an infusion of ECP-treated splenocytes one day after a T cell replete HCT. The authors found that control GVHD mice experienced approximately 25% weight loss, a marker of GVHD severity, compared to the attenuated 10–15% weight loss in the ECP treatment groups, and no weight loss in the ECP prophylaxis group [54].

6.3.3 Targeting Dendritic Cells and Regulatory T Cells

It is important to recognize that these two potential mechanisms, generation of tolerogeneic DCs and regulatory T cells, may not be independent pathways, but in fact, complementary. It is known that Tregs recognize alloantigen presented on MHC class II molecules, and it is this interaction that is critical for their activation and survival [55]. A recent murine model demonstrated that host APCs are essential for donor Treg-induced GVHD suppression. This was observed in both MHC-matched and mismatched models. Using several different chimeric backgrounds, the authors were able to demonstrate that MHC class II expression specifically on host APCs was necessary and sufficient to promote donor Treg suppression of GVHD [56]. In another murine model, Sela et al. expanded inducibile antigen specific Tregs ex vivo by combining DCs and T cells in an mixed lymphocyte reaction (MLR) that were MHC mismatched in the presence of TGF-β and all-trans retinoic acid (ATRA). This approach yielded a 70% increase in the induction of Treg. When these inducible Treg were infused simultaneously with MHC mismatched T cell replete HCT, the animals had markedly improved

GVHD survival and decreased GVHD associated weight loss. The transferred Tregs were able to be identified 2.5 months following HCT, indicating that these cells were long-lived [57].

There is also evidence to support that a pharmacologic approach to GVHD prevention, possibly through direct effects on cytokine production of DCs, results in expansion of the Treg population. Tawara et al analyzed the outcomes of a murine haploidentical HCT model in which the experimental recipients also received Alpha-1-antitrypsin (AAT) monotherapy starting just before HCT, and continuing through day 13 post-HCT. This approach resulted in 100% survival of AAT treated recipients, compared to 50% survival in the GVHD control mice (p<0.02). Administration of AAT resulted in reduced expansion of T effector cells, but expansion of Tregs. In order to further elucidate potential mechanisms of Treg expansion, the authors incubated BM-derived DCs from B6 mice overnight with AAT, then stimulated the treated DCs with LPS. They found significant reductions in pro-inflammatory cytokines, including TNF-α, IL-1β and IL-6, while levels of the anti-inflammatory cytokine IL-10 were markedly increased [58].

Finally, in a murine model of cardiac allograft rejection, Zheng et al. investigated ECP as a potential treatment. First the authors analyzed recipient DC maturation in the presence of donor splenocytes that did or did not undergo ECP treatment. Those DCs exposed to ECP treated donor splenocytes demonstrated lower expression of DC maturation markers such as CD40, CD86 and MHC-II, and also resulted in higher levels of IL-10. Infusion of ECP-splenocyte exposed DCs into cardiac allograft recipients resulted in prolonged allograft survival (32 days versus 8 days, p<0.01) [59].

6.4 Extracorporeal Photopheresis during HCT Preparative Regimens

Addition of ECP to HCT preparative regimens was initially attempted to help overcome graft failure following NMA conditioning. Since ECP treatment induces tolerogeneic DCs, treatment with ECP prior to HCT may result in less rejection of donor hematopoietic elements by residual host DCs. Therefore, one early strategy in NMA HCT explored a regimen that combined ECP, pentostatin and low-dose TBI in order to decrease DC function and therefore promote donor chimerism. Miller et al performed a total of 55 NMA HCT using ECP (given on two consecutive days), followed by 48 hours of continuous infusion of pentostatin (4 mg/m^2/day × 2 days), and TBI of 200 cGy × 3 doses (600 cGy total) [60]. All patients also received CSA, MTX and MMF as GVHD prophylaxis. Forty-four patients received sibling donor HCT (80%) using this preparative regimen, and it was well tolerated. Consistent with the hypothesis that the regimen would promote donor engraftment, high rates of donor chimerism (98%) and low rates (11%) of NRM at 100 days post HCT were observed. An unanticipated outcome was that patients treated with this regimen had lower than expected rates of both acute and chronic GVHD. Grades

II–IV GVHD were seen in 9% of patients, and severe grades III-IV in only 4%. However, chronic GVHD developed in 43% of patients. The two-year event free survival (EFS) was 47%. Given that malignancy was the indication for transplant in this study, most patients had received several lines of therapy prior to HCT, which may have immunosuppressed the recipients such that the NMA conditioning was sufficient to support engraftment. Further studies to better elucidate the role ECP during conditioning may play in facilitating engraftment following NMA HCT have not yet been published.

Based on these results, a phase II multi-institutional study evaluated the role of ECP pre-HCT using a myeloablative preparative regimen [61]. All 62 patients received CY (60 mg/kg/day × 2 days) and TBI (10-13.5 Gy over 3–4 days) and were treated with two days of ECP within four days of starting the preparative regimen. Standard GVHD prophylaxis included CSA and MTX. Half of the study participants received a sibling donor HCT. The 100 day cumulative incidence (CI) of acute GVHD grades II-IV was 35%, and the one year CI of chronic GVHD was 38%, with a one year DFS of 69%. Data from the Center for International Blood and Marrow Transplant Research (CIBMTR) formed a historic control. Compared to 347 matched historical controls, the ECP treated group had a lower rate of grades II-IV acute GVHD (relative risk 0.61; 95% CI, 0.38–0.97; p=0.04). While far from definitive, these findings support further investigation into ECP as a GVHD prevention strategy.

6.5 ECP for Prevention of Solid Organ Rejection

Solid organ rejection is a clinical model for GVHD because similar processes of allorecognition are operative. Acute rejection following solid organ transplantation has been successfully treated with ECP [62]. More recently, clinical investigators have explored the possibility of adding ECP to upfront strategies for prevention of acute rejection. These studies further support ECP for GVHD prophylaxis. In a recent publication, Kusztal et al. performed a randomized study investigating the use of standard immunosuppression with MMF, a CNI and prednisone ± ECP given for the first three months post renal allograft (total of 12–16 treatments given). Twenty patients received renal allografts from 10 cadaveric donors, and were randomly assigned to the ECP group or the control group. There were no episodes of acute rejection in the ECP treated patients and one in the control group. There was a non-significant trend toward improved kidney function in the ECP group at three months post-allograft which correlated with a higher percentage of Tregs among CD3+ cells (9.4% ± 15% vs 3% ± 1%; p=0.01). An increased percentage of immature myeloid DCs was also observed in the ECP treatment group at 6 months after completion of the study (89% vs 69%, p=0.08) [63]. These findings support the hypothesis that early post-allograft ECP treatments promote a tolerogenic shift in the immune environment through increases in Tregs and immature DCs. Although the data is preliminary, ECP treatment may result in fewer episodes of acute rejection.

6.6 ECP for GVHD Prevention: Tolerogeneic DC and Treg Induction

Currently, a clinical trial at the University of Michigan is testing a novel approach to GVHD prevention that combines TNF-α inhibition with etanercept and Treg induction with ECP, added to standard MMF and CNI following a reduced intensity unrelated donor transplant (URD). Etanercept is given twice weekly starting on the day of transplant for 16 total doses to provide blockade of known GVHD pathways prior to and following early engraftment, when ECP cannot be reliably delivered. Weekly ECP initiation begins at d +28, after adequate engraftment has been achieved, and is given on a tapering schedule through d +180 for a total of 11-12 treatments. The rationale for this design is that broad, multipathway coverage for GVHD is provided through d +56, when patients are most at risk for developing severe early acute GVHD, and double coverage continues from d +56 through d +180 since late onset acute GVHD and classic chronic GVHD continue to be problematic, and may be prevented or attenuated with this prophylactic approach. This trial will finish accrual by mid-2012.

There are several factors that are important to consider when designing a clinical trial that will incorporate ECP for GVHD prevention. One of the most critical is the time to engraftment. Until the white blood count is reliably greater than 1×10^9/L, it is not possible to deliver effective ECP treatments. Therefore, in order to have an impact on very early GVHD prevention, it will likely be necessary to utilize a highly effective regimen for the first 2–4 weeks post-HCT. In the University of Michigan approach, etanercept was added based on our previous experience using this agent plus tacrolimus and MTX following full intensity HCT [64]. Another potential approach may be to add complementary treatments to enhance Treg induction such as sirolimus [65] or low dose IL-2 [66], as both have been shown to increase the numbers of Tregs.

Patient selection is also a critical factor to the success of ECP for GVHD prevention. Adequate venous access is essential for delivery of consistent ECP treatments. Patients with poor venous access, such as a history of recurrent deep venous thromboses (DVTs) or very young patients who might not be able to have appropriate catheter placement, will likely not be candidates for such interventions. Another important consideration is the stability of the patients' hematocrit and platelet count following HCT. Patients unlikely to respond well to transfusions, such as those with a known history of splenomegaly or platelet refractoriness will likely have challenges to reliably adhering to a set ECP schedule. In addition, patients receiving a major ABO-incompatible HCT may face similar challenges to meet the hematocrit parameters for safe ECP administration.

Finally patient comorbidities will also have a major impact on the safety of ECP delivery. Patients with a known cardiac history may have a poor tolerance for the fluid shifts associated with ECP treatment, and may be at increased risk for ischemic events. Also, patients with known hemostatic disorders such as recurrent DVTs or a history of increased bleeding risk such as a hemorrhagic stroke will likely have a higher than expected risk associated with the anticoagulation provided during a routine ECP administration.

6.7 Conclusions

Despite many improvements in GVHD prevention strategies, this post-HCT complication remains one of the main contributors to morbidity and mortality following allogeneic HCT. Future strategies that focus on promoting tolerance through a variety of mechanisms such as inhibition of DC function or alteration toward a tolerogeneic phenotype may promote the expansion of Tregs in vivo. There is an ever expanding body of evidence to support that ECP may be an important modality to impact both of these sensors and mediators of the GVHD pathway that would result in less alloreactivity, and therefore, less GVHD (Figure 6.1b). In addition, since ECP is felt to be immunomodulating, rather than immunosuppressive, this potential decreased GVHD will not come at the expense of higher infectious complications. Moving forward, clinical investigators will need to focus on the challenges of delivering ECP treatments during the most critical period for GVHD development.

References

[1] Ferrara JL, Levine JE, Reddy P, Holler E. Graft-versus-host disease. Lancet 2009;373(9674): 1550–61.
[2] Ram R, Gafter-Gvili A, Yeshurun M, Paul M, Raanani P, Shpilberg O. Prophylaxis regimens for GVHD: systematic review and meta-analysis. Bone Marrow Transplant 2009;43:643–53.
[3] Storb R, Epstein RB, Graham TC, Thomas ED. Methotrexate regimens for control of graft-versus-host disease in dogs with allogeneic marrow grafts. Transplantation 1970;9:240–6.
[4] Thomas E, Storb R, Clift RA, et al. Bone-marrow transplantation (first of two parts). N Engl J Med 1975;292:832–43.
[5] Storb R, Prentice RL, Buckner CD, et al. Graft-versus-host disease and survival in patients with aplastic anemia treated by marrow grafts from HLA-identical siblings. Beneficial effect of a protective environment. N Engl J Med 1983;308:302–7.
[6] Brodsky RA, Jones RJ. Aplastic anaemia. Lancet 2005;365(9471):1647–56.
[7] Jones RJ, Barber JP, Vala MS, et al. Assessment of aldehyde dehydrogenase in viable cells. Blood 1995;85:2742–6.
[8] Luznik L, Engstrom LW, Iannone R, Fuchs EJ. Posttransplantation cyclophosphamide facilitates engraftment of major histocompatibility complex-identical allogeneic marrow in mice conditioned with low-dose total body irradiation. Biol Blood Marrow Transplant 2002;8: 131–8.
[9] Luznik L, Bolanos-Meade J, Zahurak M, et al. High-dose cyclophosphamide as single-agent, short-course prophylaxis of graft-versus-host disease. Blood 2010;115:3224–30.
[10] Hess A, Fuchs EJ, Luznik L, et al. Rapid reconstitution of the regulator T cell compartment after high dose Cy prevents the development of GVHD after allogeneic BMT. Biol Blood Marrow Transplant 2010;16:S168.
[11] Storb R, Deeg HJ, Fisher L, et al. Cyclosporine v methotrexate for graft-v-host disease prevention in patients given marrow grafts for leukemia: long-term follow-up of three controlled trials. Blood 1988;71:293–8.
[12] Storb R, Deeg HJ, Farewell V, et al. Marrow transplantation for severe aplastic anemia: methotrexate alone compared with a combination of methotrexate and cyclosporine for prevention of acute graft-versus-host disease. Blood 1986;68:119–25.

[13] Storb R, Deeg HJ, Whitehead J, et al. Methotrexate and cyclosporine compared with cyclosporine alone for prophylaxis of acute graft versus host disease after marrow transplantation for leukemia. N Engl J Med 1986;314:729–35.

[14] Sorror ML, Leisenring W, Deeg HJ, Martin PJ, Storb R. Re: Twenty-year follow-up in patients with aplastic anemia given marrow grafts from HLA-identical siblings and randomized to receive methotrexate/cyclosporine or methotrexate alone for prevention of graft-versus-host disease. Biol Blood Marrow Transplant 2005;11:567–8.

[15] Sorror ML, Leisenring W, Deeg HJ, Martin PJ, Storb R. Twenty-year follow-up of a controlled trial comparing a combination of methotrexate plus cyclosporine with cyclosporine alone for prophylaxis of graft-versus-host disease in patients administered HLA-identical marrow grafts for leukemia. Biol Blood Marrow Transplant 2005;11:814–5.

[16] Hansen JA, Gooley TA, Martin PJ, et al. Bone marrow transplants from unrelated donors for patients with chronic myeloid leukemia. N Engl J Med 1998;338:962–8.

[17] Ratanatharathorn V, Nash RA, Przepiorka D, et al. Phase III study comparing methotrexate and tacrolimus (prograf, FK506) with methotrexate and cyclosporine for graft-versus-host disease prophylaxis after HLA-identical sibling bone marrow transplantation. Blood 1998;92:2303–14.

[18] Nash RA, Antin JH, Karanes C, et al. Phase 3 study comparing methotrexate and tacrolimus with methotrexate and cyclosporine for prophylaxis of acute graft-versus-host disease after marrow transplantation from unrelated donors. Blood 2000;96:2062–8.

[19] McSweeney PA, Niederwieser D, Shizuru JA, et al. Hematopoietic cell transplantation in older patients with hematologic malignancies: replacing high-dose cytotoxic therapy with graft-versus-tumor effects. Blood 2001;97:3390–400.

[20] Maris MB, Niederwieser D, Sandmaier BM, et al. HLA-matched unrelated donor hematopoietic cell transplantation after nonmyeloablative conditioning for patients with hematologic malignancies. Blood 2003;102:2021–30.

[21] Nieto Y, Patton N, Hawkins T, et al. Tacrolimus and mycophenolate mofetil after nonmyeloablative matched-sibling donor allogeneic stem-cell transplantations conditioned with fludarabine and low-dose total body irradiation. Biol Blood Marrow Transplant 2006;12:217–25.

[22] Nash RA, Johnston L, Parker P, et al. A phase I/II study of mycophenolate mofetil in combination with cyclosporine for prophylaxis of acute graft-versus-host disease after myeloablative conditioning and allogeneic hematopoietic cell transplantation. Biol Blood Marrow Transplant 2005;11:495–505.

[23] Perkins J, Field T, Kim J, et al. A randomized phase II trial comparing tacrolimus and mycophenolate mofetil to tacrolimus and methotrexate for acute graft-versus-host disease prophylaxis. Biol Blood Marrow Transplant 2010;16:937–47.

[24] Bensinger SJ, Walsh PT, Zhang J, et al. Distinct IL-2 receptor signaling pattern in CD4+CD25+ regulatory T cells. J Immunol 2004;172:5287–96.

[25] Battaglia M, Stabilini A, Roncarolo MG. Rapamycin selectively expands CD4+CD25+FoxP3+ regulatory T cells. Blood 2005;105:4743–8.

[26] Cutler C, Li S, Ho VT, et al. Extended follow-up of methotrexate-free immunosuppression using sirolimus and tacrolimus in related and unrelated donor peripheral blood stem cell transplantation. Blood 2007;109:3108–14.

[27] Rodriguez R, Nakamura R, Palmer JM, et al. A phase II pilot study of tacrolimus/sirolimus GVHD prophylaxis for sibling donor hematopoietic stem cell transplantation using 3 conditioning regimens. Blood 2010;115:1098–105.

[28] Cutler C, Stevenson K, Kim HT, et al. Sirolimus is associated with veno-occlusive disease of the liver after myeloablative allogeneic stem cell transplantation. Blood 2008;112:4425–31.

[29] Antin JH, Ferrara JL. Cytokine dysregulation and acute graft-versus-host disease. Blood 1992;80:2964–8.

[30] Reddy P, Ferrara JL. Immunobiology of acute graft-versus-host disease. Blood Reviews 2003;17:187–94.

[31] Cooke KR, Olkiewicz K, Erickson N, Ferrara JL. The role of endotoxin and the innate immune response in the pathophysiology of acute graft versus host disease. J Endotoxin Research 2002; 8:441–8.
[32] Shlomchik WD, Couzens MS, Tang CB, et al. Prevention of graft versus host disease by inactivation of host antigen-presenting cells. Science 1999;285(5426):412–5.
[33] Matte CC, Liu J, Cormier J, et al. Donor APCs are required for maximal GVHD but not for GVL. Nat Med 2004;10:987–92.
[34] Reddy P, Maeda Y, Liu C, Krijanovski OI, Korngold R, Ferrara JL. A crucial role for antigen-presenting cells and alloantigen expression in graft-versus-leukemia responses. Nat Med 2005; 11:1244–9.
[35] Reddy P, Maeda Y, Hotary K, et al. Histone deacetylase inhibitor suberoylanilide hydroxamic acid reduces acute graft-versus-host disease and preserves graft-versus-leukemia effect. Proc Nat Acad Sci U.S.A. 2004;101:3921–6.
[36] Reddy P, Sun Y, Toubai T, et al. Histone deacetylase inhibition modulates indoleamine 2,3-dioxygenase-dependent DC functions and regulates experimental graft-versus-host disease in mice. J Clin Invest 2008;118:2562–73.
[37] Lamioni A, Parisi F, Isacchi G, et al. The immunological effects of extracorporeal photopheresis unraveled: induction of tolerogenic dendritic cells in vitro and regulatory T cells in vivo. Transplantation 2005;79:846–50.
[38] Lucas M, Stuart LM, Savill J, Lacy-Hulbert A. Apoptotic cells and innate immune stimuli combine to regulate macrophage cytokine secretion. J Immunol 2003;171:2610–5.
[39] Fadok VA, Bratton DL, Konowal A, Freed PW, Westcott JY, Henson PM. Macrophages that have ingested apoptotic cells in vitro inhibit proinflammatory cytokine production through autocrine/paracrine mechanisms involving TGF-beta, PGE2, and PAF. J Clin Invest 1998;101:890–8.
[40] Steinman RM, Turley S, Mellman I, Inaba K. The induction of tolerance by dendritic cells that have captured apoptotic cells. J Exp Med 2000;191:411–6.
[41] Barker RN, Erwig L, Pearce WP, Devine A, Rees AJ. Differential effects of necrotic or apoptotic cell uptake on antigen presentation by macrophages. Pathobiol :J Immunopat Mol Cell Biol 1999; 67:302–5.
[42] Huynh ML, Fadok VA, Henson PM. Phosphatidylserine-dependent ingestion of apoptotic cells promotes TGF-beta1 secretion and the resolution of inflammation. J Clin Invest 2002; 109: 41–50.
[43] Edinger M, Hoffmann P, Ermann J, et al. CD4+CD25+ regulatory T cells preserve graft-versus-tumor activity while inhibiting graft-versus-host disease after bone marrow transplantation. Nat Med 2003;9:1144–50.
[44] Taylor PA, Lees CJ, Blazar BR. The infusion of ex vivo activated and expanded CD4(+)CD25(+) immune regulatory cells inhibits graft-versus-host disease lethality. Blood 2002;99:3493–9.
[45] Hoffmann P, Ermann J, Edinger M, Fathman CG, Strober S. Donor-type CD4(+)CD25(+) regulatory T cells suppress lethal acute graft-versus-host disease after allogeneic bone marrow transplantation. J Exp Med 2002;196:389–99.
[46] Shin HJ, Baker J, Leveson-Gower DB, Smith AT, Sega EI, Negrin RS. Rapamycin and IL-2 reduce lethal acute graft-versus-host disease associated with increased expansion of donor type CD4+CD25+Foxp3+ regulatory T cells. Blood 2011;118:2342–50.
[47] Magenau JM, Qin X, Tawara I, et al. Frequency of CD4(+)CD25(hi)FOXP3(+) regulatory T cells has diagnostic and prognostic value as a biomarker for acute graft-versus-host-disease. Biol Blood Marrow Transplant 2010;16:907–14.
[48] Brunstein CG, Miller JS, Cao Q, et al. Infusion of ex vivo expanded T regulatory cells in adults transplanted with umbilical cord blood: safety profile and detection kinetics. Blood 2011;117: 1061–70.
[49] Di Ianni M, Falzetti F, Carotti A, et al. Tregs prevent GVHD and promote immune reconstitution in HLA-haploidentical transplantation. Blood 2011;117:3921–8.

[50] Gatza E, Rogers CE, Clouthier SG, et al. Extracorporeal photopheresis reverses experimental graft-versus-host disease through regulatory T cells. Blood 2008;112:1515–21.
[51] Biagi E, Di Biaso I, Leoni V, et al. Extracorporeal photochemotherapy is accompanied by increasing levels of circulating CD4+CD25+GITR+Foxp3+CD62L+ functional regulatory T-cells in patients with graft-versus-host disease. Transplantation 2007;84:31–9.
[52] Tsirigotis P, Kapsimalli V, Baltadakis I, et al. Extracorporeal photopheresis in refractory chronic graft-versus-host disease: The influence on peripheral blood T cell subpopulations. A study by the Hellenic Association of Hematology. Transfus Apher Sci 2012;46:181–8.
[53] Meloni F, Cascina A, Miserere S, Perotti C, Vitulo P, Fietta AM. Peripheral CD4(+)CD25(+) TREG cell counts and the response to extracorporeal photopheresis in lung transplant recipients. Transplant Proc 2007;39:213–7.
[54] Capitini CM, Davis JP, Larabee SM, Herby S, Nasholm NM, Fry TJ. Extracorporeal photopheresis attenuates murine graft-versus-host disease via bone marrow-derived interleukin-10 and preserves responses to dendritic cell vaccination. Biol Blood Marrow Transplant 2011;17:790–9.
[55] Picca CC, Larkin J, 3rd, Boesteanu A, Lerman MA, Rankin AL, Caton AJ. Role of TCR specificity in CD4+ CD25+ regulatory T-cell selection. Immunol Rev 2006;212:74–85.
[56] Tawara I, Shlomchik WD, Jones A, et al. A crucial role for host APCs in the induction of donor CD4+CD25+ regulatory T cell-mediated suppression of experimental graft-versus-host disease. J Immunol 2010;185:3866–72.
[57] Sela U, Olds P, Park A, Schlesinger SJ, Steinman RM. Dendritic cells induce antigen-specific regulatory T cells that prevent graft versus host disease and persist in mice. J Exp Med 2011; 208:2489–96.
[58] Tawara I, Sun Y, Lewis EC, et al. Alpha-1-antitrypsin monotherapy reduces graft-versus-host disease after experimental allogeneic bone marrow transplantation. Proceed Nat Acad Sci U.S. A. 2012;109:564–9.
[59] Zheng DH, Dou LP, Wei YX, et al. Uptake of donor lymphocytes treated with 8-methoxypsoralen and ultraviolet A light by recipient dendritic cells induces CD4+CD25+Foxp3+ regulatory T cells and down-regulates cardiac allograft rejection. Biochem Biophys Res Commun 2010;395: 540–6.
[60] Miller KB, Roberts TF, Chan G, et al. A novel reduced intensity regimen for allogeneic hematopoietic stem cell transplantation associated with a reduced incidence of graft-versus-host disease. Bone Marrow Transplant 2004;33:881–9.
[61] Shaughnessy PJ, Bolwell BJ, van Besien K, et al. Extracorporeal photopheresis for the prevention of acute GVHD in patients undergoing standard myeloablative conditioning and allogeneic hematopoietic stem cell transplantation. Bone Marrow Transplant 2010;45:1068–76.
[62] Hivelin M, Siemionow M, Grimbert P, Lantieri L. Extracorporeal photopheresis: from solid organs to face transplantation. Transplant Immunol 2009;21:117–28.
[63] Kusztal M, Koscielska-Kasprzak K, Gdowska W, et al. Extracorporeal photopheresis as an antirejection prophylaxis in kidney transplant recipients: preliminary results. Transplant Proceed 2011;43:2938–40.
[64] Choi SS, P.; Cooke, K.; Ferrara, J.;et al. TNF-inhibition with etanercept for graft versus host disease prevention in high risk HCT: Lower TNFR1 levels correlate with better outcomes. Biol Blood Marrow Transplant 2012; Accepted for publication March 25 (YBBMT-D-12-00063R1).
[65] Hippen KL, Riley JL, June CH, Blazar BR. Clinical perspectives for regulatory T cells in transplantation tolerance. Semin Immunol 2011;23:462–8.
[66] Koreth J, Matsuoka K, Kim HT, et al. Interleukin-2 and regulatory T cells in graft-versus-host disease. N Engl J Med 2011;365:2055–66.

Section 7: ECP in Cutaneous T Cell Lymphoma

Julia Scarisbrick and Chalid Assaf
7 ECP in Cutaneous T Cell Lymphoma

Primary cutaneous lymphomas (PCL) represent a heterogeneous group of extranodal non-Hodgkin's lymphomas (NHLs) primarily localised in the skin without evidence of extracutaneous disease at the time of diagnosis. In contrast to lymphomas of nodal origin, PCL differ in regard to clinical picture, outcome and therapy [1]. PCLs are malignant clonal proliferations often of skin-homing T or B lymphocytes with a wide range of immunologic and clinicopathologic changes, which are classified according to the recent WHO classification (Table 7.1). Cutaneous T cell lymphoma (CTCL), namely mycosis fungoides (MF) and Sézary syndrome (SS) are the most common type of PCL representing about 70% of all cutaneous lymphoma cases [2–5]. MF is a rare disease showing an annual incidence of 0.5–1 case per 100.000 population [6, 7]. It is twice as common in men as it is in women and black people are affected with a twofold higher incidence than whites [6, 7]. Most frequently, the timepoint of diagnosis is in the fifth and sixth decade of life. Clinically MF is characterised by erythematous scaling patches and plaques, which in the minority of cases may progress into the tumour stage. These tumours may present with a mushroom-like appearance being responsible for the disease name first described by Alibert, a French dermatologist in 1806. The classical histological picture shows epidermotropism of the malignant T cells in early stages. In advanced stage MF the epidermotropism is often lost and tumor cells may spread to lymph nodes, blood or visceral organs. SS, the leukemic variant of CTCL is defined by erythroderma, generalised lymphadenopathy and circulating atypical malignant T lymphocytes with cerebriform nuclei (Sézary cells) in the peripheral blood from diagnosis. Associated clinical features are intense pruritus, alopecia and palmoplantar hyperkeratosis [1, 3]. While life-expectancy for patients with limited skin involvement is excellent and closely comparable to a healthy population (stage IA and IB 5-year survival rates are 100% and 96%, respectively), the 5-year survival rate for patients with lymph node involvement drops to 40% in cases of MF and it is only 30% in patients with SS [8–10].

7.1 ECP for Treatment of CTCL

As there is no curative therapy hitherto the treatment of CTCL is performed stage-adapted [11]. Extracorporeal photopheresis (ECP) is a widely accepted type of photochemotherapy used for the treatment of CTCL, especially in patients with MF with erythroderma (stage III) or SS. Therapy with ECP has been shown an effective treatment modality with induction of clinical remission in early and late stages of MF as well as in SS as demonstrated in a large number of clinical studies (summarized in Table 7.2).

Classification

Cutaneous T cell and NK cell lymphomas
- Mycosis fungoides
- Mycosis fungoides variants and subtypes
    - Folliculotropic mycosis fungoides
    - Pagetoid reticulosis
    - Granulomatous slack skin
- Sézary Syndrome
- Adult T cell leukaemia/lymphoma
- Primary cutaneous CD30+ lymphoproliferative disorders
    - Primary cutaneous anaplastic large cell lymphoma
    - Lymphomatoid papulosis
- Subcutaneous panniculitis-like T cell lymphoma
- Extranodal NK/T cell lymphoma, nasal type
    - Primary cutaneous aggressive epidermotropic CD8+ T cell lymphoma (provisional)
    - Cutaneous γ/δ T cell lymphoma (provisional)
    - Primary cutaneous CD4+ small/medium-sized pleomorphic T cell lymphoma (provisional)

Cutaneous B cell lymphomas
- Primary cutaneous marginal zone B cell lymphoma
- Primary cutaneous follicle center lymphoma
- Primary cutaneous diffuse large cell B cell lymphoma, leg type
- Primary cutaneous diffuse large cell B cell lymphoma, other
    - Intravascular large B cell lymphoma

Precursor haematological neoplasm
- CD4+/CD56+ haematodermic neoplasm (formerly blastic NK cell lymphoma)

Table 7.1. WHO-EORTC Classification of Cutaneous Lymphomas.

In the pivotal multicentre trial for ECP reported by Edelson et al. of 37 patients 27 (73%) responded to treatment, with an average 64% decrease in cutaneous involvement with no adverse effects [12]. Following the publication by Edelson et al. in 1987 the FDA approved ECP as a medical device for treatment of CTCL. Since then, numerous studies have been conducted. A meta-analysis of 19 studies in more than 400 patients at all stages of CTCL reported a combined overall response (OR) rate of 55.5% with ECP used as monotherapy and 55.7% when used in combination with other agents, of which 14.8% and 17.6%, respectively, were complete responses (CRs). For erythrodermic disease, the OR rate was 57.6% and CR rate was 15.3%. Importantly, ECP was effective in SS, showing an OR rate of 42.9% with 9.5% CRs.

However, response rates to ECP have been shown to vary widely between different study groups. A systematic review of non-randomised and mostly retrospective studies of extracorporeal photopheresis in CTCL from over 650 patients from 30 published studies showed a mean response rate of 63%, ranging from 43% to 100% [13]. Response rates were higher in those with erythrodermic CTCL. Complete responses were recorded in 27 studies involving 527 patients with a mean CR rate of 20 %. The differences in response rates between centres may relate to different patient selection for treatment with ECP such as the presence of a peripheral T cell clone, stage of disease, prior treatment, ECP protocol, duration of ECP and definition of response (see also "predictors of response"). Similar considerations need to be applied when reporting on survival in patients with erythrodermic CTCL receiving ECP.

7.1.1 Treatment Schedule

In most of the studies till now treatment modalities and schedules were performed according to the initial study as reported by Edelson et al [12]. In general, treatment is conducted on two consecutive days every 4 weeks. Improvement may begin as early as 6 weeks into therapy, and yet some patients have a complete response 12 months after starting therapy. There are occasional temporary responses immediately following a 2-day cycle of therapy. Typically, after 4 to 6 months there is a gradual and permanent decrease in erythema (Figure 7.1), scaling, and pruritus accompanied by a reduction of tumor burden in the peripheral blood [14, 15]. Patients often notice more subtle changes such as the return of body hair, loss of rigors, and a return of the ability to

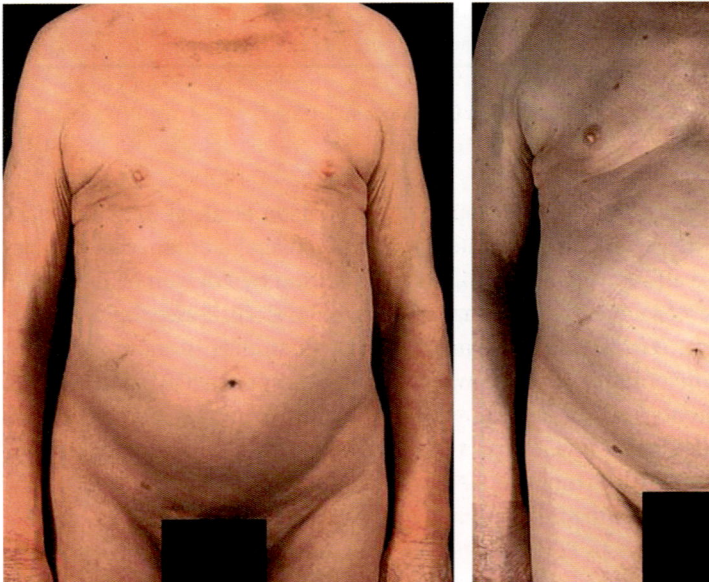

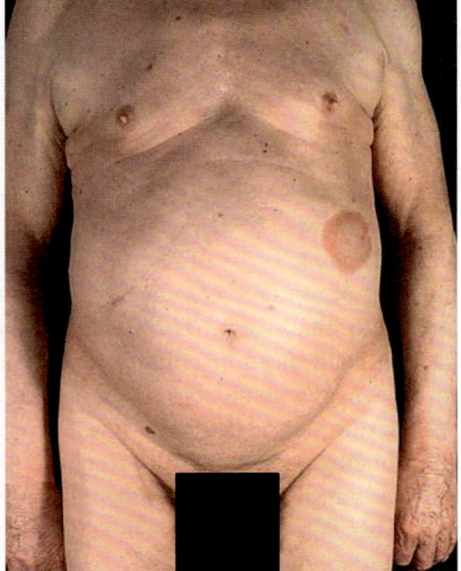

Fig. 7.1. (left) Patient with Sezary syndrome demonstrating severe erythroderma; (right) same patient after six months of monotherapy with extracorporeal photopheresis showing resolution of the erythroderma.

sweat. Partial responses may also decrease the morbidity of these patients e.g. in terms of infectious complications. More heavily involved and inflamed skin is more readily colonized, providing both a reservoir and access point for microbes to invade the host. Thus, cutaneous improvement can already minimize complications of CTCL. The ECP therapy typically continues until loss of response. The median number of treatments varies between centres from 10–32 [13]. The range is wide with some patients continuing on ECP for more than 5 years.

7.1.2 Recommendations

ECP is a recommended therapy for erythrodermic CTCL in the European Organisation for the Treatment and Research in Cancer (EORTC) mycosis fungoides/Sezary Guidelines [11] and in the Joint British Association of Dermatologists and UK Cutaneous Lymphoma Group guidelines [16]. The latter is endorsed in the Improving Outcomes Guidance in Skin Cancer by the National Institute of Clinical Excellence (NICE) [17]. ECP is also recommended for erythrodermic CTCL in the National Comprehensive Cancer Network clinical guidelines (2011) [18], the National Cancer Institute (2007) [19] and the United States Cutaneous Lymphoma Consortium [20].

However, besides the recommendations for the use of ECP in erythrodermic CTCL ("intermediate risk") there exist some data of its use – alone or in combination therapy – in low risk patients (MF stage IA-IIA) and high risk CTCL patients (MF stages IVA/IVB).

A review of the current literature of ECP in CTCL by Miller et al in 2007 reports on 124 early-stage patients treated with ECP or ECP plus adjuvant therapy from 16 published studies between 1987–2007 [21]. Response rates with ECP and ECP plus adjuvant therapy ranged from 33–88%. A recent study of 19 patients all with early-stage MF (IA (n=3), IB (n = 14), and IIA (n=2) showed an overall response rate of 42% (8/19; including 7 partial response, 1 complete response), with a median of 12 ECP sessions (range, 3–32) given over a median of 12 (range, 3–32) months and with an overall duration of response of 6.5 (range, 1–48) months. Quality of life questionnaires also showed an improvement in emotional scores [22]. Based on these data and given the excellent safety profile of ECP compared with other systemic therapies for CTCL and its demonstrated efficacy, this treatment modality is possibly beneficial for patients with earlier stages of CTCL. However in early disease comparative high costs of ECP to alternative therapies may restrict the use of ECP. Randomized trials comparing ECP to other standard therapies are needed to determine if there is a role for ECP in early stages of CTCL.

In more advanced stages ECP is recommended first line therapy for erythrodermic CTCL [23–25]. It is an effective and well tolerated therapy for patients with erythrodermic mycosis fungoides and Sézary syndrome stages III and IVA. However, ECP is not a primary effective treatment for tumour stage mycosis fungoides [26, 27].

	Patients	Overall response	CR	PR	MR
Edelson et al. 1987	Total 37 (erythrodermic 29)	73 % (27/37) 83 % (24/29)	24 % (9/37)	35 % (13/37)	14 % (5/37)
Heald et al. 1989	Total 32 (erythrodermic 22)	NK 86 % (19/22)	23 % (5/22)	45 % (10/22)	18 % (4/22)
Nagatani et al. 1990	Total 7	43 % (3/7)	NK	NK	
Zic et al. 1992	Total 20	55 % (11/20)	25 % (5/20)	30 % (6/20)	
Stevens et al. 1996	Total 17 (erythrodermic)	53 % (9/17)	29 % (5/17)	24 % (4/17)	
Koh et al. 1994	Total 34 (erythrodermic 31)	53 % (18/34)	15 % (5/34)	38 % (13/34)	
Gottlieb et al. 1996	Total 28 (erythrodermic NK)	71 % (20/28)	25 % (7/28)	46 % (13/28)	
Prinz et al. 1995	Total 17 (erythrodermic 3)	70 % (12/17)	0 % (0/17)	41 % (7/17)	29 % (5/17)
Duvic et al. 1996	Total 34 (erythrodermic 28)	50 % (17/34)	18 % (6/34)	32 % (11/34)	
Zic et al. 1996	Total 20 (erythrodermic 3)	50 % (10/20)	25 % (5/20)	25 % (5/20)	
Russell-Jones et al. 1997	Total 19 (erythrodermic)	53 % (10/19)	16 % (3/19)	37 % (7/19)[b]	
Konstantinow 1997	Total 12 (erythrodermic 6)	67 % (8/12) 50 % (3/6)	8 % (1/12) 0 % (0/6)	42 % (5/12) 50 % (3/6)	17 % (2/12)
Miracco et al. 1997	Total 7	86 % (6/7)	14 % (1/7)	71 % (5/7)	
Vonderheid et al. (1998)	Total 36 (erythrodermic 29)	33 % (12/36) 31 % (9/29)	14 % (5/36) 10 % (3/29)	19 % (7/36) 21 % (6/29)	
Zouboulis et al. 1998	Total 20	65 % (13/20)	NK	NK	
Fritz et al. 1999	Total 17	70 % (12/17)	0 % (0/17)	41 % (7/17)	29 % (5/17)
Jiang et al. 1999	Total 25 (erythrodermic)	80 % (20/25)	20 % (5/25)	60 % (15/25)	

	Patients	Overall response	CR	PR	MR
Bisaccia et al. 2000	Total 37	54% (20/37)	14% (5/37)	41% (15/37)	
Crovetti et al. 2000	Total 30 (erythrodermic 9)	73% (22/30) 66% (6/9)	33% (10/30) 33% (3/9)	40% (12/30) 33% (3/9)	
Wollina et al. 2000	Total 20	65% (13/20)	50% (10/20)	15% (3/20)	
Wollina et al. 2001	Total 14	50% (7/14)	29% (4/14)	21% (3/14)	
Bouwhuis et al. 2002	Total 55 (SS 55)	80%	62% (34/55)	18% (10/55)	
Knobler et al. 2002	Total 20 (erythrodermic 13)	50% (10/20) 85% (11/13)	15% (3/20) 15% (2/13)	54% (7/13)	15% (2/13)
Stevens et al. 2002	Total 17 (SS 15)				
Suchin et al. 2002	Total 47	79% (37/47)	26% (12/47)	53% (25/47)	
Quaglino et al. 2004	Total 19	63% (12/19)	NK	NK	
De Misa et al. 2005	Total 10 (advanced SS)	60% (6/10)	10% (1/10)	13% (1/8)	
Wain et al. 2005	Total 14 (erythrodermic) (8 used ECP)				
Rao et al. 2006	Total 16	44% (7/16)	NK	NK	
Gasova et al. 2007	Total 8 (2 CTCL patients)	100% (2/2)	NK	NK	

SS: Sezary syndrome; CR, complete response; PR, partial response (>50% improvement in skin scores); MR, minor response (>25% improvement in skin scores); NK, not known. a: Abstract/letter; b: combined PR and MR.

Table 7.2. Summary of studies of Extracorporeal Photopheresis (ECP) for the Treatment of CTCL [13].

7.2 Predictors of Response

Several pre-treatment parameters have been identified as good predictors of response to ECP therapy by different study groups. There is some consensus of opinion amongst these groups and the presence of erythroderma, those patients within 2 years of diagnosis, a leukocyte count of less than 20×10^9/L, the presence of 10–20% circulating Sezary cells (suggesting a minimum peripheral circulating tumour burden may be required), the absence of bulky lymphadenopathy or visceral disease and lack of prior intensive chemotherapy have all been repeatedly shown to be reliable indicators for a good response to ECP as either monotherapy or as combination therapy [28–31]. Other parameters such as a normal level of cytotoxic (CD8-positive) T cells has been suggested as a good predictor of response for erythrodermic CTCL in some centres [32, 33] but other studies have not confirmed these results [29]. Rao et al found an increased number of T regulatory (Treg) cells following ECP and significant rise in transforming growth factor (TGF)-beta but no discernible pattern for interleukins-4, 6, 10, and 17 or interferon-gamma [34]. A study by the same group looking at serum markers including interleukin-2R, neopterin, beta 2 microglobulin and granzyme B also did not find pretreatment levels to correlate with likelihood of response to ECP [35].

7.3 Adjuvant Therapy

ECP treatment may be initiated as monotherapy or with adjuvant therapy that is most frequent with interferon-alpha and/or bexarotene but may be safely used in combination with a variety of therapies [5–10]. Adjuvant therapy may also be added safely to improve response in those patients receiving ECP and some may benefit from combination ECP regimens [24, 42].

7.4 Monitoring during ECP Therapy

Monitoring of patients receiving ECP is recommended to be done every 3 months based on formal assessments. Responses should be measured in skin, blood and lymph nodes [22–24]. Quality of life questionnaires should be available and have shown a positive response to ECP. Where possible patients should be entered into randomised controlled trials and studies should comply with the clinical endpoints and response criteria recently published [43].

7.5 Conclusion

Beside the low-side effect profile it was shown that ECP alone or in combination with an adjuvant therapy is an effective and safe treatment modality for patients with CTCL. The overall response is about 58 % in CTCL patients which may be enhanced by adjuvant therapy including interferon alpha and/or bexarotene.

References

[1] Willemze R, Jaffe ES, Burg G et al. WHO-EORTC classification for cutaneous lymphomas. Blood 2005;105:3768–85.
[2] Diamandidou E, Colome-Grimmer M, Fayad L, et al. Transformation of mycosis fungoides/Sezary syndrome: clinical characteristics and prognosis. Blood 1998;92:1150–59.
[3] Siegel RS, Pandolfino T, Guitart J, et al. Primary cutaneous T-cell lymphoma: review and current concepts. J Clin Oncol 2000;18:2908–25.
[4] Girardi M, Heald PW, Wilson LD. The pathogenesis of mycosis fungoides. N Engl J Med 2004;350:1978–88.
[5] Paulli M, Berti E. Cutaneous T-cell lymphomas (including rare subtypes). Current concepts. II. Haematologica 2004;89:1372–88.
[6] Criscione VD, Weinstock MA. Incidence of cutaneous T-cell lymphoma in the United States, 1973-2002. Arch Dermatol 2007;143:854–95.
[7] Groves FD, Linet MS, Travis LB, et al. Cancer surveillance series: non-Hodgkin's lymphoma incidence by histologic subtype in the United States from 1978 through 1995. J Natl Cancer Inst 2000;92:1240–51.
[8] Kim YH, Liu HL, Mraz-Gernhard S, et al. Long-term outcome of 525 patients with mycosis fungoides and Sezary syndrome: clinical prognostic factors and risk for disease progression. Arch Dermatol 2003;139:857–66.
[9] Kim YH, Jensen RA, Watanabe GL, et al. Clinical stage IA (limited patch and plaque) mycosis fungoides. A long-term outcome analysis. Arch Dermatol 1996;132:1309–13.
[10] Kim YH, Chow S, Varghese A, et al. Clinical characteristics and long-term outcome of patients with generalized patch and/or plaque (T2) mycosis fungoides. Arch Dermatol 1999;135:26–32.
[11] Trautinger F, Knobler R, Willemze R. et al. EORTC consensus recommendations for the treatment of mycosis fungoides/ Sezary syndrome. Eur J Cancer 2006; 42:1014–30.
[12] Edelson R, Berger C, Gasparro F et al. Treatment of cutaneous T-cell lymphoma by extracorporeal photochemotherapy. Preliminary results. N Engl J Med 1987;316:297–303.
[13] Scarisbrick JJ, Taylor P, Holtick U, et al. U.K. consensus statement on the use of extracorporeal photopheresis for treatment of cutaneous T-cell lymphoma and chronic graft-versus-host disease. Br J Dermatol 2008;158:659–78.
[14] Assaf C, Hummel M, Zemlin M, Steinhoff M, Geilen CC, Stein H, Orfanos CE. Transition of Sézary syndrome into mycosis fungoides after complete clinical and molecular remission under extracorporeal photopheresis. J Clin Pathol 2004;57:1325–8.
[15] Gollnick HP, Owsianowski M, Ramaker J, Chun SC, Orfanos CE. Extracorporeal photopheresis-a new approach for the treatment of cutaneous T cell lymphomas. Recent Results Cancer Res 1995;139:409–15.
[16] Whittaker SJ, Marsden JR, Spittle M, et al. Joint British Association of Dermatologists and U.K. Cutaneous Lymphoma Group guidelines for the management of primary cutaneous T-cell lymphomas, Br J Dermatol, 2003 149:1095–1107.

[17] National Institute for Clinical Excellence (NICE), Improving Outcomes for people with skin tumours including melanoma, Guidance on Cancer Services, Feb 2006.
[18] National Comprehensive Cancer Network. NCCN clinical practice guidelines in oncology: Non-Hodgkin's lymphomas. Version 1 2011;Available at: www.nccn.org.
[19] US National Institutes of Health NCI. Mycosis fungoides and the Sezary syndrome treatment (PDQ). 2007;Available at http://www.nci.nih.gov/cancertopics/pdq/treatment/mycosisfungoides/healthprofessional/allpages.
[20] Olsen EA, Rook AH, Zic J, et al. Sezary syndrome: Immunopathogenesis, literature review of therapeutic options, and recommendations for therapy by the United States Cutaneous Lymphoma Consortium (USCLC). J Am Acad Dermatol 2011;64:352–404.
[21] Miller JD, Kirkland EB, Domingo DS, et al. Review of extracorporeal photopheresis in early-stage (IA, IB, and IIA) cutaneous T-cell lymphoma. Photodermatol Photoimmunol Photomed 2007;23:163–71.
[22] Talpur R, Demierre M, Geskin L, et al. Mulitcenter photopheresis intervention trial in early stage mycosis fungoides. Clin Lymphoma Myeloma Leuk 2011;11:219–27.
[23] Crovetti G, Carabelli A, Berti E, et al. Photopheresis in cutaneous T-cell lymphoma: five-year experience. Int J Artif Organs 2000;23:55–62.
[24] McKenna KE, Whittaker S, Rhodes LE, et al. Evidence-based practice of photopheresis 1987–2001: a report of a workshop of the British Photodermatology Group and the U.K. Skin Lymphoma Group. Br J Dermatol 2006;154:7–20.
[25] Scarisbrick JJ, Taylor P, Holtick U, et al. U.K. consensus statement on the use of extracorporeal photopheresis for treatment of cutaneous T-cell lymphoma and chronic graft-versus-host disease. Br J Dermatol 2008;158:659–78.
[26] Zic JA. The treatment of cutaneous T-cell lymphoma with photopheresis. Dermatol Ther 2003; 16:337–46.
[27] Knobler R, Jantschitsch C. Extracorporeal photochemoimmunotherapy in cutaneous T-cell lymphoma. Transfus Apher Sci 2003;28:81–9.
[28] Stevens SR, Baron ED, Masten S, Cooper KD. Circulating CD4+CD7- lymphocyte burden and rapidity of response: predictors of outcome in the treatment of Sezary syndrome and erythrodermic mycosis fungoides with extracorporeal photopheresis. Arch Dermatol 2002;138:1347–50.
[29] Gottlieb SL, Wolfe JT, Fox FE, et al. Treatment of cutaneous T-cell lymphoma with extracorporeal photopheresis monotherapy and in combination with recombinant interferon alfa: a 10-year experience at a single institution. J Am Acad Dermatol 1996;35:946–57.
[30] Vonderheid EC, Zhang Q, Lessin SR, et al. Use of serum soluble interleukin-2 receptor levels to monitor the progression of cutaneous T-cell lymphoma. J Am Acad Dermatol 1998;38: 207–20.
[31] Evans AV, Wood BP, Scarisbrick JJ, et al. Extracorporeal photopheresis in Sezary syndrome: hematologic parameters as predictors of response. Blood 2001;98:1298–301.
[32] Heald P, Rook A, Perez M et al. Treatment of erythrodermic cutaneous T-cell lymphoma with extracorporeal photochemotherapy. J Am Acad Dermatol 1992;27:427–33.
[33] Gasova Z, Spisek R, Dolezalova L, Marinov I, Vitek A. Extracorporeal photochemotherapy (ECP) in treatment of patients with c-GVHD and CTCL. Transfus Apher Sci 2007;36:149–58.
[34] Rao V, Saunes M, Jørstad S, Moen T. Cutaneous T cell lymphoma and graft-versus-host disease: a comparison of in vivo effects of extracorporeal photochemotherapy on Foxp3+ regulatory T cells. Clin Immunol 2009;133:303–13.
[35] Rao V, Ryggen K, Aarhaug M, Dai HY, Jorstad S, Moen T. Extracorporeal photochemotherapy in patients with cutaneous T-cell lymphoma: is clinical response predictable? J Eur Acad Dermatol Venereol 2006;20:1100–7.
[36] Dippel E, Schrag H, Goerdt S, Orfanos CE. Extracorporeal photopheresis and interferon-alpha in advanced cutaneous T-cell lymphoma. Lancet 1997;350:32–3.

[37] Suchin KR, Junkins-Hopkins JM, Rook AH. Treatment of stage IA cutaneous T-cell lymphoma with topical application of the immune response modifier imiquimod. Arch Dermatol 2002a;138:1137–9.
[38] Fritz TM, Kleinhans M, Nestle FO, Burg G, Dummer R. Combination treatment with extracorporeal photopheresis, interferon alfa and interleukin-2 in a patient with the Sezary syndrome. Br J Dermatol 1999;140:1144–7.
[39] Quaglino P, Fierro MT, Rossotto GL, Savoia P, Bernengo MG. Treatment of advanced mycosis fungoides/Sezary syndrome with fludarabine and potential adjunctive benefit to subsequent extracorporeal photochemotherapy. Br J Dermatol 2004;150:327–36.
[40] Tsirigotis P, Pappa V, Papageorgiou S, et al. Extracorporeal photopheresis in combination with bexarotene in the treatment of mycosis fungoides and Sezary syndrome. Br J Dermatol 2007;156:1379–81.
[41] Booken N, Weiss C, Utikal J, Felcht M, Goerdt S, Klemke CD. Combination therapy with extracorporeal photopheresis, interferon-alpha, PUVA and topical corticosteroids in the management of Sezary syndrome. J Dtsch Dermatol Ges 2010;8:428–38.
[42] Bisaccia E, Gonzalez J, Palangio M, Schwartz J, Klainer AS. Extracorporeal photochemotherapy alone or with adjuvant therapy in the treatment of cutaneous T-cell lymphoma: a 9-year retrospective study at a single institution. J Am Acad Dermatol 2000;43:263–71.
[43] Olsen EA, Whittaker S, Kim YH, et al. Clinical end points and response criteria in mycosis fungoides and Sézary syndrome: a consensus statement of the International Society for Cutaneous Lymphomas, the United States Cutaneous Lymphoma Consortium, and the Cutaneous Lymphoma Task Force of the European Organisation for Research and Treatment of Cancer. J Clin Oncol 2011;29:2598–607.

Section 8: ECP in Scleroderma and Other Skin Diseases

Ulrike Just and Robert Knobler
8 ECP in Scleroderma and Other Skin Diseases

8.1 Systemic Sclerosis

Systemic sclerosis (SSc) is a chronic autoimmune connective tissue disease characterised by excessive deposition of collagen in the skin, subcutaneous tissue and various internal organs including the kidneys, heart, lungs and gastrointestinal tract [1,2]. The clinical manifestations in SSc result from immune activation, fibrosis development, and damage of small blood vessels. Although the precise mechanisms of SSc pathophysiology are not yet fully understood the underlying pathogenesis involves a complex interplay of immunological activity resulting in inflammation, progressive fibrosis and obliterative vasculopathy [1]. There is evidence to suggest that autoantibodies specific to receptors on fibroblasts and endothelial cells activate both cell types and cause tissue damage [3]. In contrast to other fibrotic disorders, vasculopathy and autoimmunity occur prior to tissue fibrosis in SSc [4]. When severe and progressive, systemic sclerosis can cause severe morbidity that is associated with a significant increase in mortality [5]. Long-term prognosis is difficult to predict and varies with the extent of skin thickening, rate of disease progression and visceral organ involvement.

Since SSc is inherently difficult to diagnose due to its complex pathology the diagnosis of SSc invariably occurs late during the course of the disease. Over the past three decades there has been little improvement. The establishment of a definition and new criteria for early diagnosis of SSc may enable treatment to commence before irreversible organ damage occurs, improving the long-term outcomes for patients with SSc [6].

8.1.1 ECP in Systemic Sclerosis

As SSc is a relatively uncommon and highly heterogeneous condition, few treatments have been tested systematically. Soon after the successful use of extracorporeal photopheresis (ECP) for the treatment of cutaneous T cell lymphoma initial reports suggested that ECP provided also benefit to patients with systemic sclerosis [7, 8] and could normalise collagen synthesis in the skin [9], reduce dermal edema [10] and improve skin elasticity [8] without evidence of improvement in internal organ involvement.

A study of long-term treatment of five patients over a mean of 59 months with monthly treatments indicated improvement or stabilization not only of skin thickening, but also in joint mobility, oral aperture, and in symptoms such as Raynaud's phenomenon and digital ulcers in the majority of patients over the course of therapy [11]. Even stabilization of the pulmonary function could be demonstrated in selected patients with early disease [11, 12].

In a prospective clinical trial published in 1992 comparing ECP treatments with treatment with D-penicillamine, seventy-nine patients with systemic sclerosis of recent onset and progressive skin involvement during the preceding 6 months entered a randomized, single-blinded clinical trial [13]. Blinded clinical examiners evaluated skin thickness, percentage surface area involvement, oral aperture, and hand closure. Serial skin biopsies and pulmonary function studies were also performed. Skin severity score, percentage of skin involvement, and oral aperture measurements as well as hand closure measurements were significantly improved from baseline among those who received ECP treatment. By comparison, among the patients treated with D-penicillamine, none of the parameters of cutaneous disease had improved significantly after 6 months of therapy. Skin biopsy studies revealed a correlation between clinical improvement and decreased thickness of the dermal layer. The authors concluded that for patients with systemic sclerosis of recent onset ECP is a well-tolerated treatment that may partially reverse the process that results in cutaneous sclerosis [13].

In contrast, in a second prospective trial of ECP versus no treatment in 19 patients with progressive systemic sclerosis of less than five years' duration the improvement in skin scores with ECP was insufficient to reach statistical significance [14]. However, in both of these preceeding studies, a placebo effect associated with ECP could not be ruled out. Therefore, a multicentre randomized, placebo-controlled, double-blind trial was undertaken, comparing ECP with a sham procedure in 64 patients with systemic sclerosis of recent onset [15]. A statistically significant improvement in skin scores when compared to baseline was observed after treatment at 6 and 12 months among those who received active ECP, but not among those who received sham ECP (Figures 8.1 and 8.2). However, statistical significance was not achieved when comparing the outcomes in the two treatment groups with each other. The authors considered the latter to be a result of the small number of patients in each study arm hence lacking statistical power to show such a difference. Nevertheless, in the absence of effective side-effect-free treatment alternatives, they stated that these results justify serious consideration of ECP as an initial treatment for systemic sclerosis [15]. The suggestion being that ECP therapy is implemented during the early stages of the disease either alone or combined with other immunomodulatory drugs, which may lead to better long-term outcome and response.

It also seems that the presence of circulating clonal populations of T cells detectable in a subgroup of patients with SSc may be associated with responsiveness to ECP [16]. Recently it could be demonstrated in 16 patients with SSc receiving 12 ECP treatments in total that dermal thickness was reduced, mobility of joints improved and internal organ involvement did not deteriorate during ECP therapy [17]. The percentages and numbers of peripheral Th17 cells decreased, the values of regulatory T cells increased with an improvement of their suppressor capacity. Interestingly, there was a positive correlation between the reduction of IL-17 levels and skin thickness measured by ultrasound. ECP treatments contribute to the restoration of disproportional autoimmune responses and attenuate fibrotic processes, thus decelerating the disease progression [17].

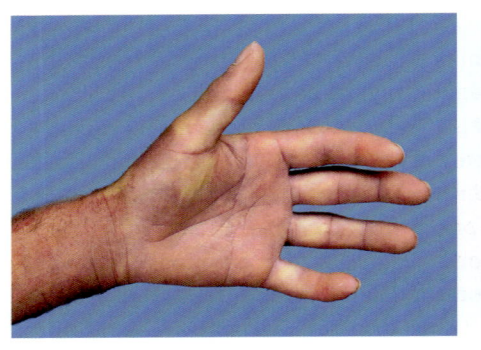

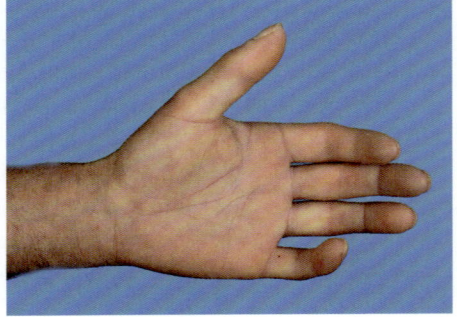

Fig. 8.1. Improvement of Skin of a Patient With Systemic Sclerosis.
(a) Before and **(b)** After 6 Months of ECP Treatment. (from Knobler RM et al.; J Am Acad Dermatol 2006;54:793–9).

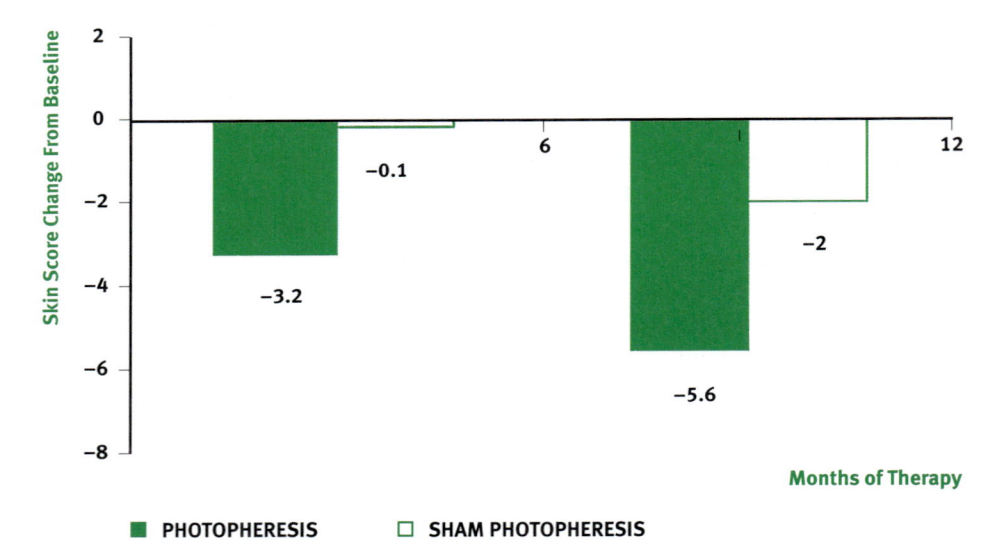

Fig. 8.2. Effect of Active and Sham Photopheresis on Skin Involvement.
Shown is average intrapatient change from baseline by treatment assignment. (from Knobler RM et al. J Am Acad Dermatol 2006;54:793–9).

8.2 ECP in Localized Scleroderma/Morphea

So far, there is limited experience in the use of ECP for treatment of certain clinical variants of localized scleroderma. Clinical observation shows that significant improvement may be obtained in recalcitrant disease progression. Further research is needed to gather more information on the immunomodulatory effects ECP treatment exerts on localized scleroderma [18].

8.3 ECP in Autoimmune Bullous Diseases

ECP as an adjuvant therapy in bullous diseases may obtain a significant reduction in immunosuppressive drugs needed. In some cases even long-term remission can be achieved. The mechanism of action in the treatment of bullous diseases is not yet fully understood. Presumably, a T cell mediated suppression of the immune response with consecutive reduction of antibody production is the underlying process. In therapy-refractory patients the effectiveness as well as the balanced risk–benefit ratio compared with long-term immunosuppressive medication makes ECP a recommendable long term treatment modality for drug-resistant autoimmune bullous diseases [19–21].

8.4 Atopic Dermatitis

The results of ECP treatment in patients suffering from therapy-refractory atopic dermatitis show an overall positive clinical effect. Patients especially reported good effect on pruritus. Patients with initially very high levels of IgE seem to respond even better [22]. In some observations the course of ECP treatment has been extended up to more than 80 months and the effect of the treatment was stable and persistent. No signs or symptoms of severe adverse events have been recorded. However, some studies have a clear selection bias, in the sense that the treatment was continued on a long-term basis only in patients experiencing a beneficial effect [23].

A recent study in seven patients with severe recalcitrant atopic dermatitis evaluated the role of ECP in long-term treatment of the disease. It was shown that with ECP not only a long-term stabilization was obtained in four out of seven patients but also an immunosuppressant sparing effect could be demonstrated. When used as a long-term treatment in patients with severe atopic dermatitis resistant to previous therapies ECP offers a safe, effective therapy [24].

References

[1] Denton CP, Black CM. Targeted therapy comes of age in scleroderma. Trends Immunol 2005; 26:596–602.
[2] Mouthon L, Guillevin L, Humbert M. Pulmonary arterial hypertension: an autoimmune disease? Eur Respir J 2005;26:986–8.
[3] Varga J Abraham D. Systemic sclerosis: a prototypic multisystem fibrotic disorder. J Clin Invest 2007;117:557–67.
[4] Korn JH. Scleroderma: a treatable disease. Cleve Clin J Med 2003;70:954–68.
[5] Barnet AJ, Miller M, Littlejohn GO. The diagnosis and classification of scleroderma (systemic sclerosis). Postgrad Med J 1998;64:121–5.
[6] Matucci-Cerinic M, Allanore Y, Czirják L, et al. The challenge of early systemic sclerosis for the EULAR Scleroderma Trial and Research group (EUSTAR) community. It is time to cut the Gordian knot and develop a prevention or rescue strategy. Ann Rheum Dis 2009;68:1377–80.

[7] Rook AH, Freundlich B, Nahass GT, et al. Treatment of autoimmune disease with extracorporeal photochemotherapy: progressive systemic sclerosis. Yale J Biol Med 1989;62:639–45.
[8] Fimiani M, Rubegni P, Flori mL, Mazzatenta C, D'Ascenzo G, Andreassi L. Three cases of progressive systemic sclerosis treated with extracorporeal photochemotherapy. Arch Dermatol Res 1997;289:120–2.
[9] Ohtsuka T, Okita H, Yamakage A, Yamazaki S. The effect of extracorporeal photochemotherapy on alpha1(I) and alpha1(III) procollagen mRNA expression in systemic sclerosis skin tissue. Arch Dermatol Res 2002;293:642–5.
[10] Hashikabe M, Ohtsuka T, Yamazaki S. Quantitative echographic analysis of photochemotherapy on systemic sclerosis skin. Arch Dermatol Res 2005;296:522–7.
[11] Schwartz J, Gonzalez J, Palangio M, KlainerAS, Bisaccia E. Extracorporeal photochemotherapy in progressive systemic sclerosis: a follow-up study. Int J Dermatol 1997;36:380–5.
[12] Di Spaltro FX, Cottrill C, Cahill C, et al. Extracorporeal photochemotherapy in progressive systemic sclerosis. Int J Dermatol 1993;32:417–21.
[13] Rook AH, Freundlich B, Jegasothy BV, et al. Treatment of systemic sclerosis with extracorporeal photochemotherapy: results of a multicenter trial. Arch Dermatol 1992;128:337–46.
[14] Enomoto DN, Mekkes JR, Bossuyt PM, et al. Treatment of patients with systemic sclerosis with extracorporeal photochemotherapy (photopheresis). J Am Acad Dermatol 1999;41:915–22.
[15] Knobler RM, French LE, Kim Y, et al. A randomized, double-blind, placebo-controlled trial of photopheresis in systemic sclerosis. J Am Acad Dermatol 2006;54:793–9.
[16] French LE, Rook AH. T cell clonality and the effect of photopheresis in systemic sclerosis and graft versus host disease. Transfus Apher Sc 2002;26:191–6.
[17] Papp G, Horvath IF, Barath S, Gyimesi E, Vegh J, Szodoray P, Zeher M. Immunomodulatory effects of extracorporeal photochemotherapy in systemic sclerosis. Clin Immunol. 2012; 142:150–9.
[18] Neustadter JH, Samarin F, Carlson KR, Girardi M. Extracorporeal photochemotherapy for generalized deep morphea. Arch Dermatol 2009;145:127–30.
[19] Kaiser J, Kaatz M, Elsner P, Ziemer M. Complete remission of drug-resistant Pemphigus vegetans treated by extracorporeal photopheresis. JEADV 2007;21:843–4.
[20] Sanli H, Akay BN, Ayyildiz E, Anadolu R, Ilhan O. Remission of severe autoimmune bullous disorders induced by long-term extracorporeal photochemotherapy. Transfus Apher Sci 2010;43:353–9.
[21] Saraceno R, Ruzzetti M, Lanti A, Marinacci M, Chimenti S. Therapeutic options in an immunocompromised patient with pemphigus vulgaris: potential interest of plasmapheresis and extracorporeal photochemotherapy. Eur J Dermatol 2008;18:354–6.
[22] Sand M, Bechara FG, Sand D, et al. Extracorporeal photopheresis as a treatment for patients with severe, refractory atopic dermatitis. Dermatology 2007;215:134–8.
[23] Hjuler KP, Vestergaard C, Deleuran M. A retrospective study of six cases of severe recalcitrant atopic dermatitis treated with long-term extracorporeal photopheresis. Acta Derm Venereol 2010;90:635–6.
[24] Rubegni P, Poggiali S, Cevenini G, et al. Long term follow-up results on severe recalcitrant atopic dermatitis treated with extracorporeal photochemotherapy. J Eur Acad Dermatol Venereol 2012 April 28. doi: 10.1111/j.1468–3083.2012.04552.x.

Section 9: ECP in Crohn's Disease

Walter Reinisch
9 ECP in Crohn's Disease

Crohn's disease is a chronic progressive inflammatory disorder of the gastrointestinal tract, which can affect any of its segments, but mostly involves the terminal ileum and colon. Stricturing and penetrating complications arise as sequelae of destruction, necessitating intestinal surgery in the majority of patients [1]. Evidence suggests that Crohn's disease derives from perturbations at the interface between the intestinal microbiota and the innate immune system, based on genetic predisposition, which result in a hyperresponsiveness of the mucosal immune system and chronic inflammation [2]. Thus, current treatment strategies almost exclusively harness immunosuppressive mechanisms of action, and include steroids, thiopurines, methotrexate and anti-tumour necrosis factor (TNF)-alpha agents. Such treatment strategies are associated with an increased risk of infection, however, and recently advocated strategies combining thiopurines and anti-TNF-alpha agents may even increase this risk further [3].

9.1 Results on ECP in Crohn's Disease

Extracorporeal photopheresis (ECP) is thought to engage an alternative mechanism of therapeutic action [4, 5]. Activation of a counterbalancing regulatory response induced by T regulatory (T_{reg}) cells directed against the hyperactive adaptive arm of the immune system, as described in Crohn's disease, could mitigate the inflammatory response without compromising general immunity against pathogenic danger signals. Murine models of inflammatory bowel disease have provided information on the potential therapeutic role of T_{reg} cells in overcoming the disease in humans [2]. Re-infusion of apoptotic leukocytes generated by ECP is hypothesized to generate a tolerogenic response in treated patients via T_{reg} cells; indeed, re-circulation of DNA-adduct-positive cells to the intestinal mucosa has been described following photopheresis [6, 7]. However, data on the efficacy and mode of action of photopheresis in Crohn's disease remain scarce and uncontrolled.

A small prospective single-centre study evaluated the use of photopheresis in patients with steroid-dependent Crohn's disease evaluated at predefined time points during treatment [7]. Photopheresis was administered as two treatments every 2 weeks, for a total of 24 weeks. In four out of nine patients (44.4%), steroid therapy could be completely withdrawn during photopheresis, without recurrence of symptoms of Crohn's disease; in another four patients, the dose of steroids could be reduced by at least 50%; only one patient with a long disease duration and a high baseline steroid dose experienced therapeutic failure.

In a subsequent multicentre study, CD1, patients with steroid-dependent Crohn's disease received two treatments every other week, for a 24-week steroid-tapering period, and underwent a forced steroid-tapering protocol [8]. Steroid-free remission was achieved in seven out of 31 patients (22.6%). In general, steroid-free remission is an endpoint which is difficult to achieve in patients with steroid-dependent Crohn's disease that is refractory to, or intolerant of, other therapies, including immunosuppressive medication or anti-TNF-alpha agents. From the literature a steroid-free remission rate of maximum 25% is expected to be achieved by switch to a second line anti-TNF alpha inhibitor, whereas the placebo steroid-free remission rate is expected to be less than 10% [9].

The CD2 study followed a different approach. Patients with moderate-to-severe active Crohn's disease refractory to immunomodulators and/or anti-TNF-alpha agents received photopheresis twice weekly for 4 weeks, tapering to twice every other week for another 6 weeks [10]. Among the 28 patients included, there was a marked reduction in the Crohn's Disease Activity Index score during the 12-week treatment period, with 14 patients (50%) being classified as responders, and seven patients (25%) achieving a remission.

9.2 Conclusions

Existing data show some promise for the use of photopheresis in Crohn's disease. To date, two indications have been investigated in open-label trials, namely steroid-dependent Crohn's disease and moderate-to-severe active Crohn's disease. Most patients included in these trials had shown no benefit following previous exposure to the available standard of care, including immunosuppressive medications and anti-TNF-alpha agents. Currently, data are lacking on a patient population less progressed in disease and therefore, possibly more sensitive to a tolerogenic response. Photopheresis is generally considered a safe procedure. However, we are still waiting for a final proof of its efficacy from sham-controlled clinical trials as well as a delineation of those patients who could gain most of benefit from ECP. In clinical practice ECP should, therefore, be primarily used in patients with Crohn's disease not responding to or being intolerant of standard of care.

References

[1] Cosnes J, Cattan S, Blain A, et al. Long-term evolution of disease behavior of Crohn's disease. Inflamm Bowel Dis 2002;8:244–50.
[2] Garrett WS, Gordin JI, Glimcher LH. Homeostasis and inflammation in the intestine. Cell 2010; 140:859–70.
[3] Dignass A, Van Assche G, Lindsay JO, et al. European Crohn's and Colitis Organisation (ECCO). The second European evidence-based consensus on the diagnosis and management of Crohn's disease: current management. J Crohns Colitis 2010;4:28–62.
[4] Greinix HT, Socie G, Bacigalupo A, et al. Assessing the potential role of photopheresis in hematopoietic stem cell transplantation. Bone Marrow Transplant 2006;38:265–73.

[5] Marshall SR. Technology insight: ECP for the treatment of GVHD – can we offer selevtive immune control without generalized immunosuppression? Nat Clin Pract Oncol 2006;3:302–14.
[6] Maeda A, Schwarz A, Bullinger A, Morita A, Peritt D, Schwarz T. Experimental extracorporeal photopheresis inhibits the sensitization and effector phases of contact hypersensitivity via two mechanisms: generation of IL-10 and induction of regulatory T cells. J Immunol. 2008;181:5956–62.
[7] Reinisch W, Nahavandi H, Santella R, et al. Extracorporeal photochemotherapy in patients with steroid-dependent Crohn's disease: a prospective pilot study. Aliment Pharmacol Ther 2001;15:1313–22.
[8] Reinisch W, Knobler R, Rutgeerts P, et al. Extracorporeal photopheresis in patients with steroid-dependent Crohn's disease: An open-label, multi-center, prospective trial. Inflamm Bowel Dis 2012: accepted for publication 2012.
[9] Danese S, Fiorino G, Reinisch W. Review article: causative factors and clinical management of patients with Crohn's disease who lose response to anti-TNF-α therapy. Aliment Pharmacol Ther. 2011. doi: 10.1111/j.1365–2036.2011.04679.x [Epub ahead of print].
[10] Abreu MT, von Tirpitz C, Hardi R, et al. Extracorporeal photopheresis for the treatment of refractory Crohn's disease: results of an open-label pilot study. Inflamm Bowel Dis 2009;15:829–36.

Section 10: Extracorporeal Photopheresis after Solid Organ/Tissue Transplantation

10 Extracorporeal Photopheresis after Solid Organ/Tissue Transplantation

John A. Zic

10.1 Prevention and Treatment of Solid Organ Transplant Rejection

10.1.1 Introduction

The first attempt, albeit unsuccessful, to transplant a solid organ into a human being was performed by Mathieu Jaboulay, professor of surgery in Lyon, France in 1906 [1]. Two patients with life-threatening renal failure received renal xenografts from a goat and a pig. Over the next fifty years refinement of surgical technique and improved understanding of transplant immunology eventually led to the first successful organ transplant on December 23, 1954. Led by the clinical team of John Merrill, Joseph Murray, and Hartwell Harrison at the Peter Bent Brigham Hospital in Boston a kidney was transplanted from one healthy identical twin to his twin who was dying of renal disease [1, 2].

Attempts at transplanting other organs followed. Initial attempts at liver transplantation in 1963 by Thomas E. Starzl [3] in Denver were unsuccessful, but following a move to Pittsburgh in 1967, his results improved [2]. The first lung transplant was performed by Hardy, in 1964. Unfortunately, the patient succumbed to renal failure three weeks later [2]. The pioneer in cardiac transplantation was the American surgeon Norman Shumway working in Palo Alto, California [2]. However, it was Christiaan Barnard, having visited Shumway's unit, who performed the first human heart transplant in 1967 at the Groote Schuur Hospital in Cape Town [2, 4].

If these early transplant patients survived the immediate post-operative risks of the procedure they faced inevitable rejection despite treatment with high dose corticosteroids. It was not until the discovery of the immunosuppressive effects of the purine analogue 6-mercaptopurine and, more importantly, its less toxic derivative azathioprine by Gertrude Elion and George Hitchings that renal transplant patients saw meaningful increases in survival. Azathioprine offered more specific immunosuppression than corticosteroids by allowing engraftment of the transplanted organ while maintaining the integrity of most other immune functions [1, 2]. This remarkable addition to transplant medicine led to what some have called the azathioprine era (mid-1960s to early 1980s) [1].

The discovery of cyclosporine in the mid-1970s heralded the emergence of the modern immunosuppressive era. Sir Roy Calne, the British pioneer in transplantation, introduced cyclosporine, a calcineurin inhibitor with more targeted T cell suppression, into clinical practice in 1978 [5]. When cyclosporine was introduced into the clinic in the early 1980s it led to a marked reduction in the loss of kidneys from acute rejection, as well as a dramatic improvement in the outcome of liver and cardiac transplantation [1].

From the 1990s emerged other immunosuppressive drugs with unique safety profiles and mechanisms of action. Tacrolimus, another calcineurin inhibitor, offers deeper immunosuppression than cyclosporine and has proven superior in most forms of organ transplantation [2]. Sirolimus (formerly rapamycin) and everolimus are inhibitors of the mammalian target of rapamycin (mTOR), a serine/threonine protein kinase involved in the regulation of cell growth, cell proliferation, protein synthesis and ribosome biogenesis. They are generally used as alternatives to calcineurin inhibitors in patients with impaired renal function, but may show other benefits in heart transplantation [2]. Mycophenolate mofetil (MMF) blocks DNA synthesis in lymphocytes through inhibition of inosine monophosphate dehydrogenase, an enzyme required for the *de novo* synthesis of guanosine nucleotides. MMF shows immunosuppressive potency between that of azathioprine and the more potent calcineurin and mTOR inhibitors [2]. The rapid development of novel biologic agents entering clinical trials has yielded several that may be promising for immunomodulation in transplantation [6].

The International Society for Heart and Lung Transplantation estimates that from 1980 to 2010 over 100,000 heart transplants and over 35,000 lung transplants have been performed [7, 8]. The Organ Procurement and Transplantation Network estimates that from 1998 to 2010 over 180,000 renal transplants were performed in the United States [9].

Though advances in immunosuppression have reduced the rates of acute rejection, the incidence of chronic immune damage in any organ has not been affected [2, 10]. The exception may be everolimus which shows promise in preventing, but not treating, coronary allograft vasculopathy in heart transplant recipients [11–13]. In addition to potential organ toxicities from modern immunosuppressive agents, there is an increased risk for serious infections and malignancies that may have devastating consequences for patients. Many malignancies are substantially more frequent after organ transplantation with squamous cell carcinoma of the skin being increased 65- to 100-fold [14].

10.1.2 Immune Mechanisms of Acute and Chronic Allograft Rejection

In order to understand how photopheresis may help manage the complications of solid organ transplantation it is necessary to summarize our present understanding of transplant immunology. Though T cell mediated immune mechanisms may dominate the rejection of a transplanted organ, activation of the innate immune system and antibody mediated mechanisms may also play key roles. As a consequence of tissue injury sustained during organ retrieval and ischemia reperfusion, the damaged cells within the allograft produce molecules (Hsp70, fibrinogen, etc.) known as damage-associated molecular patterns (DAMPS). Pattern recognition receptors (toll-like receptors, C-type lectin receptors, etc.) expressed by cells of the recipient's innate immune system recognize DAMPS [15]. The now activated leukocytes rapidly release inflammatory mediators and chemoattractant cytokines or chemokines attracting other leukocytes into the graft causing further damage. Though it is rare for the innate immune system to reject an allograft on its own, the activated innate immune system does signal the activation of the adaptive arm of the immune response against the allograft [16].

Alloantibody binding to allograft tissue and subsequent complement activation provide the primary path of antibody mediated immunity in the transplant setting. Antibodies may target donor human leukocyte antigen (HLA) molecules, minor histocompatibility antigens, endothelial cells, red blood cells (RBCs), or autoantigens. Though the majority of B cells require help from T cells to initiate antibody production, through these mechanisms early and late rejection may emerge and contribute significantly to graft loss after transplantation [10, 16].

T cells require a minimum of two signals for activation: antigen recognition and costimulation. Once activated, transduction of signals delivered by interleukin-2 (IL-2) promotes cell cycle progression and initiates the clonal expansion and differentiation of activated T cells. As a result of heterologous immunity, memory T cells are present in the majority of transplant recipients. Alloantigen-specific CD4 T cells (typically T helper 1 cells) contribute to the effector phase of allograft rejection by a delayed-type hypersensitivity response. Proinflammatory cytokines interleukin-1 (IL-1), interferon (IFN)γ, and tumor necrosis factor (TNF)α lead to cellular damage as a result of the ensuing infiltration of activated leukocytes and the production of non-specific mediators, such as nitric oxide, reactive oxygen species, and arachidonic acid derivatives (prostaglandin E2, thromboxane, and leukotrienes).

Chronic allograft rejection continues to be the most important cause of long-term graft failure and current immunosuppressive regimens have not significantly reduced its incidence [10]. Fibrosis primarily affecting the blood vessels and tubular structures in the allograft characterize chronic rejection which ultimately leads to decreased physiological function. This manifests as chronic allograft nephropathy (CAN) in kidney, cardiac allograft vasculopathy (CAV) in heart and bronchiolitis obliterans syndrome (BOS) in lung allografts [10]. Recent studies suggest that alloimmune damage to the allograft may expose self-antigens such as collagen or epithelial surface antigens leading to an autoimmune response [10, 17].

Further evidence that autoimmune responses play a role in chronic rejection comes from several reports that reveal the association of loss of regulatory T cells (Treg) and the development of chronic rejection [10, 18]. Treg cells characterized by $CD4^+$ $CD25^+$ $Foxp3^+$ expression have been shown to play an important role in maintaining tolerance towards self-antigens [10]. Treg cells directly attenuate dendritic cells and also directly kill or suppress the activation of T cells (Figure 10.1) [19]. A reduction in either Treg cell number or function potentiates autoimmune responses [20]. Therefore, although current immunosuppressive agents may prevent acute rejection, they may increase the risk of chronic rejection by decreasing the population of Treg cells in allograft recipients [10, 20]. The importance of Treg cells in modulating alloimmune responses has led to several clinical trials including The European Union-funded multicenter clinical trial 'The ONE Study', which will test the safety of Treg cell transfer in solid-organ transplant patients [19, 21]. However, this therapy is complicated by the discovery that Treg cells can be converted into pro-inflammatory and pro-fibrotic Th17 cells in the presence of inflammatory cytokines [22, 23]. These discoveries indicate that the complex integration and molecular signaling of the many facets of the immune system lead to acute and chronic allograft rejection [10, 16].

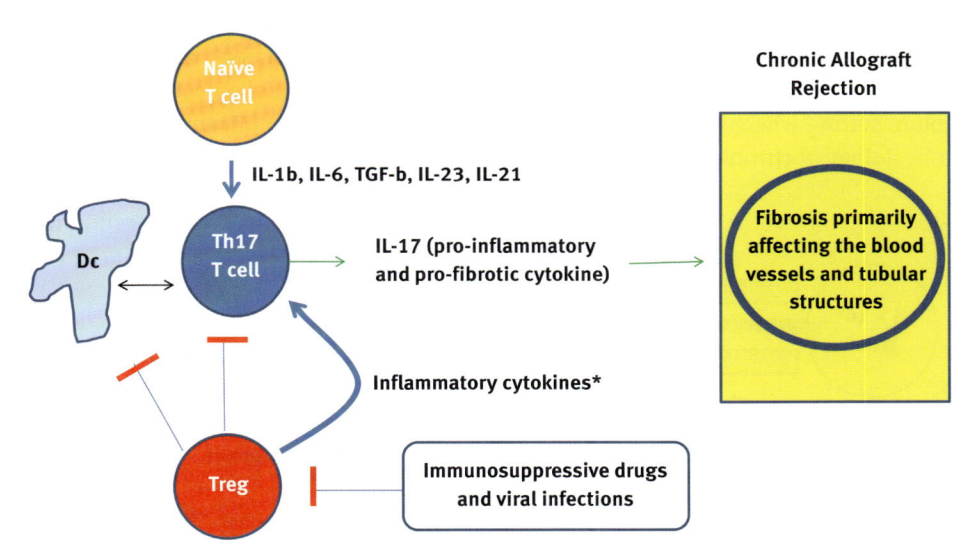

Fig. 10.1. T Cell Mechanisms of Chronic Allograft Rejection (Tiriveedhi, Sarma et al. 2012; *Mitchell, Afzali et al. 2009). DC=dendritic cell; Treg=regulatory T cell; IL-1b=interleukin-1b; IL-6=interleukin-6; TGF-b=transforming growth factor-b; IL-23=interleukin-23; IL-21=interleukin-21; IL-17=interleukin-17.

10.1.3 Potential Mechanisms of Action of Photopheresis in the Treatment of Allograft Rejection

Other chapters have detailed the potential mechanism of action of extracorporeal photopheresis (ECP) in the treatment of cutaneous T cell lymphoma and graft-versus-host disease. The photoactivation phase of ECP leads to the induction of apoptosis in up to 60% of the 5 billion leukocytes treated each session representing only 10% of the total body leukocyte pool [24, 25]. Upon re-infusion the treated cells become sequestered in the liver and spleen where over the next 24 to 48 hours apoptosis ensues [25, 26]. There, immature dendritic cells (Dc) engulf the apoptotic cells and differentiate into tolerogenic dendritic cells (Figure 10.2) [27, 28].

The apoptosis of alloreactive T cells directed against the transplanted organ does not adequately explain how ECP may attenuate allograft rejection. This stems from only 10% of leukocytes and thus, only 10% of alloreactive T cells being exposed to the ECP device each session. Therefore, other mechanisms of action must be at work. Along with the induction of tolerogenic Dc, Voss and colleagues summarize the following general mechanisms of action of ECP: 1. decreased production of pro-inflammatory cytokines and increased production of anti-inflammatory cytokines; 2. reduced ability of antigen presenting cells to stimulate T cell responses; 3. enhanced production and function of Treg cells and T suppressor cells [25]. In the transplant setting it is possible that different mechanisms of action may explain how ECP attenuates acute rejection and chronic rejection because of their different pathophysiology.

There is mounting evidence that ECP enhances the production and function of Treg cells in a number of diseases [27, 29–42]. This is particularly relevant in the transplant setting where loss of Treg cell number and function is implicated in the pathophysiology of chronic allograft rejection [10, 18].

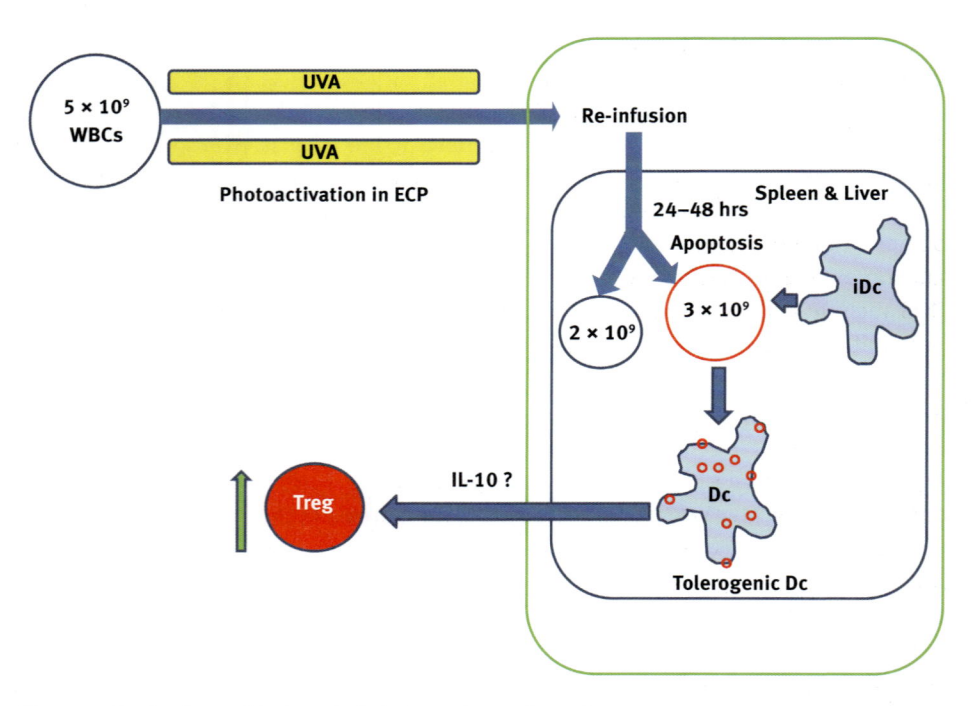

Fig. 10.2. Mechanisms of Action of ECP in Organ Transplantation.
UVA=ultraviolett A; WBC=white blood cell; Treg=regulatory T cell; IL-10= interleukin 10; Dc=dendritic cell; iDc=immature dendritic cell; hrs=hours.

10.1.4 ECP in Lung Transplantation

Based on recent International Society of Heart and Lung Transplantation (ISHLT) registry data, more than 2,700 lung transplantation procedures were performed in 2010 with over 35,000 procedures since 1980 [7, 8]. The shift towards more potent immunosuppressive regimens in lung transplantation, particularly those containing Tacrolimus and MMF or azathioprine along with corticosteroids, has reduced the prevalence of acute rejection of the allograft to 30–40 % of recipients in the first year post transplant [7, 8]. Nevertheless, treatment-related adverse events and persistently high risk of chronic graft rejection remain major obstacles to long-term survival after lung transplantation [43, 44]. Chronic lung allograft rejection manifests as bronchiolitis obliterans syndrome and occurs in more than 50 % of lung transplant survivors within 10 years post transplant. It remains the leading cause of death of lung transplant recipients after the first year post transplant representing 20 % to 30 % of all deaths [7, 8].

10.1.4.1 Bronchiolitis Obliterans Syndrome

Bronchiolitis obliterans primarily affects small airways and can be difficult to diagnose by transbronchial biopsy [45]. Therefore, diagnosis is made on the basis of graft deterioration due to persistent airflow obstruction measured by spirometry. BOS pathogenesis may be linked to ischemia induced by a transient loss of airway microvasculature [45, 46]. Acute rejection is a primary risk factor for BOS and a recent study demonstrated that a therapy that enhances vascular integrity during acute rejection may promote graft health and prevent chronic rejection [45, 47]. Other risk factors for BOS include cytomegalovirus (CMV) pneumonitis, HLA-mismatching, lymphocytic bronchitis/bronchiolitis, noncompliance with medications, and primary graft dysfunction [48]. As noted previously, several studies suggest that alloimmune damage to the lung allograft, perhaps through acute rejection, may expose self-antigens such as collagen or epithelial surface antigens leading to an autoimmune response [10, 17]. This autoimmune response may emerge as a critical step in the development of chronic graft rejection in the lung transplant setting.

Clinically, BOS is characterized by progressive dyspnea and unexplained declining forced expiratory volume in 1 second (FEV1). According to the ISHLT staging system for BOS, stage 0 signifies no significant abnormality and FEV1 > 90 % of best postoperative value, while stage 3 signifies severe BOS with FEV1 ≤ 50 % [49]. Potential BOS (stage 0-p), defined as FEV1 81–90 %, was added to detect early changes in graft function that might predict the onset of stage 1 (Table 10.1). Salama and colleagues discovered that elevated serum endothelin-1 (ET-1) concentrations were predictive of BOS, and the assessment of circulating ET-1 might be beneficial in diagnosing and monitoring of BOS [50]. Although the most precipitous decline in airflow typically occurs in the first six months following a diagnosis of BOS, the time of onset and rate of decline of FEV1 are highly variable [51]. Irrespective of whether BOS developed early or late, Burton and colleagues found that the development and progression of BOS grades 2 and 3 is associated with a 3-fold increase in the risk of death at each stage [52].

BOS Stage	Classification
0	$FEV_1 > 90\%$ of baseline & $FEF_{25-75\%} > 75\%$ of baseline
0–p	FEV_1 81–90 % of baseline &/or $FEF_{25-75\%} \leq 75\%$ of baseline
1	FEV_1 66–80 % of baseline
2	FEV_1 51–65 % of baseline
3	$FEV_1 \leq 50\%$ of baseline

Hayes D, Jr. A review of bronchiolitis obliterans syndrome and therapeutic strategies. J Cardiothoracic Surgery 2011;6:92.

Table 10.1. Classification of Bronchiolitis Obliterans Syndrome (BOS).

10.1.4.2 Treatment of Bronchiolitis Obliterans Syndrome

The initial treatment of BOS usually consists of repeated pulses of high-dose methylprednisolone followed by augmentation of existing regimens [48]. Without treatment, patients with BOS will experience progressive pulmonary decline and eventual death. Realistic goals of therapy are "stabilization" or "slowing" of FEV1 decline rather than normalization of airflow [53]. Refractory BOS management may include possible salvage immunosuppressive regimens using methotrexate, antithymocyte globulin (ATG), muromonab-CD3 (OKT3) or alemtuzumab [45, 48]. Recently, the antibiotic azithromycin has shown efficacy in improving FEV1 in lung transplant recipients suffering from BOS [54, 55].

ECP has been utilized as a salvage therapy for the treatment of acute and chronic lung transplant rejection when conventional therapies fail. Unlike immunosuppressant drugs, ECP is not associated with an increased risk of infection. The first use of ECP in human lung transplantation was reported in 1995 for treatment of an acute rejection episode in a patient with a severe infection. The patient improved clinically after three weeks and histologically after 4 weeks ultimately living a normal life at twenty-two months [56]. During the same year, the first use of ECP to treat chronic lung rejection was reported from Vanderbilt University in Nashville. Three patients with steroid refractory BOS received monthly ECP leading to stabilization of their rapidly declining pulmonary function [57].

In 1999 O'Hagan and colleagues described five patients with severe refractory bronchiolitis obliterans treated with adjunctive ECP who demonstrated temporary stabilization of the airflow obstruction in four of the five patients [58]. This cohort suffered a high rate of complications reported to be a consequence of the augmented immunosuppression rather than ECP including a lymphoproliferative disease in one patient and opportunistic infections in three others that resulted in two deaths [58]. In the same year Salerno and colleagues reported their ECP experience in 8 patients with progressively decreasing lung graft function of whom 7 demonstrated grade 3 BOS. Five patients improved on ECP with a histological reversal of rejection in two. Four patients remained in stable condition after follow-up of over 36 months without any ECP-related complications [59]. ECP plus the moderate reduction of immunosuppressive agents resulted in the complete disappearance of Epstein-Barr virus-associated lymphoma in a patient with post-transplantation lymphoproliferative disorder after lung transplantation [60].

Villanueva and colleagues reported their lung transplant experience in a cohort of 14 patients with BOS who received 3 to 13 (median 6) ECP treatments [61]. ECP led to the resolution of concurrent acute rejection in three patients. Of the eight patients with BOS stage 1 or less, two progressed to grade 2, one died of lung cancer and the other five stabilized. Unfortunately, the six patients with BOS stage 2 or 3 progressed despite ECP therapy: five died and one was re-transplanted [61]. These data suggest that early use of ECP is preferable, as low-grade BOS is more amenable to treatment than high-grade BOS.

A direct relationship of increased CD4 (+)CD25(high) cells with in vitro features of Treg cells and improved lung function was reported in 5 patients with BOS following lung transplant treated with ECP [37]. Stabilization of lung function was observed in 3 of 5 patients with an accompanying slight increase or stabilization of the number of peripheral blood Treg cells. In contrast, the other 2 non-responsive patients with BOS showed a decline in the peripheral Treg subset (Figure 10.3) [37]. Additional evidence of the positive role of Treg cells was reported recently by Nakagiri and colleagues who showed that the frequency of Treg cells was positively correlated with good lung function in the early period after lung transplantation [62].

Further evidence that ECP can impact the rapid decline in lung function in patients with BOS was reported by Benden and colleagues [63]. Their single-center experience with ECP for BOS (n=12) after lung transplantation showed a decline in FEV1 of 112 mL/month before the start of ECP and 12 mL/month after 12 cycles of treatment ($P=0.011$). ECP, thus, reduced the rate of lung function decline in recipients with BOS and was well tolerated. In addition, other patients with recurrent acute rejection (n=12) experienced clinical stabilization [63].

In the largest single-center series to date, Morrel and colleagues at Barnes-Jewish Hospital in St. Louis analyzed the efficacy and safety of ECP for progressive BOS in a total of 60 lung allograft recipients [64]. Over 90% of the patients had stage 2 or 3 BOS. The ECP protocol required five 2-day ECP cycles (10 treatments) during the first month, biweekly for the next 2 months (8 treatments), and then monthly for the remaining 3 months (6 treatments). During the 6-month period *before* the initiation of ECP, the average rate of decline in FEV1 was −116.0 mL/month, but the slope decreased to −28.9 during the 6-month period *after* the initiation of ECP. The mean difference in the rate of decline was 87.1 mL/month (95% confidence interval, 57.3–116.9; p<0.0001). In addition, FEV1 improved in 25% of patients after the initiation of ECP, with a mean increase of 20.1 mL/month (Figure 10.4).

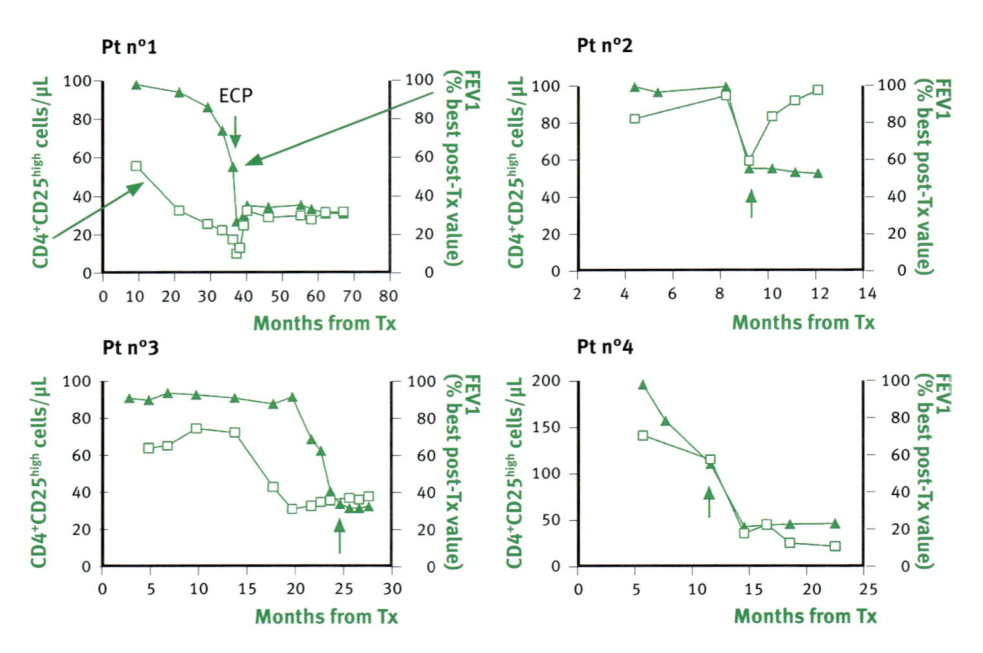

Fig. 10.3. Peripheral CD4(+)CD25(+) Treg Cell Counts and Response to Extracorporeal Photopheresis in Lung Transplant Recipients. Arrow indicates onset of ECP; square = number of Treg cells; triangle = FEV1 level
(Meloni F., Cascina A., et al. (2007), Transplant Proc 39(1): 213–217).

10.1.4.3 Conclusions

In summary, there have been several retrospective studies on the use of ECP in just over one-hundred lung transplant recipients. Most of the patients received ECP to treat BOS and a smaller number of acute rejection episodes were treated successfully. Few patients with BOS experienced improvement of lung function after initiating ECP, but the majority experienced stabilization or a decline in the rate of deterioration of lung function which is impressive in light of the refractory nature of their disease. There are no studies addressing the prophylactic effect of ECP for lung transplantation. The potential for ECP to increase Treg cells holds promise in treating chronic allograft rejection in the lung transplant setting. Despite a lack of robust evidence, ECP should be considered as therapy for the treatment of refractory lung transplant rejection due to its efficacy and excellent side effect profile.

10.1.5 ECP in Cardiac Transplantation

Based on recent International Society of Heart and Lung Transplantation (ISHLT) registry data, more than 3700 cardiac transplantation procedures were performed in 2010. It is estimated that acute rejection of the transplanted heart occurs in more than

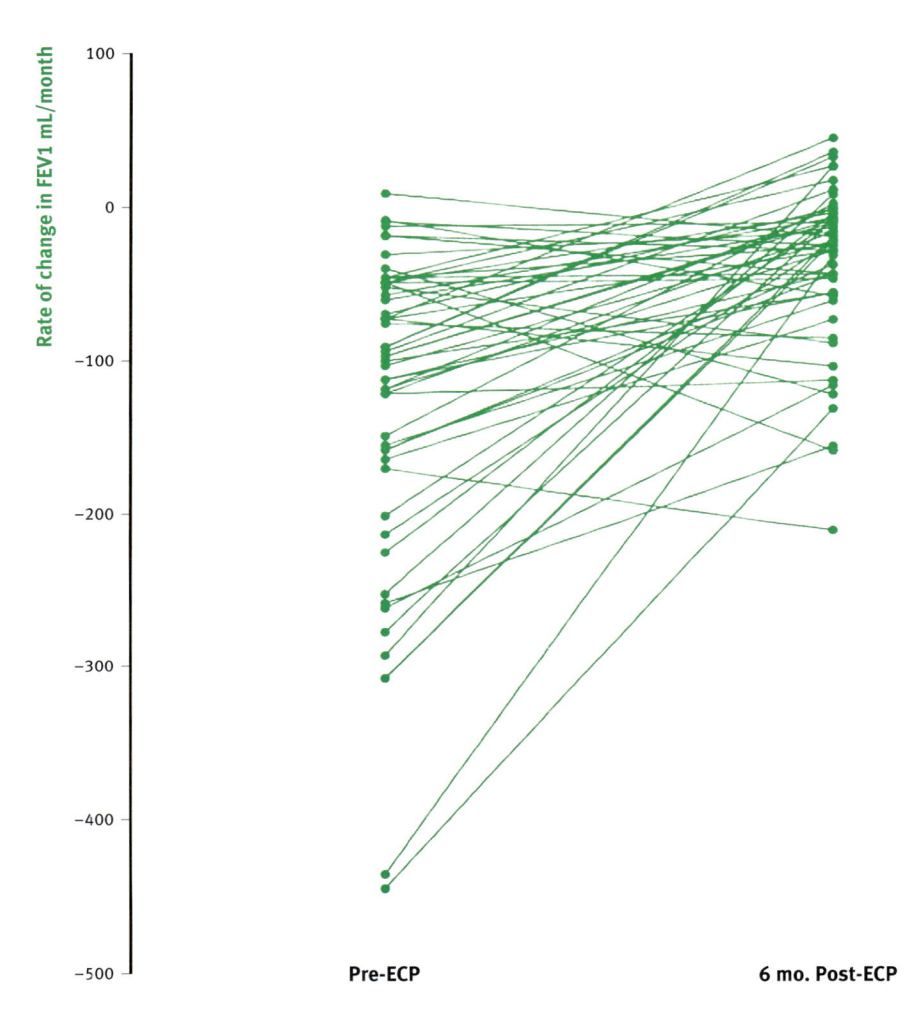

Fig. 10.4. Change in the Rate of Decline of Forced Expiratory Volume in 1 Second (FEV1) in mL/ Months in the 6-Month Period Before ECP and the 6-Month Period after Initiation of ECP.
Each decline represents one patient (Morrell M. R., Despotis G. J., et al. (2010), J Heart Lung Transplant 29(4): 424–431).

25–40 % of recipients within the first year and approximately 5 % will result in severe hemodynamic compromise [8].

Although major improvements have been made in the prevention and treatment of acute transplant rejection, accelerated cardiac allograft vasculopathy still limits the long-term success of heart transplantation [65, 66]. After the first year, CAV is the second most common cause of death, after malignancy. Its pathogenesis, although not fully understood, is characterized by a fibroproliferative process affecting all cardiac arteries and resulting in concentric narrowing, obliteration and, ultimately, allograft failure [65]. CAV is detectable by angiography in 5% of survivors within the first year and in over 27% within the first 5 years [67]. Patient survival after report of CAV is diminished significantly, and CAV and graft failure (most likely undetected CAV) are, in addition to malignancy, the most important causes of death in patients who survive the first year after transplantation [65, 68].

10.1.5.1 Treatment of Cardiac Allograft Vasculopathy

The first reports of ECP therapy for cardiac transplant rejection surfaced in 1992. These early reports showed rapid biopsy-proven reversal of acute cardiac rejection after 2 to 4 ECP treatments [69–72]. By 1998 the first multicenter randomized prospective clinical trial was published [73]. In this study 60 cardiac transplant recipients were randomized post transplant to receive standard triple immunosuppressive therapy versus standard triple immunosuppressive therapy plus ECP. After six months of follow up it was clear that the addition of ECP (10 treatments in month 1, 4 treatments in months 2, 3 and 2 treatments in months 4, 5, 6) resulted in significantly fewer cardiac rejection episodes (p=0.03) [73]. There was no significant difference in the time to a first episode of rejection, the incidence of rejection associated with hemodynamic compromise, or survival at 6 and 12 months [73].

Shortly thereafter, a pilot, prospective, randomized study was published to determine whether the addition of prophylactic photopheresis to a triple immunosuppressive regimen in cardiac transplant recipients resulted in decreased levels of panel reactive antibodies (PRA) and CAV [74]. Twenty-three cardiac transplant recipients were randomized to receive standard triple immunosuppressive therapy versus standard triple immunosuppressive therapy plus ECP (2 treatments per month × 12, 2 treatments every 6–8 weeks in months 12–24). Though there was no difference between the two groups in regard to infection or acute rejection incidence, the ECP group had a significant reduction in PRA levels and coronary artery intimal thickness (CAV) at 12 and 24 months [74].

In 2006 Kirklin and colleagues, published a retrospective review of 13 years of experience with managing cardiac transplant rejection [75]. The group compared the fate of 36 patients that received at least 3 months of ECP for hemodynamically compromised (HC) or recalcitrant rejection to 307 patients that did not receive ECP. Survival and risk factors were analyzed using multivariate hazard function modulated renewal function. After 3 months of ECP, rejection risk was decreased (p=0.04) and the hazard for subsequent HC rejection or rejection death was significantly reduced toward the risk-adjusted level of lower-risk non-ECP patients (p=0.006) [75]. This study was the first to suggest that ECP reduces the risk of subsequent HC rejection and death in patients with high rejection risk.

The mechanism by which ECP modulates cardiac rejection was studied using a murine model of ECP [33]. Splenocytes exposed to 8-MOP + UVA were injected into syngeneic mice both before and after heterotopic cardiac allograft transplant. None of the mice received immunosuppressive agents. The treatment group showed extended cardiac allograft survival and increased levels of FoxP3 expressing $CD4^+CD25^+$ Treg cells as compared to controls. The authors concluded that in this murine model ECP extended graft survival in fully histoincompatible strain combinations with no immunosuppression [33].

10.1.5.2 Conclusions

In summary, there have been several retrospective studies and case series on the use of ECP in well over one-hundred cardiac transplant recipients. In addition, there are two prospective randomized clinical trials addressing the prophylactic use of ECP to prevent acute rejection and chronic rejection as manifested as CAV. The impact of ECP on acute cardiac rejection is rapid requiring 2 to 4 treatments to see biopsy proven remission, though the effect on reducing the hazard for subsequent HC rejection or rejection death may take several months of ECP. The potential for ECP to increase Treg cells holds promise in the treatment of chronic allograft rejection in the cardiac transplant setting. Despite a lack of robust evidence, ECP should be considered as therapeutic option for the treatment of refractory cardiac transplant rejection due to its efficacy and excellent side effect profile.

10.1.6 ECP in Renal Transplantation

The Organ Procurement and Transplantation Network estimates that from 1998 to 2010 over 180,000 renal transplants were performed in the United States [9]. Chronic allograft nephropathy remains a leading cause of graft loss [76]. In a large cohort of 872 renal allograft recipients 55.5% of patients presented CAN after approximately 8 years from renal transplantation [77]. Unlike cardiac and lung transplant recipients, graft failure in renal transplant recipients may not be life-threatening due to the availability of hemodialysis. However all three solid organ recipients must deal with the adverse effects of immunosuppression.

10.1.6.1 Treatment of Chronic Allograft Nephropathy

The first formal report of ECP use to reverse renal allograft rejection was published in 1996 by Wolfe and colleagues at the Hospital of the University of Pennsylvania in Philadelphia [78]. Using an ECP protocol with once weekly ECP during the first month, at 2-week intervals during the second and third months, and then monthly for another 3 months, Dall'Amico and colleagues successfully reversed uncontrolled rejection episodes in four adolescent patients after renal transplantation [79]. Furthermore, clinical improvement allowed progressive reduction of oral steroids in three of four patients treated [79].

Lamioni and colleagues studied the induction of regulatory T cells after prophylactic treatment with photopheresis in two pediatric renal transplant recipients who received six ECP treatments over three weeks post transplantation [35]. When compared with four transplanted control patients, the ECP-treated ones showed lower TNFα serum levels in the short-term and a marked increase of Treg cells that were still higher than in the controls 1 year after transplantation. The authors suggested that the addition of ECP to standard immunosuppressive therapy induced a tolerogenic shift in the immune system of kidney transplanted patients [35].

The long-term outcome of a cohort of ten renal transplant recipients following the use of ECP therapy for treatment-resistant rejection was reported by Jardine and colleagues [80]. Median follow-up was 66.7 months following photopheresis commencement and rejection resolved concurrently with photopheresis in all 10 patients. Six patients continued to have stable graft function (median serum creatinine: 191.5 micromol/L) at a median follow-up of 71.0 months. There were three reported deaths due to sepsis (n=1) and malignancy (n=2) [80]. The authors concluded that ECP may have a role as an adjuvant or salvage anti-rejection therapy in solid organ transplantation, but that evaluation in randomized controlled clinical trials is required to evaluate its potential [80].

10.1.6.2 Conclusions

In summary, fewer renal transplant patients have been reported to receive ECP for treatment of acute and chronic rejection than cardiac or lung transplant recipients. This may be due to the availability of hemodialysis should renal graft failure occur. Nonetheless, ECP shows promise in reversing uncontrolled acute renal graft rejection. Further studies are warranted to explore the potential role of ECP in the management of CAN.

References

[1] Morris PJ. Transplantation – a medical miracle of the 20th century. New Engl J Med 2004; 351:2678–80.

[2] Watson CJ, Dark JH. Organ transplantation: historical perspective and current practice. Brit J Anaesthesia 2012;108 Suppl 1:i29–42.

[3] Starzl TE, Marchioro TL, Huntley RT, et al. Experimental and clinical homotransplantation of the liver. Ann N Y Acad Sci 1964;120:739–65.

[4] Barnard CN. Human cardiac transplantation. An evaluation of the first two operations performed at the Groote Schuur Hospital, Cape Town. Am J Cardiol 1968;22:584–96.

[5] Calne R. Courage and character, leaders and legends: an interview with Sir Roy Calne, FRS. Interview by Linda Ohler. Prog Transplant 2010;20:201–2.

[6] Page EK, Dar WA, Knechtle SJ. Biologics in organ transplantation. Transplant Int doi:10.1111/j.1432-2277.2012.01456.x

[7] Christie JD, Edwards LB, Kucheryavaya AY, et al. The Registry of the International Society for Heart and Lung Transplantation: twenty-seventh official adult lung and heart-lung transplant report--2010. J Heart Lung Transplant 2010;29:1104–18.

[8] Stehlik J, Edwards LB, Kucheryavaya AY, et al. The Registry of the International Society for Heart and Lung Transplantation: twenty-seventh official adult heart transplant report--2010. J Heart Lung Transplant 2010;29:1089–103.
[9] Organ Procurement and Transplantation Network and Scientific Registry of Transplant Recipients 2010 data report. Am J Transplant 2012;12 Suppl 1:1–156.
[10] Tiriveedhi V, Sarma N, Mohanakumar T. An important role for autoimmunity in the immunopathogenesis of chronic allograft rejection. Int J Immunogenet doi:10.1111/j.1744-313X.2012.01112.x.
[11] Eisen HJ, Tuzcu EM, Dorent R, et al. Everolimus for the prevention of allograft rejection and vasculopathy in cardiac-transplant recipients. New Engl J Med 2003;349:847–58.
[12] Arora S, Ueland T, Wennerblom B, et al. Effect of everolimus introduction on cardiac allograft vasculopathy--results of a randomized, multicenter trial. Transplantation 2011;92:235–3.
[13] Patel JK, Kobashigawa JA. Everolimus for cardiac allograft vasculopathy--every patient, at any time? Transplantation 2011;92:127–8.
[14] Hofbauer GF, Freiberger SN, Iotzova-Weiss G, Shafaeddin B, Dziunycz PJ. Organ transplantation and skin--principles and concepts. Current Problems Dermatol 2012;43:1–8.
[15] Nace G, Evankovich J, Eid R, Tsung A. Dendritic cells and damage-associated molecular patterns: endogenous danger signals linking innate and adaptive immunity. J Innate Immunity 2012;4:6–15.
[16] Wood KJ, Goto R. Mechanisms of rejection: current perspectives. Transplantation 2012;93:1–10.
[17] Saini D, Weber J, Ramachandran S, et al. Alloimmunity-induced autoimmunity as a potential mechanism in the pathogenesis of chronic rejection of human lung allografts. J Heart Lung Transplant 2011;30:624–31.
[18] Bhorade S, Ahya VN, Baz MA, et al. Comparison of sirolimus with azathioprine in a tacrolimus-based immunosuppressive regimen in lung transplantation. Am J Respir Crit Care Med 2011;183:379–87.
[19] Schliesser U, Streitz M, Sawitzki B. Tregs: application for solid-organ transplantation. Current Opin Organ Transplant 2012;17:34–41.
[20] Sakaguchi S, Sakaguchi N. Regulatory T cells in immunologic self-tolerance and autoimmune disease. Int Rev Immunol 2005;24:211–26.
[21] Tang Q, Bluestone JA, Kang SM. CD4(+)Foxp3(+) regulatory T cell therapy in transplantation. J Mol Cell Biol 2012;4:11–21.
[22] Mitchell P, Afzali B, Lombardi G, Lechler RI. The T helper 17-regulatory T cell axis in transplant rejection and tolerance. Current Opin Organ Transplant 2009;14:326–31.
[23] Nakagiri T, Inoue M, Minami M, Shintani Y, Okumura M. Immunology Mini-review: The basics of T(H)17 and interleukin-6 in transplantation. Transplant Proc 2012;44:1035–40.
[24] Szodoray P, Papp G, Nakken B, Harangi M, Zeher M. The molecular and clinical rationale of extracorporeal photochemotherapy in autoimmune diseases, malignancies and transplantation. Autoimmunity Rev 2010;9:459–64.
[25] Voss CY, Fry TJ, Coppes MJ, Blajchman MA. Extending the horizon for cell-based immunotherapy by understanding the mechanisms of action of photopheresis. Transfus Med Rev 2010;24:22–32.
[26] Ward DM. Extracorporeal photopheresis: how, when, and why. J Clin Apher 2011;26:276–85.
[27] Lamioni A, Parisi F, Isacchi G, et al. The immunological effects of extracorporeal photopheresis unraveled: induction of tolerogenic dendritic cells in vitro and regulatory T cells in vivo. Transplantation 2005;79:846–50.
[28] Berger C, Hoffmann K, Vasquez JG, et al. Rapid generation of maturationally synchronized human dendritic cells: contribution to the clinical efficacy of extracorporeal photochemotherapy. Blood 2010;116:4838–47.
[29] Biagi E, Di Biaso I, Leoni V, et al. Extracorporeal photochemotherapy is accompanied by increasing levels of circulating CD4+CD25+GITR+Foxp3+CD62L+ functional regulatory T-cells in patients with graft-versus-host disease. Transplantation 2007;84:31–9.

[30] Bladon J, Taylor P. Extracorporeal photopheresis normalizes some lymphocyte subsets (including T regulatory cells) in chronic graft-versus-host-disease. Therap Apher Dial 2008;12:311–8.
[31] Di Biaso I, Di Maio L, Bugarin C, et al. Regulatory T cells and extracorporeal photochemotherapy: correlation with clinical response and decreased frequency of proinflammatory T cells. Transplantation 2009;87:1422–5.
[32] Gatza E, Rogers CE, Clouthier SG, et al. Extracorporeal photopheresis reverses experimental graft-versus-host disease through regulatory T cells. Blood 2008;112:1515–21.
[33] George JF, Gooden CW, Guo L, Kirklin JK. Role for CD4(+)CD25(+) T cells in inhibition of graft rejection by extracorporeal photopheresis. J Heart Lung Transplant 2008;27:616–22.
[34] Jonson CO, Pihl M, Nyholm C, Cilio CM, Ludvigsson J, Faresjo M. Regulatory T cell-associated activity in photopheresis-induced immune tolerance in recent onset type 1 diabetes in children. Clin Exp Immunol 2008;153:174–81.
[35] Lamioni A, Carsetti R, Legato A, et al. Induction of regulatory T cells after prophylactic treatment with photopheresis in renal transplant recipients. Transplantation 2007;83:1393–6.
[36] Maeda A, Schwarz A, Bullinger A, Morita A, Peritt D, Schwarz T. Experimental extracorporeal photopheresis inhibits the sensitization and effector phases of contact hypersensitivity via two mechanisms: generation of IL-10 and induction of regulatory T cells. J Immunol 2008;181:5956–62.
[37] Meloni F, Cascina A, Miserere S, Perotti C, Vitulo P, Fietta AM. Peripheral CD4(+)CD25(+) Treg cell counts and the response to extracorporeal photopheresis in lung transplant recipients. Transplant Proc 2007;39:213–7.
[38] Quaglino P, Comessatti A, Ponti R, et al. Reciprocal modulation of circulating CD4+CD25+bright T cells induced by extracorporeal photochemotherapy in cutaneous T-cell lymphoma and chronic graft-versus-host-disease patients. Int J Immunopath Pharmacol 2009;22:353–62.
[39] Rubegni P, Sbano P, Cevenini G, et al. CD4+CD25+ lymphocyte subsets in chronic graft versus host disease patients undergoing extracorporeal photochemotherapy. Int J Immunopath Pharmacol 2007;20:801–7.
[40] Schmitt S, Johnson TS, Karakhanova S, Naher H, Mahnke K, Enk AH. Extracorporeal photopheresis augments function of CD4+CD25+FoxP3+ regulatory T cells by triggering adenosine production. Transplantation 2009;88:411–6.
[41] Xia CQ, Campbell KA, Clare-Salzler MJ. Extracorporeal photopheresis-induced immune tolerance: a focus on modulation of antigen-presenting cells and induction of regulatory T cells by apoptotic cells. Current Opin Organ Transplant 2009;14:338–43.
[42] Zheng DH, Dou LP, Wei YX, et al. Uptake of donor lymphocytes treated with 8-methoxypsoralen and ultraviolet A light by recipient dendritic cells induces CD4+CD25+Foxp3+ regulatory T cells and down-regulates cardiac allograft rejection. Biochem Biophys Research Commun 2010;395:540–6.
[43] Ioreth T, Bhorade SM, Ahya VN. Conventional and novel approaches to immunosuppression. Clin Chest Med 2011;32:265–77.
[44] Treede H, Glanville AR, Klepetko W, et al. Tacrolimus and cyclosporine have differential effects on the risk of development of bronchiolitis obliterans syndrome: Results of a prospective, randomized international trial in lung transplantation. J Heart Lung Transplant dx.doi.org/10.1016/j.healun.2012.03.008
[45] Knoop C, Estenne M. Chronic allograft dysfunction. Clinics in Chest Medicine 2011;32:311–26.
[46] Pettersson GB, Budev M. The role of ischemia in postlung transplantation complications. Current Opin Organ Transplant 2010;15:549–51.
[47] Jiang X, Khan MA, Tian W, et al. Adenovirus-mediated HIF-1 alpha gene transfer promotes repair of mouse airway allograft microvasculature and attenuates chronic rejection. J Clin Invest 2011;121:2336–49.
[48] Hayes D, Jr. A review of bronchiolitis obliterans syndrome and therapeutic strategies. J Cardiothoracic Surg 2011;6:92.

[49] Cooper JD, Billingham M, Egan T, et al. A working formulation for the standardization of nomenclature and for clinical staging of chronic dysfunction in lung allografts. International Society for Heart and Lung Transplantation. J Heart Lung Transplant 1993;12:713–6.

[50] Salama M, Jaksch P, Andrukhova O, Taghavi S, Klepetko W, Aharinejad S. Endothelin-1 is a useful biomarker for early detection of bronchiolitis obliterans in lung transplant recipients. J Thoracic Cardiovascular Surg 2010;140:1422–7.

[51] Finkelstein SM, Snyder M, Stibbe CE, et al. Staging of bronchiolitis obliterans syndrome using home spirometry. Chest 1999;116:120–6.

[52] Burton CM, Carlsen J, Mortensen J, Andersen CB, Milman N, Iversen M. Long-term survival after lung transplantation depends on development and severity of bronchiolitis obliterans syndrome. J Heart Lung Transplant 2007;26:681–6.

[53] Huppmann P, Neurohr C, Leuschner S, et al. The Munich-LTX-Score: predictor for survival after lung transplantation. Clin Transplant 2012;26:173–83.

[54] Vos R, Vanaudenaerde BM, Verleden SE, et al. A randomised controlled trial of azithromycin to prevent chronic rejection after lung transplantation. Eur Respir J 2011;37:164–72.

[55] Jain R, Hachem RR, Morrell MR, et al. Azithromycin is associated with increased survival in lung transplant recipients with bronchiolitis obliterans syndrome. J Heart Lung Transplant 2010;29:531–7.

[56] Andreu G, Achkar A, Couetil JP, et al. Extracorporeal photochemotherapy treatment for acute lung rejection episode. J Heart Lung Transplant 1995;14:793–6.

[57] Slovis BS, Loyd JE, King LE, Jr. Photopheresis for chronic rejection of lung allografts [letter]. New Engl J Med 1995;332:962.

[58] O'Hagan AR, Stillwell PC, Arroliga A, Koo A. Photopheresis in the treatment of refractory bronchiolitis obliterans complicating lung transplantation. Chest 1999;115:1459–62.

[59] Salerno CT, Park SJ, Kreykes NS, et al. Adjuvant treatment of refractory lung transplant rejection with extracorporeal photopheresis. J Thoracic Cardiovascular Surg 1999;117:1063–9.

[60] Schoch OD, Boehler A, Speich R, Nestle FO. Extracorporeal photochemotherapy for Epstein-Barr virus-associated lymphoma after lung transplantation. Transplantation 1999;68:1056–8.

[61] Villanueva J, Bhorade SM, Robinson JA, Husain AN, Garrity ER, Jr. Extracorporeal photopheresis for the treatment of lung allograft rejection. Ann Transplant 2000;5:44–7.

[62] Nakagiri T, Warnecke G, Avsar M, et al. Lung function early after lung transplantation is correlated with the frequency of regulatory T cells. Surg Today 2012;42:250–8.

[63] Benden C, Speich R, Hofbauer GF, et al. Extracorporeal photopheresis after lung transplantation: a 10-year single-center experience. Transplantation 2008;86:1625–7.

[64] Morrell MR, Despotis GJ, Lublin DM, Patterson GA, Trulock EP, Hachem RR. The efficacy of photopheresis for bronchiolitis obliterans syndrome after lung transplantation. J Heart Lung Transplant 2010;29:424–31.

[65] Schmauss D, Weis M. Cardiac allograft vasculopathy: recent developments. Circulation 2008;117:2131–41.

[66] Avery RK. Cardiac-allograft vasculopathy. New Engl J Med 2003;349:829–30.

[67] Hertz MI, Aurora P, Benden C, et al. Scientific Registry of the International Society for Heart and Lung Transplantation: introduction to the 2011 annual reports. J Heart Lung Transplant 2011;30:1071–7.

[68] Wang SS. Treatment and prophylaxis of cardiac allograft vasculopathy. Transplant Proc 2008;40:2609–10.

[69] Costanzo-Nordin MR, McManus BM, Wilson JE, EJ OS, Hubbell EA, Robinson JA. Efficacy of photopheresis in the rescue therapy of acute cellular rejection in human heart allografts: a preliminary clinical and immunopathologic report. Transplant Proc 1993;25:881–3.

[70] Macey WH, DeNardo B, Rook AH, Singh A, Bromley P. Use of extracorporeal photochemotherapy in heart transplant recipients during acute rejection: a case study. Am J Crit Care 1994;3:452–6.

[71] Heshmati F, Guillemain R, Achkar A, et al. Treatment of organ graft rejection by extracorporeal photochemotherapy. Ann Med Interne (Paris) 1994;145:312–5.
[72] Wieland M, Thiede VL, Strauss RG, et al. Treatment of severe cardiac allograft rejection with extracorporeal photochemotherapy. J Clin Apher 1994;9:171–5.
[73] Barr ML, Meiser BM, Eisen HJ, et al. Photopheresis for the prevention of rejection in cardiac transplantation. Photopheresis Transplantation Study Group. New Engl J Med 1998;339:1744–51.
[74] Barr ML, Baker CJ, Schenkel FA, et al. Prophylactic photopheresis and chronic rejection: effects on graft intimal hyperplasia in cardiac transplantation. Clin Transplant 2000;14:162–6.
[75] Kirklin JK, Brown RN, Huang ST, et al. Rejection with hemodynamic compromise: objective evidence for efficacy of photopheresis. J Heart Lung Transplant 2006;25:283–8.
[76] Manfro RC. Management of chronic allograft nephropathy. Jornal brasileiro de nefrologia 2011;33:485–92.
[77] Grinyo JM, Saval N, Campistol JM. Clinical assessment and determinants of chronic allograft nephropathy in maintenance renal transplant patients. Nephrol Dial Transplant 2011;26:3750–5.
[78] Wolfe JT, Tomaszewski JE, Grossman RA, et al. Reversal of acute renal allograft rejection by extracorporeal photopheresis: a case presentation and review of the literature. J Clin Apher 1996;11:36–41.
[79] Dall'Amico R, Murer L, Montini G, et al. Successful treatment of recurrent rejection in renal transplant patients with photopheresis. J Am Soc Nephrol 1998;9:121–7.
[80] Jardine MJ, Bhandari S, Wyburn KR, Misra AK, McKenzie PR, Eris JM. Photopheresis therapy for problematic renal allograft rejection. J Clin Apher 2009;24:161–9.

Mauricette Michallet and Mohamad Sobh

10.2 ECP after Facial Transplantation

10.2.1 Introduction

Extracorporeal photopheresis (ECP) is a technique of modulating white blood cells (WBCs) ex vivo in a way that, when they are reinfused into the patient, a down-regulation of T-lymphocyte activity is achieved. The principle of ECP is to induce leukocyte apoptosis with UVA radiation after incubation with psoralen. Following apoptosis, leukocytes are engulfed by dendritic cells without co-stimulatory molecules leading to anti-inflammatory cytokine secretion, a switch from TH1 to TH2 CD4+ lymphocytes inducing anergy, and deletion of effector T cells that responded to the presented antigens. An increase in regulatory T cells has also been observed after ECP and may contribute to allograft acceptance by the recipient.

ECP was first developed for the treatment of cutaneous T cell lymphoma by Edelson and colleagues [1]. Advances in molecular biology and immunology have allowed a better understanding of the mechanisms involved in ECP. As a result, it has been increasingly considered as a safe and promising immunomodulatory therapy with diverse clinical applications. ECP has been used in the treatment of patients following acute allograft rejection in cardiac, lung, renal or liver transplantation, graft-versus-host disease (GVHD), systemic lupus erythematosus, systemic scleroderma, rheumatoid arthritis and pemphigus vulgaris [2]. However, the exact mechanism by which ECP exerts its effects in different fields remains not very well elucidated yet. Important questions regarding the use of ECP in the clinical setting, such as length of therapy or design of specific protocols, concomitant use of immunosuppressive therapy, patient eligibility criteria, long-term side effects, assessment of therapeutic efficacy and cost effectiveness continue to remain unanswered. Nevertheless, future clinical studies with ECP can be done with the objective of designing more appropriate treatment protocols based on expected patient response and with a side effect profile that is fairly tolerable. The advantage of ECP is its minimal toxicity and side effects, compared with other immmunomodulatory therapies. This well tolerated therapy is not associated with increased incidence of infections or malignancies. Moreover, with this treatment the use of systemic corticosteroids and other immunosuppressant agents can be reduced in many cases, thus positively affecting long-term morbidity and mortality of patients.

10.2.2 Immunosuppression in Organ and Tissue Transplantation

One of the recent experimental fields of application of ECP is composite tissue allotransplantation (CTA). The main aim of CTA is to restore structure and function in patients with devastating injuries and therefore, improve their quality of life [3]. As opposed to a solid organ allotransplant, CTA contains several cadaveric tissues such as skin, mucosa, muscle, tendon, cartilage, bone, nerves, vessels, and/or immune cells. These multiple tissues represent a different antigenic load than a typical solid organ allograft [4]. Because CTAs are derived from genetically disparate cadaveric donors, recipients require immunosuppression for life to prevent rejection of the transplant [5, 6].

Although skin is thought to be more highly antigenic, the current immunosuppressive protocols applied to CTA are extrapolated from regimens used in solid organ transplantation [5, 7–9]. The most common maintenance immunosuppressant treatment consists of a triple therapy combining tacrolimus, mycophenolate mofetil (MMF), and corticosteroids [6]. Moreover, this maintenance therapy is preceded by a potent induction protocol, including diverse combinations of drugs, eg, cyclosporine, tacrolimus, MMF, prednisolone, polyclonal anti-thymocyte globulins, anti-interleukin-2 receptor antibodies, and anti-CD3 monoclonal antibodies [3, 9].

Improvements in immunosuppression have allowed the transition of CTA from research models to clinical reality, but immunosuppressive therapy still has many disadvantages and risks, mainly infection, organ toxicity, and malignancy [10]. Furthermore, modern maintenance therapy aims to elicit synergistic effects of drugs to reduce dosages and minimize individual side effects [3, 11]. Chimerism is known to be a prerequisite for tolerance induction, and bone marrow is critical to establishing it [12]. CTAs contain immunocompetent elements such as bone marrow and lymph nodes that may hasten the rejection processes or result in GVHD [13]. However, it is believed that high doses of bone marrow cells, infused in the absence of recipient conditioning with irradiation, do not induce GVHD [6, 14]. Immunomodulatory strategies with potential ECP and mesenchymal stem cell-based protocols are still under consideration, including donor bone marrow stem cells [15–17], while cell-based therapy including regulatory T cells appears to be another promising immunomodulative strategy [6, 18].

Our centre was the first to perform the human hand transplantation in 1998 by Dubernard and colleagues [19] and later in 2005, we were the pioneers in using ECP in the first face transplantation in the modern immunosuppressive era [15, 20]. We describe in this chapter our experience in using ECP in the first human partial face transplantation.

10.2.3 Case Description

The recipient was a 38-year-old woman who had been previously severely bitten by her dog, resulting in amputation of her distal nose, both lips, her entire chin, and the adjacent parts of her right and left cheeks [15, 20, 21]. The immunosuppressive regimen included anti-thymocyte globulins from day 0 to day 10, tacrolimus, MMF, and prednisone. Valgancyclovir prophylaxis was prescribed for cytomegalovirus (CMV) infection and cotrimoxazole was administered for prevention of bacterial infections. Donor bone marrow hematopoietic cells were infused into the recipient on days 1 and 11 after surgery. Sequential biopsies were taken from the oral mucosa, the facial skin, and, particularly in this case, from a sentinel skin graft (a free radial forearm flap from the donor, anastomosed to the thoracodorsal vessels of the recipient and located in the left submammary fold, as a means of taking skin biopsies and therefore, limiting damage to the grafted face).

Sensory recovery was achieved before motor after 6 and 10 months, respectively. Psychological acceptance of the graft progressed as function improved, and psychological support was continuously provided, as well as physical therapy, which was started on the second day after surgery. Rejection episodes occurred on days 18 and 214 after transplantation and were reversed with intravenous boluses of corticosteroids and increases in the doses of oral prednisone, tacrolimus, and MMF, as well as corticoid mouthwashes. On day 185, a herpes simplex virus type 1 (HSV1) infection of the patient's lip was documented and was treated by systemic valgancyclovir and topical acyclovir.

10.2.3.1 ECP Treatment and Side Effects

ECP was performed at 10 months to prevent recurrence of rejection. The ECP interest for this patient has been raised in view of clinical benefits in treatment of cardiac and renal rejection, treatment of GVHD and of the histological similarities between lesions of GVHD and the ones observed on the graft biopsies. ECP was performed using the Spectra blood cell separator (Gambro BCT, Denvers, USA) and an UV-irradiator (Vilbert-Lourmat, Marne-la-Vallée, France). At each session, mononuclear cells were extracted, liquid methoxsalen (Uvadex°, Therakos, Exton, PA) was added ex vivo at 200 ng/mL and then mononuclear cells were UVA-irradiated at 2 Jcm^{-2}, and finally reinfused into the patient. ECP was performed twice a week for the 4 initial weeks, then once a week for 8 weeks, and then sessions were decreased progressively to once every 4 weeks.

Clinical follow-up and clinical tolerance were performed at each ECP session. Peripheral blood cells, blood chemistry with renal and hepatic function, total serum protein, and albumin were evaluated. Mononuclear cells' response to Phytohemagglutinin (PHA) was studied at the first ECP session. Absolute CD4+ and CD8+ cell count and CD4+/CD8+ ratio were quantified in fresh blood samples every 2 weeks. The tolerance of treatment was excellent. The patient received 34 ECP sessions, the last one was in December 2008. She did not have hypotension, pyrexia or infectious complications. Her lymphocyte count was already low at the initiation of ECP (370/mm^3), and remained low during the treatments. CD4+ T Lymphocytes were especially low at 106/mm^3 at the beginning of the treatment and further decreased to 84/mm^3 later on. The median WBCs collected was 33×10^9/L (range, 11.9 to 61.5×10^9/L). The median percentage of mononuclear cells was 83% (range, 61–99%). After thymoglobulin induction, T and NK cell subsets were rapidly and profoundly depleted and remained at low levels over time. Immune reconstitution was characterized by a large expansion of memory CD4+ and CD8+ T cell subsets. Regulatory T cells that were initially increased decreased to stable normal values, whereas activated CD4+DR+ and CD8+DR+ T cell subsets were preferentially increased during the follow-up.

Starting from 12 months after transplantation, the immunosuppressive regimen consisted of sirolimus (targeted trough level: 6–12 ng/mL), MMF (1500 mg/day), and prednisone (5 mg/day). Sirolimus was introduced 11 months after transplantation to slowly reduce tacrolimus. However, when the immunosuppressive drugs were combined, the patient developed mild thrombotic thrombocytopenic purpura (TTP); consequently, both drugs were stopped for 15 days and then only sirolimus was reintroduced. The TTP episode was not related to the ECP procedure. The mechanism of TTP is the abnormal secretion of ultralarge von Willebrand factor (VWF) multimers from activated endothelial cells associated with a deficiency of VWF-cleaving protease (ADAMTS-13) [22–24]. These multimers promote platelet-dependent microvascular thrombosis and disseminated potentially life-threatening thrombotic microangiopathy. TTP occurred sometimes in association with autoimmune diseases, metastatic cancer, pregnancy, infection, use of drugs such as cyclosporine A, tacrolimus, ticlopidin, stem cell and solid organ transplantation.

The main side effect of the immunosuppressive treatment in our patient was a progressive decrease in renal function. Indeed, measured creatinine clearance was 90 mL/min before transplantation and dropped to 59 and 43 mL/min at 6 and 12 months post-transplant, respectively. Renal function improved slowly after tacrolimus withdrawal. This further decrease in renal function was correlated to the uncontrolled arterial hypertension. Fifty months after transplantation, the patient developed cervical in situ carcinoma due to papilloma virus that was treated by conization.

In September 2010, the patient presented a bacterial bilateral pneumopathy (without germ identification), which was successfully treated with antibiotics. At the last follow-up and after more than 5 years post face allotransplantation, the patient is able to smile normally, and she is satisfied with the aesthetic and functional results.

10.2.4 Conclusions

Face composite tissue allogeneic transplantation is currently a feasible therapeutic strategy able to reconstruct severe facial disfigurements, and it may become the new gold standard for full-face reconstruction. Improvements in the immunosuppressive regimens, innovative and ongoing research on immune tolerance, along with the potential use of stem cells to decrease the risks associated with lifelong immunosuppressive drugs and improve functional and cosmetic outcomes, may facilitate its future use. ECP seems to be an interesting option as an additional therapy for acute rejection episodes, as it does not have the adverse effects of immunosuppressive treatment,

10.2 ECP after Facial Transplantation — 195

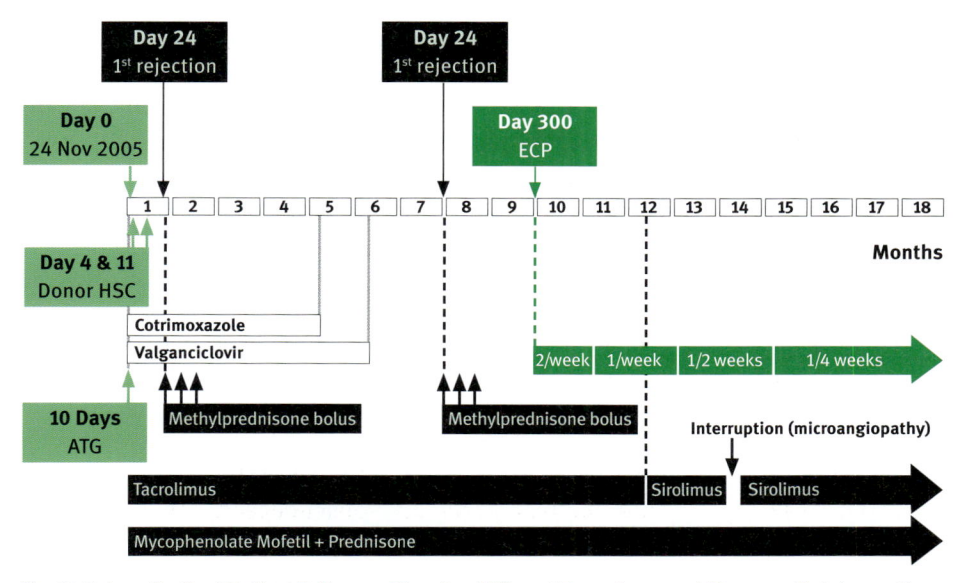

Fig. 10.5. Longitudinal Patient Follow-up Showing Different Procedures and Therapeutic Interventions.
HSC=hematopoietic stem cells; ATG=antithymocyte globulin.

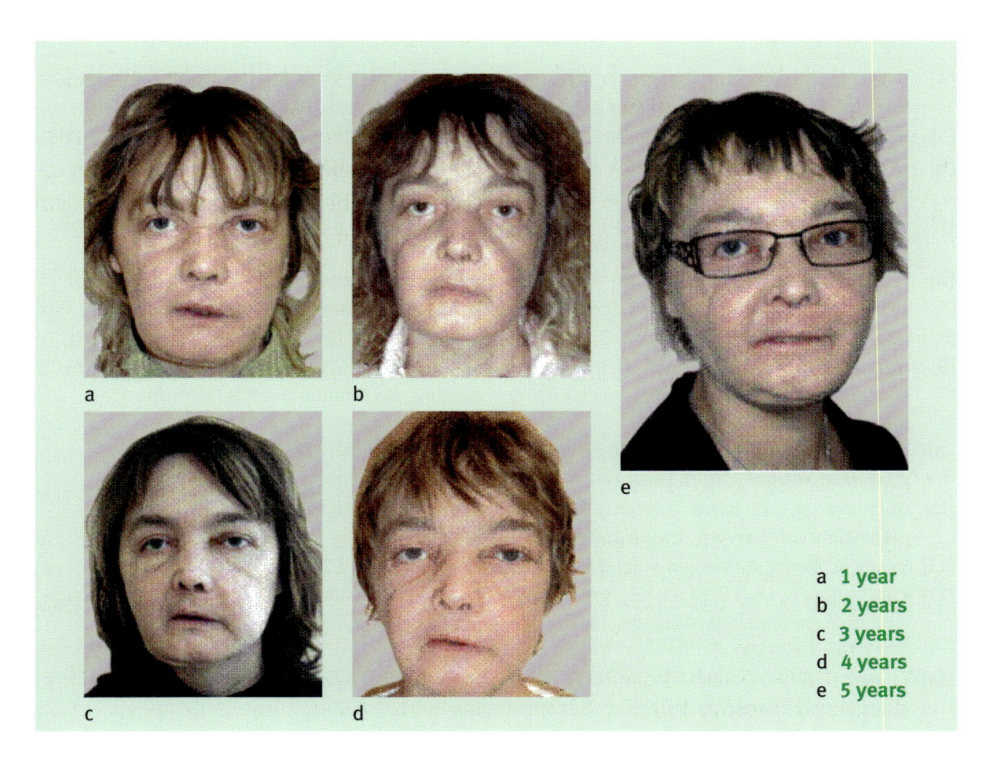

a 1 year
b 2 years
c 3 years
d 4 years
e 5 years

Fig. 10.6. Facial Composite Tissue Allotransplantation Results in Our Patient During 5 Years of Follow-up.

such as corticosteroids, which still seem to be required for grade 2 rejection episodes. Further uses in face CTA are needed in order to validate actual results and try to improve treatment administration by decreasing the type and dosages of concomitant immunosuppressive medications.

Acknowledgments

We would like to thank J.-M. Dubernard, B. Devauchelle, O. Hequet, V. Dubois, I. Parnat and E. Morelon for their main contribution in achieving this case and permission to publish these data.

References

[1] Edelson R, Berger C, Gasparro F, et al. Treatment of cutaneous T-cell lymphoma by extracorporeal photochemotherapy. Preliminary results. N Engl J Med 1987;316:297–303.
[2] Szczepiorkowski ZM, Winters JL, Bandarenko N, et al. Guidelines on the use of therapeutic apheresis in clinical practice--evidence-based approach from the Apheresis Applications Committee of the American Society for Apheresis. J Clin Apher 2010;25:83–177.
[3] Madani H, Hettiaratchy S, Clarke A, Butler PE. Immunosuppression in an emerging field of plastic reconstructive surgery: composite tissue allotransplantation. J Plast Reconstr Aesthet Surg 2008;61:245–9.
[4] Petruzzo P, Kanitakis J, Badet L, et al. Long-term follow-up in composite tissue allotransplantation: in-depth study of five (hand and face) recipients. Am J Transplant 2011;11:808–16.
[5] Brandacher G, Gorantla VS, Lee WP. Hand allotransplantation. Semin Plast Surg 2010;24(1):11–7.
[6] Schneeberger S, Landin L, Jableki J, et al. Achievements and challenges in composite tissue allotransplantation. Transpl Int 2011;24:760–9.
[7] Petruzzo P, Lanzetta M, Dubernard JM, et al. The International Registry on Hand and Composite Tissue Transplantation. Transplantation 2010;90:1590–4.
[8] Whitaker IS, Duggan EM, Alloway RR, et al. Composite tissue allotransplantation: a review of relevant immunological issues for plastic surgeons. J Plast Reconstr Aesthet Surg 2008;61: 481–92.
[9] Gorantla VS, Barker JH, Jones JW, Jr., Prabhune K, Maldonado C, Granger DK. Immunosuppressive agents in transplantation: mechanisms of action and current anti-rejection strategies. Microsurgery 2000;20:420–9.
[10] Cendales L, Hardy MA. Immunologic considerations in composite tissue transplantation: overview. Microsurgery 2000;20:412–9.
[11] Golshayan D, Pascual M. Tolerance-inducing immunosuppressive strategies in clinical transplantation: an overview. Drugs 2008;68:2113–30.
[12] Sykes M. Mixed chimerism and transplant tolerance. Immunity 2001;14:417–24.
[13] Ramsamooj R, Llull R, Black KS, Hewitt CW. Composite tissue allografts in rats: IV. Graft-versus-host disease in recipients of vascularized bone marrow transplants. Plast Reconstr Surg 1999;104:1365–71.
[14] Ciancio G, Miller J, Garcia-Morales RO, et al. Six-year clinical effect of donor bone marrow infusions in renal transplant patients. Transplantation 2001;71:827–35.
[15] Dubernard JM, Lengele B, Morelon E, et al. Outcomes 18 months after the first human partial face transplantation. N Engl J Med 2007;357:2451–60.

[16] Kuo YR, Goto S, Shih HS, et al. Mesenchymal stem cells prolong composite tissue allotransplant survival in a swine model. Transplantation 2009;87:1769–77.
[17] Popp FC, Renner P, Eggenhofer E, et al. Mesenchymal stem cells as immunomodulators after liver transplantation. Liver Transpl 2009;15:1192–8.
[18] Li XC, Turka LA. An update on regulatory T cells in transplant tolerance and rejection. Nat Rev Nephrol 2010;6:577–83.
[19] Dubernard JM, Owen E, Herzberg G, et al. Human hand allograft: report on first 6 months. Lancet 1999;353(9161):1315–20.
[20] Petruzzo P, Testelin S, Kanitakis J, et al. First human face transplantation: 5 years outcomes. Transplantation 2012;93:236–40.
[21] Devauchelle B, Badet L, Lengele B, et al. First human face allograft: early report. Lancet 2006;368(9531):203–9.
[22] Furlan M, Robles R, Solenthaler M, Wassmer M, Sandoz P, Lammle B. Deficient activity of von Willebrand factor-cleaving protease in chronic relapsing thrombotic thrombocytopenic purpura. Blood 1997;89:3097–103.
[23] Furlan M, Robles R, Solenthaler M, Lammle B. Acquired deficiency of von Willebrand factor-cleaving protease in a patient with thrombotic thrombocytopenic purpura. Blood 1998;91:2839–46.
[24] Fujikawa K, Suzuki H, McMullen B, Chung D. Purification of human von Willebrand factor-cleaving protease and its identification as a new member of the metalloproteinase family. Blood 2001;98:1662–6.

Section 11: ECP in Diabetes Mellitus

Gösta Berlin and Johnny Ludvigsson
11 ECP in Diabetes Mellitus

11.1 Introduction

Type 1 diabetes mellitus (T1D) is a common and serious disease with an increasing incidence worldwide. It is regarded as an autoimmune disease mediated by self-reactive T cells against pancreatic insulin-producing beta cells. Genetic predisposition plays a role but environmental factors are crucial for the pathogenesis as illustrated by the rapidly increasing incidence and migration studies showing that children coming from low-incidence countries get the T1D incidence of their new country. Despite multiple insulin therapy or insulin pumps and regular self-monitoring of blood glucose, T1D has substantial morbidity and mortality [1, 2]. It has been shown that preservation of even modest residual insulin secretion may reduce long-term complications [3] and studies have also indicated that beta cells may regenerate [4]. These findings give new hope for prevention and treatment of T1D.

It is not known what precipitates or stimulates the autoimmune process against beta cells. Viral infections may be important as well as nutritional agents. It has also been suggested that increased demand for insulin (because of e. g. rapid growth, increased weight, reduced physical exercise, psychological stress) may precipitate an autoimmune reaction in genetically predisposed individuals whose immune system has less balance. This could be due to factors such as too high hygiene with lack of exogenous enemies, or changes in the gut flora. Mononuclear cells, mainly T cells, are thought to kill beta cells. Auto-antibodies are usually found in T1D, but are regarded more as markers of the process rather than causing the beta cell destruction. The auto-antibodies react against different islet cell related auto-antigens such as insulin, tyrosine phosphatase or glutamic acid decarboxylase (GAD) [5]. These antigens are attacked by the own immune system, and an insufficient immune regulation is thought to allow a self-destructive process.

Already in 1983 it was shown that plasma exchange seemed to preserve the beta-cell function at onset of the T1D [6]. Several other immune interventions have been tested such as immunosuppression by cyclosporine [7, 8], anti-CD3 antibodies [9, 10], linomide [11] and B cell depleting agents [12]. However, all these interventions were only associated with minor and/or transient benefit and in some cases unacceptable adverse effects were observed. Recent studies with anti-CD3 monoclonal antibodies [13] or GAD-vaccinations [14, 15] have shown unsatisfactory efficacy even though encouraging results in subgroups support these treatment concepts.

It was therefore relevant to try another type of immune modulation. Thus, with the aim to slow down the autoimmune process involved in T1D we performed a clinical trial using extracorporeal photopheresis (ECP) at onset of the disease. Since a placebo effect of ECP cannot be ruled out we decided to perform a prospective, double blind, placebo controlled study using placebo psoralen and sham pheresis in the control group. We also planned for a long-term follow-up of the clinical effects as diabetes often has a variable course after diagnosis and start of insulin treatment. This clinical trial [16] also gave us the opportunity to study the immunological response to ECP treatment in children with recent onset of diabetes regarding lymphocyte subsets [17], the balance of Th1/Th2-like cytokines [18] and T-cell-associated activity [19].

11.2 Prospective, Placebo-Controlled Clinical Study on Use of ECP

Forty-nine patients (10 to 18 years of age) were included in the study but 9 patients were withdrawn for various reasons (afraid of needles, venous access problems, "boring study", living too far away from the apheresis unit, or adverse events as mild urticaria and moderate nausea) resulting in 19 patients completing the study in the active treatment group and 21 patients in the placebo group. ECP was performed using the THERAKOS® UVAR® instrument. Patients randomised to active treatment received oral psoralen tablets (0.6 mg/kg body weight) 1 hour before ECP treatment and patients in the control group got placebo tablets. The plasma psoralen concentration was measured by a high-performance liquid chromatography (HPLC) technique and the psoralen dose was adjusted with the aim of achieving a peak plasma concentration above 100 ng/mL (mean concentration 324 ng/mL; range, 50–878 ng/mL) and a cell suspension concentration above 50 ng/mL (mean concentration 105 ng/mL; range, 10–273 ng/mL). The procedure at the apheresis unit was similar for the ECP-treated and the placebo control group. Patients could not see the ECP instrument, all put their arm through a curtain and were venepunctured. Blood was taken for analyses from all patients. ECP was performed in the standard way for actively treated patients and the control patients got a saline infusion at a slow flow rate with the ECP instrument turned on mimicking standard treatment. The procedure was blinded not only for the patients and their parents but also for all clinicians, diabetes teams and hospital personnel except the staff of the apheresis unit.

The ECP procedure (active or sham) was administered on two consecutive days 5–6 days after diagnosis when the patients had a stable glucose value without ketonuria. The treatment was then repeated after two, four, eight, and twelve weeks. Thus, all patients got five double treatments in a period of three months.

Blood samples were taken for analyses of glucose, coagulation parameters, C peptide (blood and urine), HbA1c, islet cell antibodies (ICA) and antibodies to glutamic acid decarboxylase (GAD).

For the studies on the immunological effects of ECP we also analysed a panel of lymphocyte subsets by flow cytometry as well as interferon (IFN)-gamma, interleukin-4 (IL-4) and interleukin-13 (IL-13) (spontaneous and antigen-induced response) reflecting the Th1/Th2 balance, and interleukin-10 (IL-10) reflecting the anti-inflammatory response.

11.3 Results

Despite the random allocation to active or placebo treatment, children in the actively treated group seemed to have a more severe disease at enrolment into the study, manifested by greater weight loss, tendency to lower base excess and pronounced ketonuria, and a higher HbA1c value.

The C peptide values in serum (fasting and breakfast stimulated) and in overnight urine were followed up to month 36. As shown in Figure 11.1 the actively treated patients had higher C peptide concentrations in the urine during the follow-up period compared to patients in the control group. The fasting serum C peptide values showed a similar difference while we found no difference in maximal, stimulated C peptide serum values (Figure 11.2).

There was no difference between the groups regarding HbA1c values during the treatment or follow-up period (Figure 11.3). However, to achieve stable blood glucose values the actively treated patients needed a lower insulin dose/kg body weight (Figure 11.4).

When analysing the lymphocyte populations we found no influence of a history of a previous infection, heredity or antibodies to GAD on lymphocyte subsets in samples taken before treatment. However, girls had a higher proportion and a larger number of T cells and T helper cells and a higher proportion of naïve CD4-positive cells compared to boys. Looking at the longitudinal changes in lymphocyte populations during the study we found an increase in the number of activated CD4-positive and CD8-positive cells in the placebo group which was not found in the actively treated patients. No correlation between lymphocyte subsets and the clinical outcome was found one year after the ECP treatment.

The cytokine pattern changed so that the ratio of IFN-gamma/IL-4 expression after stimulation with GAD or insulin was reduced after active ECP treatment compared to the control group.

Placebo-treated patients showed reduced T cell-associated activity in contrast to well-preserved activity in ECP-treated patients.

11.3.1 Discussion of Study Results

Despite the fact that by chance the actively treated patients were more severely ill at onset of the disease we noticed an effect of ECP treatment on preservation of residual insulin secretion. Thus, the ECP-treated patients had slightly better C peptide secretion in urine and serum, and needed significantly lower insulin doses to reach the same HbA1c values as patients in the control group. The results shown in this randomised, double blind, placebo controlled study indicate that ECP does have an effect on the disease course of diabetes. This effect, although clinically weak, was still seen after three years of follow-up.

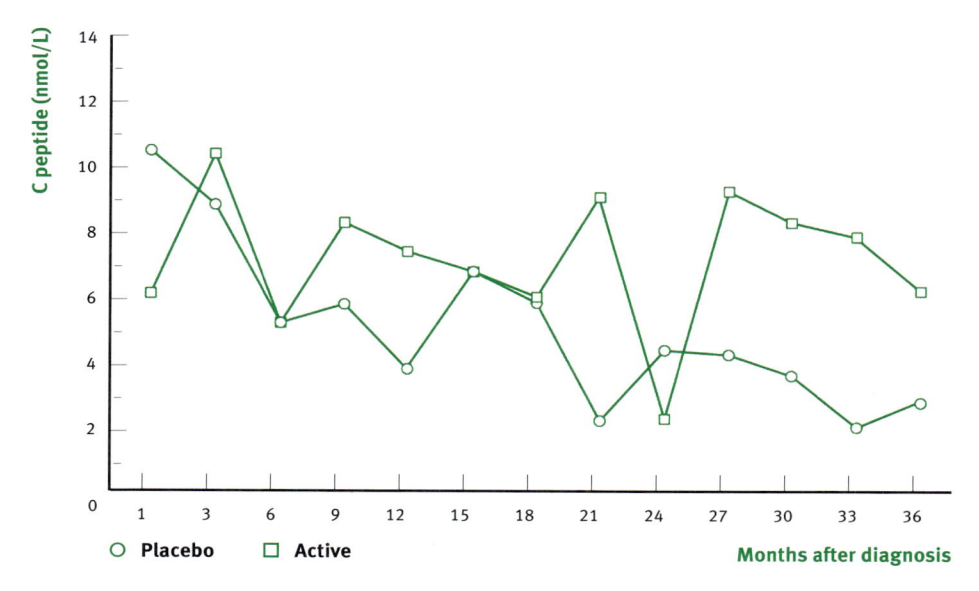

Fig. 11.1. Mean C Peptide Values in Overnight Urine.

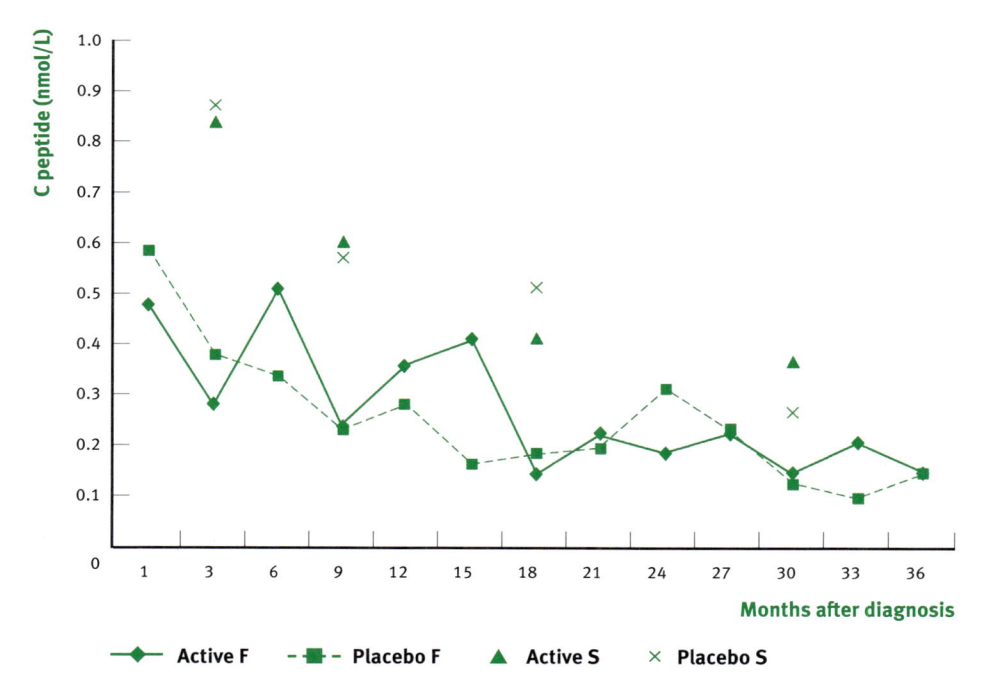

Fig. 11.2. Mean Fasting (F) and Breakfast Stimulated (S) Serum C Peptide Values.

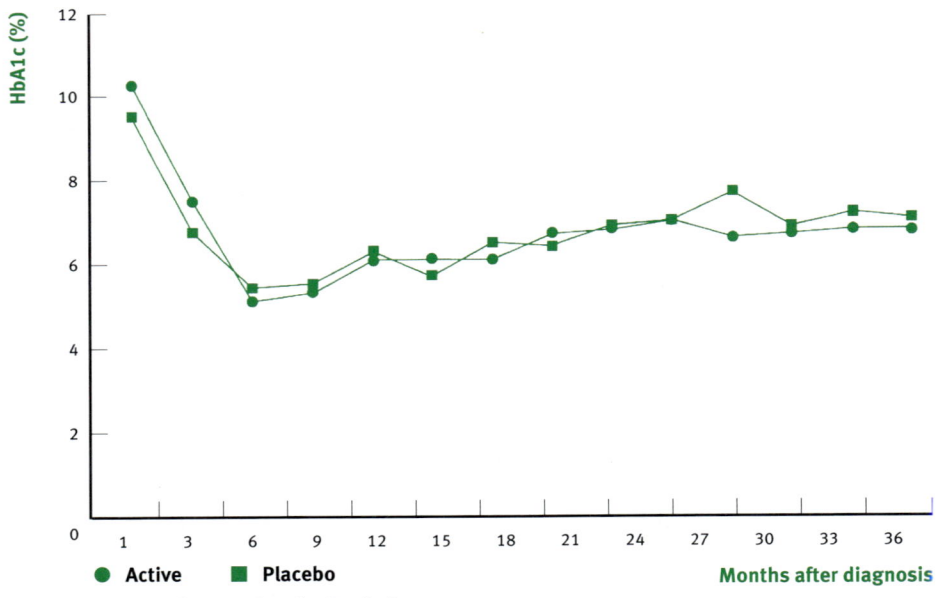

Fig. 11.3. HbA1c Values During the Study Course.

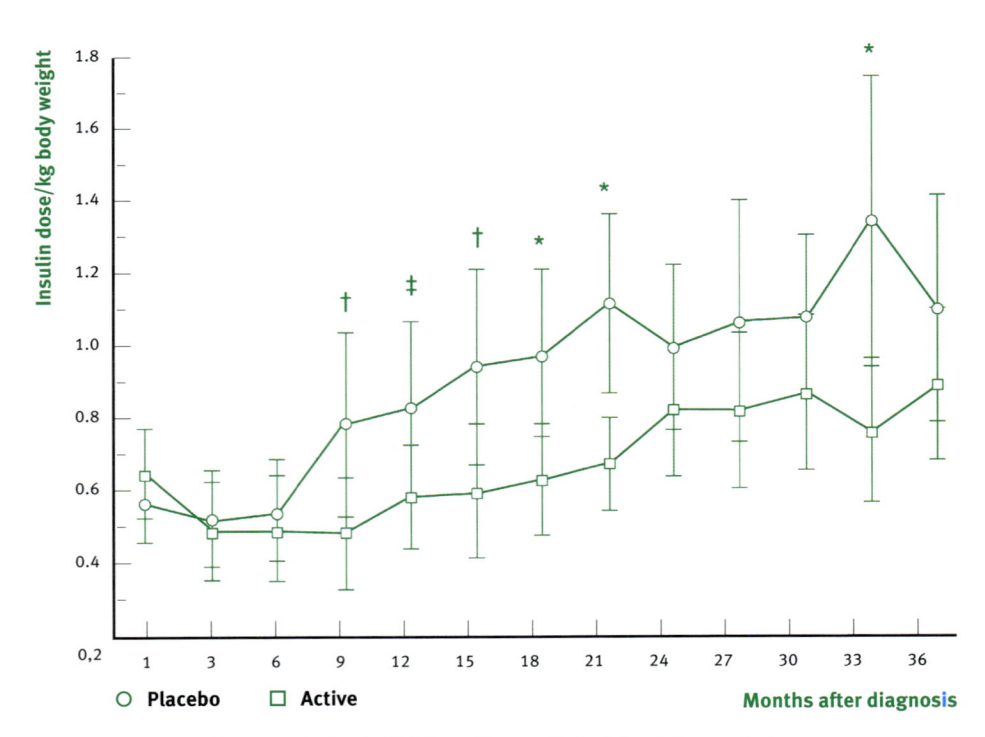

Fig. 11.4. Mean Insulin Dose/kg Body Weight to Keep a Stable Blood Glucose Value.

Looking at the immunological effects we found no major influence of ECP on lymphocyte subpopulations. However, the proportion of activated CD4-positive and CD8-positive cells increased in the placebo group, probably reflecting that activation of lymphocytes is part of the natural course of T1D. Since these changes did not occur in the actively treated group, our findings suggest that ECP may have some suppressive effects preventing lymphocyte activation. ECP also caused cytokine changes, reflecting a Th2-like deviation. The fact that ECP-treated patients showed preserved T cell activity compared to reduced activity in the control patients indicate that ECP seems to maintain regulatory T cell (Treg)-associated activity in recent onset T1D.

11.4 Conclusions

The findings reported in these studies were supported by a more recently published experimental study which showed that intravenous delivery of ECP-treated spleen cells delayed the onset of T1D in non-obese diabetic (NOD) mice [20]. The combination of ECP-treated cells with beta cell antigens appeared to improve the efficacy of ECP cell therapy. Tregs were induced by ECP treatments, suggesting that ECP provides T1D protection through promotion of immune regulation. ECP-treated spleen cells also induced suppression of the immune response to beta cell antigens. The combination of ECP-treated cells with beta cell antigens improved the protective effect. The results suggest that the protective effect of ECP against T1D includes suppression of T cell responses to the offending antigens and production of Tregs. Loss of protection might be associated with a loss of Treg activity or a rise in the number of pathogenic effector T cells. These observations also suggest that a combined therapy may be required to optimise ECP therapy in T1D. For instance, a combination of ECP with beta cell antigens might result in a more potent protective effect.

In summary, there is to date only one well-designed clinical study evaluating the effect of ECP in T1D. This study suggests that ECP might influence and delay the disease process by increasing the Treg production and by an immune suppressive effect. The results are supported by an experimental study in NOD mice suggesting that the protective ECP effect might be enhanced by combining ECP with beta cell antigens. However, the experience of ECP in the treatment of T1D is very limited and should only be used in well-designed clinical trials, which is an opinion supported by previously published guidelines [21].

References

[1] The Diabetes Control and Complications Trial Research Group. The effect of intensive treatment of diabetes on the development and progression of long-term complications in insulin-dependent diabetes mellitus. N Engl J Med 1993;329:977–86.
[2] Bojestig M, Arnqvist HJ, Hermansson G, Karlberg BE, Ludvigsson J. Declining incidence of nephropathy in insulin-dependent diabetes mellitus. N Engl J Med 1994;330:15–8.

[3] Steffes MW, Sibley S, Jackson M, Thomas W. Beta-cell function and the development of diabetes-related complications in the Diabetes Control and Complications Trial. Diabetes Care 2003;26:832-6.
[4] Winter WE, Schatz DA. Autoimmune markers in diabetes. Clin Chem 2011;57:168–75.
[5] Butler PC, Meier JJ, Butler AE, Bhushan A. The replication of beta cells in normal physiology, in disease and for therapy. Nat Clin Pract Endocrinol Metab 2007;3:758–68.
[6] Ludvigsson J, Heding L, Liedén G, Marner B, Lernmark A. Plasmapheresis in the initial treatment of insulin-dependent diabetes mellitus. Br Med J 1983;286:176–8.
[7] Mandrup-Poulsen T, Nerup J, et al. Disappearance and reappearance of islet cell cytoplasmic antibodies in cyclosporin-treated insulin-dependent diabetics. Lancet 1985;1:599–602.
[8] Bougneres PF, Carel JC, Castano L, et al. Factors associated with early remission of type I diabetes in children treated with cyclosporine. N Engl J Med 1988;318:663–70.
[9] Herold KC, Gitelman SE, Masharani U, et al. A single course of anti-CD3 monoclonal antibody hOKT3gamma1(Ala-Ala) results in improvement in C-peptide responses and clinical parameters for at least 2 years after onset of type 1 diabetes. Diabetes 2005;54:1763–9.
[10] Keymeulen B, Vandemeulebroucke E, Ziegler AG, et al. Insulin needs after CD3-antibody therapy in new-onset type 1 diabetes. N Engl J Med 2005;352:2598–608.
[11] Coutant R, Landais P, Rosilio M, et al. Low dose linomide in type 1 juvenile diabetes of recent onset: a randomised placebo-controlled double blind trial. Diabetologia 1998;41:1040–6.
[12] Pescovitz MD, Greenbaum CJ, Krause-Steinrauf H, et al. Rituximab, B-lymphocyte depletion, and preservation of beta-cell function. N Engl J Med 2009;361:2143–52.
[13] Sherry N, Hagopian W, Ludvigsson J, et al. Teplizumab for treatment of type 1 diabetes (Protégé study): 1-year results from a randomised, placebo-controlled trial. Lancet 2011;378:487–97.
[14] Ludvigsson J, Faresjö M, Hjorth M, et al. GAD treatment and insulin secretion in recent-onset type 1 diabetes. N Engl J Med 2008; 359:1909–20.
[15] Ludvigsson J, Krisky D, Casas R, et al. GAD65 antigen therapy in recently diagnosed type 1 diabetes mellitus. N Engl J Med 2012;366:433–42.
[16] Ludvigsson J, Samuelsson U, Ernerudh J, Johansson C, Stenhammar L, Berlin G. Photopheresis at onset of type 1 diabetes: a randomised, double blind, placebo controlled study. Arch Dis Child 2001;85:149–54.
[17] Ernerudh J, Ludvigsson J, Berlin G, Samuelsson U. Effect of photopheresis on lymphocyte population in children with newly diagnosed type 1 diabetes. Clin Diagn Lab Immunol 2004;11:856–61.
[18] Karlsson Faresjö M, Ernerudh J, Berlin G, Garcia J, Ludvigsson J. The immunological effect of photopheresis in children with newly diagnosed type 1 diabetes. Pediatr Res 2005;58:459–66.
[19] Jonsson CO, Pihl M, Nyholm C, Cilio CM, Ludvigsson J, Faresjö M. Regulatory T cell-associated activity in photopheresis-induced immune tolerance in recent onset type 1 diabetes children. Clin Exper Immun 2008;153:174–81.
[20] Chang-Qing X, Chernatynskaya, Lai Y, Campbell KA, Clare-Salzler MJ. Experimental extracorporeal photopheresis therapy significantly delays the development of diabetes in non-obese diabetic mice. Clin Immunol 2010;135:374–83.
[21] McKenna KE, Whittaker S, Rhodes LE, Taylor P, Lloyd L, Ibbotson S, Russell-Jones R. Evidence-based practice of photopheresis 1987-2001: a report of a workshop of the British Photodermatology Group and the U.K. Skin Lymphoma Group. Brit J Dermatol 2006;154:7–20.

Section 12: Side Effects of Extracorporeal Photopheresis

Uwe Hillen
12 Side Effects of Extracorporeal Photopheresis

Extracorporeal photopheresis (ECP) is an apheresis procedure that is based on the principles of therapy with 8-methoxypsoralen (8-MOP) and ultraviolet A irradiation (PUVA). In PUVA therapy which is used successfully by dermatologists since decades for treatment of several skin diseases (e. g. psoriasis, cutaneous T cell lymphoma) a photosensitizing drug (8-MOP) is combined with UVA light. The first clinical trial using photopheresis for treatment of advanced cutaneous T cell lymphoma (CTCL) was published in 1987 by Edelson and colleagues [1]. Photopheresis comprises three steps: (i) Collection of mononuclear cells (ii) Irradiation of the psoralen-exposed buffy coat with UVA-light, and (iii) reinfusion of the treated mononuclear cells into the patient. For ECP a venous access which allows flow rates of 50 mL/min is necessary. Peripheral venous access is preferred, however in some patients central venous access is needed to perform the therapy. Thus, side effects of ECP may result from the apheresis procedure itself and from the drugs used during therapy.

12.1 Side Effects Concerning the Apheresis Procedure

A relevant problem of the photopheresis procedure is the occurrence of fluid shifts resulting in hypo- or hypervolemia. The extracorporeal volumes observed depend on the technique and the device used for treatment. Two techniques are currently in clinical use, a closed system and an open, two step system ("off-line technique") [2]. The former was developed and is distributed by THERAKOS®. The UVAR® System was the first-generation model which was replaced by the UVAR® XTS™ System. With the UVAR® System a treatment volume consisting of 240 mL of buffy coat and 300 mL of plasma was separated. Performing ECP with the UVAR XTS® System may result in extracorporeal volumes up to 600 mL in patients with a low hematocrit even if the smaller of the two bowls available is used. The newest generation of the THERAKOS® devices, CELLEX® is based on an advanced centrifuge technology which allows a continuous cell separation and thereby reduces the extracorporeal volumes to 180mL using double-needle configuration and 236 mL in single needle configuration. In the off-line technique, leukocytes are harvested with a cell separator (e. g., Cobe Spectra), and in a second step they are transferred to UVA-light permeable bag. Finally, after liquid 8-MOP is added, the buffy coat is photo-activated in a UVA irradiation unit. In comparison to the UVAR XTS® System performing ECP with the "off-line technique" results in lower extracorporeal volumes [3] (although the extracorporeal volumes with the newer CELLEX® system and the offline techniques are more similar). However, in an open system other safety problems may be relevant, such as exchanging the treatment bags by mistake between patients, which is excluded in a closed system, and infectious complications.

To avoid clinical relevant hypovolemia, the extracorporeal volume should not exceed 15 % of the total blood volume [4]. Before starting photopheresis, the total blood volume and the tolerable extracorporeal volume, therefore, has to be calculated. If the fluid shifts are kept within the 15% margins, the risk of hypovolemia during the procedure is low, if not unforeseeable events during the procedure occur.

In over 1500 ECP procedures (THERAKOS® System) in patients with cutaneous T cell lymphoma hypotension has only rarely been observed, and the symptoms were responsive to fluid administration [5]. In a prospective phase 2 randomized study in patients with chronic graft-versus-host disease (cGVHD) no relevant hypotension was reported using the THERAKOS® System [6]. In a retrospective study of 71 patients with cGVHD given a median of 32 ECP procedures (range, 1-259 procedures) using the THERAKOS® System two patients had variations in blood pressure, which were classified as mild [7]. Salvaneschi et al. [8] reported on 720 ECP procedures, performed with the "off-line system", Kanold et al. [3] reported on 750 procedures in pediatric patients with GvHD and both did not observe blood pressure variations.

Other side effects, which have been reported, are fever (typically 4 to 12 hours after reinfusion of the treated cells), headache, chills [8, 9], and a drop in absolute neutrophil counts and platelet counts [10]. Anemia may be a relevant side effect of ECP: during the phase 2 study in patients with cGvHD anemia occurred in 24.5% of ECP patients and 6% of control patients, which was statistically significant [6].

Occurrence of side effects may depend on the underlying disease. In a study on photopheresis in pediatric patients with GvHD side effects were more frequent in children with acute than with chronic GvHD [11].

12.2 Side Effects Concerning 8-Methoxypsoralen

The effect of photopheresis is based on the interaction between 8-MOP and UVA light. In the presence of 8-MOP irradiation of the buffy coat with UVA-light results in covalent cross-linking of DNA and proliferative arrest of the treated mononuclear cells. The treated cells undergo apoptosis over a period of 48–72 hours [12]. Besides phototoxic reactions frequent side effects of 8-MOP are pruritus, nausea, vomiting, occasionally headache, dizziness, and tiredness. Nausea and headache have been observed in several studies [5, 8]. However, nausea occurs more often if 8-MOP is applied orally. In 1993 Knobler et al. [13] showed that parenteral administration of 8-MOP by injection of drug into the treatment bag before irradiation of the buffy coat cells substantially improved tolerability. For equivalent levels only a small fraction of the oral dose (1/250 to 1/500) was required. While with the use of oral 8-MOP 12 of 16 patients had side effects (nausea, vertigo, vomiting, facial edema, and sunlight-induced erythema), which led to discontinuation of the drug in one patient, none of the patients had side effects after 8-MOP had been administrated parenterally [13].

12.3 Miscellaneous

During a standard photopheresis procedure intravenous heparin is administered to prevent clotting in the extracorporeal circuit. Thus, during ECP known adverse effects of heparin, e. g. heparin induced thrombocytopenia, bleeding, elevation of liver enzymes, and osteoporosis may occur. However, heparin induced side effects during photopheresis have rarely been reported. Dittberner et al. [14] reported casuistically on heparin-induced thrombopenia. McPherson et al. [15] observed moderately severe anaphylactoid reactions in eight of 16 patients undergoing ECP. Each affected individual exhibited hypotension of sudden onset, usually with tachycardia, during the return of heparin-anticoagulated blood at the end of the first cycle of collection of leukocytes. A systematic investigation of possible contributing factors revealed that all reactions were associated with administration of a single new lot of heparin. Changing to a different manufacturer of heparin eliminated the occurrence of further hypotensive reactions [15]. In patients with contraindications to heparin ECP with acid citrate dextrose (ACD-A) may be used. ACD-A has either exclusively been used as anticoagulant or in combination with heparin. ACD-A induced side effects, e. g. electrolyte imbalances, especially hypocalcaemia and imbalances in acid-base equilibrium rarely occurred and were usually mild [16, 17]. During 404 treatments seven transient paresthesias (1.73%), five of which occurred in the first 50 treatments, were observed [16]. Bleeding complications were noted during heparin anticoagulation in 1.07 % of procedures but not during citrate anticoagulation [16]. Nedelcu et al. [17] who used exclusively ACD-A for anticoagulation observed minimal citrate toxicity (grade 1) that manifested as transient perioral tingling in 23 procedures, with an overall incidence of 24.5%. All these episodes resolved within approximately 15 minutes of additional calcium gluconate administration, indicating that the tingling was due to ACD-A-induced hypocalcaemia and not to other electrolyte imbalances.

Kanold et al. [3] observed 77 episodes of clinical adverse events concerning 17 patients in 60 sessions, one of them being a life-threatening septic shock. Bacteremia, disseminated fungal and viral infections were also reported, but were not attributed to photopheresis. Infections during ECP were also reported in adult patients with acute GvHD [9], however, the rate was not increased in comparison to patients who had not been treated with photopheresis. In the prospective phase 2 randomized study in patients with cGvHD [6] infections were the most serious adverse events, but there was no statistical significant difference between the ECP arm and the control arm. One staphylococcal endocarditis occurred in over 1500 procedures in patients with CTCL given conventional treatment [5].

One case of chorioretinitis after ECP has been reported [18]. In this 54-year-old man with Sézary syndrome therapeutic blood levels of 8-MOP persisted as long as 18 weeks after termination of therapy. The adverse effect was probably linked to impaired drug elimination. However, in the study performed by Knobler et al. [13] none of the patients treated with liquid 8-MOP had systemic plasma levels after reinfusion of the treated cells.

It has been shown that extracorporeal exposure of plasma to UVA during ECP leads to photodegradation of folic acid [19]. To date, it has not been investigated if this is of clinical relevance.

In summary, ECP is a safe therapy with a very low incidence of adverse events (< 0.003 %) [10]. ECP may also be safely used in children and patients with low body weight [3, 11, 20]. The major limiting factor of ECP is that of venous access [12], however, this is not a side effect of the therapy in the classical meaning.

References

[1] Edelson RL Berger C, Gasparro F, et al. Treatment of cutaneous T-cell lymphoma by extracorporeal photochemotherapy. N Engl J Med 1987;316: 297-303.
[2] Schooneman F. Extracorporeal photopheresis technical aspects. Transfus Apher Sci 2003;28: 51–61.
[3] Kanold J, Merlin E, Halle P, et al. Photopheresis in pediatric graft-versus-host disease after allogeneic marrow transplantation: clinical practice guidelines based on field experience and review of the literature. Transfusion 2007;47:2276–89.
[4] Kim HC. Therapeutic pediatric apheresis J Clin Apher 2000;15:129–57.
[5] Gottlieb SL, Wolfe JT, Fox FE, et al. Treatment of cutaneous T-cell lymphoma with extracorporeal photopheresis monotherapy and in combination with recombinant interferon alfa: a 10-year experience at a single institution. J Am Acad Dermatol 1996;35:946–57.
[6] Flowers ME, Apperley JF, van Besien K, et al. A multicenter prospective phase 2 randomized study of extracorporeal photopheresis for treatment of chronic graft-versus-host disease. Blood 2008;112:2667–74.
[7] Couriel DR, Hosing C, Saliba R, et al. Extracorporeal photochemotherapy for the treatment of steroid-resistant chronic GVHD. Blood 2006;107:3074–80.
[8] Salvaneschi L, Perotti C, Toretta L. Adverse effects associated with extracorporeal photochemotherapy. Transfusion 2000;40:1299–1305.
[9] Scarisbrick JJ, Taylor P, Holtick U, et al. U.K. consensus statement on the use of extracorporeal photopheresis for treatment of cutaneous T-cell lymphoma and chronic graft-versus-host disease. Br J Dermatol 2008;158:659–78.
[10] Greinix H, Volc-Platzer B, Kalhs P, et al. Extracorporeal photochemotherapy in the treatment of severe steroid-refractory acute graft-versus-host disease: a pilot study. Blood 2000;96: 2426–31.
[11] Messina C, Locatelli F, Lanino E, et al. Extracorporeal photochemotherapy for paediatric patients with graft-versus-host disease after haematopoietic stem cell transplantation. Br J Haematol 2003;122:118–27.
[12] McKenna KE, Whittaker S, Rhodes LE, et al. Evidence-based practice of photopheresis 1987–2001: a report of a workshop of the British Photodermatology Group and the U.K. Skin Lymphoma Group. Br J Dermatol 2006;154:7–20.
[13] Knobler RM, Trautinger F, Graninger W, et al. Parenteral administration of 8-methoxypsoralen in photopheresis. J Am Acad Dermatol 1993;28:580–4.
[14] Dittberner T, Schöttler E, Ranze O, et al. Heparin-induced thrombocytopenia: a complication in extracorporeal photochemotherapy (photopheresis). J Am Acad Dermatol 2002;47:452–3.
[15] McPherson RA, Buckler AG, Sanford KW, Roseff S. Investigation of heparin-related hypotensive adverse events during photopheresis: utility of a patient care database. Transfusion 2011;51:1314–20.

[16] Apsner R, Uenver B, Sunder-Plassmann G, Knobler RM. Regional anticoagulation with acid citrate dextrose-A for extracorporeal photoimmunochemotherapy. Vox Sang 2002;83:222–6.
[17] Nedelcu E, Ziman A, Fernando LP, et al.Exclusive use of acid citrate dextrose for anticoagulation during extracorporeal photopheresis in patients with contraindications to heparin: an effective protocol. J Clin Apher 2008;23:66–73.
[18] Vagace JM, Gervasini G, Morais F, et al. Retinal toxic reactions following photopheresis. Arch Dermatol 2007;143:622–5.
[19] Der-Petrossian M, Födinger M, Knobler R, et al. Photodegradation of folic acid during extracorporeal photopheresis. Br J Dermatol 2007;156:117–21.
[20] Hillen U, Meyer S, Schadendorf D, Kremens B. Photopheresis in pediatric patients with low-body weight using the UVAR XTS® System. J Dtsch Dermatol Ges 2010;8:32–7.

Section 13: Summary

Hildegard T. Greinix
13 Summary

Extracorporeal photopheresis (ECP) is a leukapheresis-based therapy incorporating ex vivo mononuclear cell incubation with the photosensitizing agent 8-methoxypsoralen followed by irradiation with ultraviolet-A light. In 1987 results of a prospective, multicentre, international clinical study on the use of ECP for treatment of cutaneous T cell lymphoma were published by Edelson and colleagues leading to FDA approval of ECP as the first cellular immunotherapy for cancer. During the following 25 years ECP has been investigated worldwide for prevention and treatment of a variety of T cell-mediated diseases including acute and chronic graft-versus-host disease (GVHD), solid organ and tissue transplantation, systemic sclerosis, systemic lupus erythematodes, rheumatoid arthritis, Crohn's disease and diabetes mellitus. Administering ECP to patients suffering of these diseases revealed promising results initially in retrospective and increasingly in recent years also in prospective single and multicentre clinical trials.

Whereas ECP for prolonged periods of time was used empirically in the clinic, recent preclinical and clinical research provides insight into its mechanisms of action revealing induction of apoptosis of treated mononuclear cells, modulation of cytokine production, effects on antigen presenting cells and T cells and generation of regulatory T cells after ECP therapy. Preclinical hypersensitivity models established by Schwarz and colleagues as well as preclinical GVHD models using donor cells mismatched at minor histocompatibility antigens and thus, resembling clinical allogeneic hematopoietic cell transplantation (HCT) as established by Ferrara and colleagues, provided important insights on the effects induced by ECP in various diseases and support clinical findings obtained in GVHD and selected autoimmune diseases excellently.

In the early years of clinical use of ECP the vast majority of patients had advanced disease refractory to a multitude of immunosuppressive agents. During the last 25 years the use of ECP has received wide and increasing acceptance from clinical investigators, policy makers and afflicted patients worldwide. Over 750,000 treatments have been performed attesting to its safety and excellent tolerance. Due to the favourable risk-benefit profile of ECP in adults and children and the increasing number of clinical trial results available to the scientific community, many clinical investigators as well as scientific organizations have agreed to recommend the use of ECP earlier in the course of selected diseases. Recently, the American Association for Blood and Marrow Transplantation recommended ECP as second-line therapy for corticosteroid unresponsive patients with acute GVHD. The German/Austrian/Swiss Consensus Conference on Clinical Practice in chronic GVHD evaluated the currently available evidence on therapeutic modalities recommending ECP as safe and beneficial second-line therapy for steroid-refractory chronic GVHD patients and mentioning a potential benefit of ECP in first-line therapy as well. The European Organisation for the Treatment and Research in Cancer (EORTC), the Joint British Association of Dermatologists and UK Cutaneous Lymphoma Group, the National Cancer Institute and the United States Cutaneous Lymphoma Consortium recommend ECP for patients with cutaneous T cell lymphoma. Thus, for some indications ECP has received sufficient acceptance so that multiple consensus statements place ECP within the accepted and recommended therapeutic modalities.

ECP's excellent safety profile and its demonstrated, important corticosteroid-sparing potential in diseases such as acute and chronic GVHD led to investigation of ECP as first-line therapy of both acute as well as chronic GVHD and for prevention of GVHD. Currently, prospective, multicentre clinical trials are on their way to address the role of ECP in clinical scenarios when no or little damage due to alloreactive cells has been observed. Well-designed prospective, multicentre clinical studies with suitable patient numbers and acceptable therapeutic control groups are highly warranted to better define the potential of ECP in selected disease categories. Existing guidelines on diagnosis, treatment and response evaluation of diseases treated by ECP allow comparison of clinical results and are the prerequisite for establishing meaningful clinical studies. International cooperations within scientific organizations enable rapid patient recruitment for clinical studies which is of utmost importance for progress in the near future. In view of the logistical challenges associated with intensified ECP schedules and the rising demands for efficient use of limited resources in costly areas such as allogeneic HCT and solid organ transplantation, biomarkers predicting response to ECP are urgently needed. First reports provide promising evidence and further studies are to be followed to increase our knowledge in this novel field of research.

The exciting scientific advances during the last years moved ECP from mere empirical treatment to a recognized and accepted immunomodulatory therapeutic modality with the potential for tolerance induction. New technical developments allow its use in small children and substantially shortened treatment times. The excitement generated by this therapeutic modality, a development and expansion from classical PUVA photomedicine, from the outset and shared by prominent and numerous preclinical and clinical researchers worldwide will hopefully enable us to further extend the value of ECP into the future. Additional knowledge gained from further understanding the complexities of its mechanisms of action as well as extension of its clinical use in the coming years should contribute to cement its safe use for the benefit of patients around the world in a multi-disciplinary manner.